POLYUNSATURATED
FATTY ACIDS IN
HUMAN NUTRITION

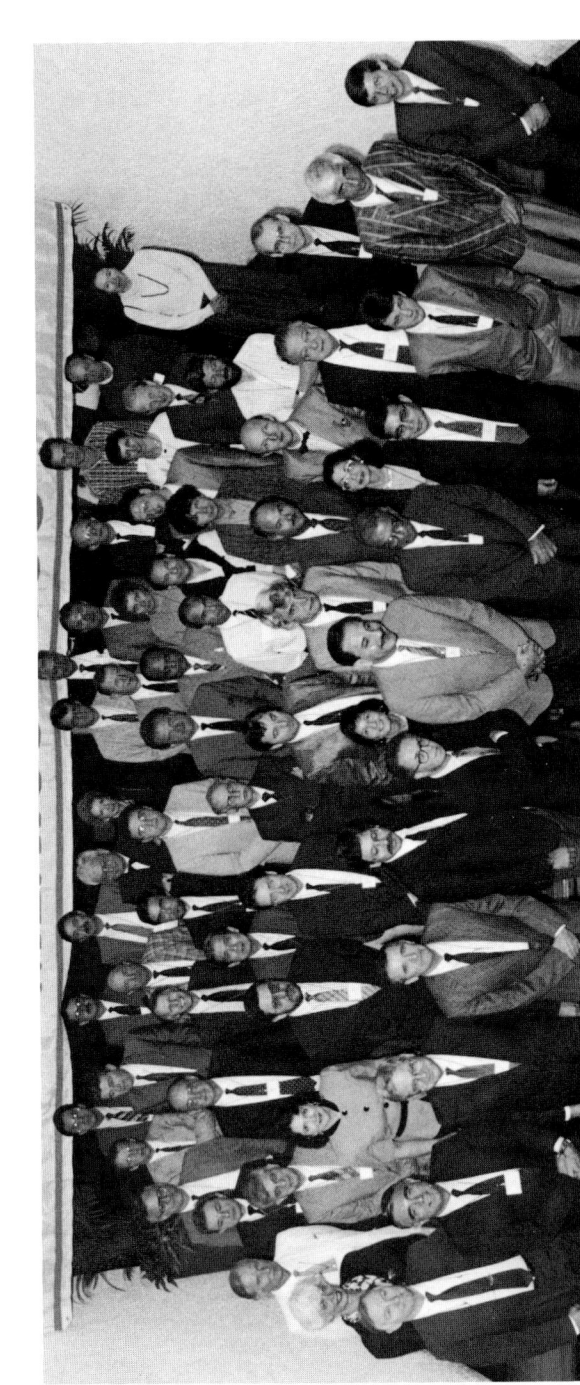

The 28th Nestlé Nutrition Workshop, Polyunsaturated Fatty Acids In Human Nutrition, was held in Mexico City, Mexico, November 27–30th, 1990.

Workshop participants (left to right, from front to back row): D. M. Small, P. R. Guesry, A. A. Spector, U. Bracco, R. J. Deckelbaum, C. Galli, N. G. Bazan, H. Sprecher, H. Okuyama, J. Y. Jeremy, O. Hernell, B. Koletzko, B. Strandvik, E. Eggermont, M. Escobedo, N. Gualde, P. Sarda, D. Spielmann, M. T. Clandinin, W. C. Heird, L. Dufour, K. Widhalm, J.-P. van Biervliet, H. W. Moser, A. H. Merrill Jr., M. A. Crawford, A. Lerdo de Tejada, W. Glinsmann, B. Duvivier, P. Tantibhedhyankul, H. Bourges Rodriguez, P.-J. Lamotte, D. Brasseur, M. Verghote, P.-P. Forget, P. Marien, G. de Bethune, K. de Block, A. Jacob, S. Cunnane, T. Heim, N. S. Bhandari, D. Lauvau, W. Laureys, L. Juhlin, V. Uzcanga Vicarte, E. Vasquez-Garibay, J. A. Garcia-Aranda, J. Timmermans, M. Stedman, L. Emmery, M. Van Eygen, G. van Paemel, F. Aguillen, J. Taveirne, H. Ingelaere, B. de Bont, B. Vanheule, J. Gigot, A. B. Moser.

Nestlé Nutrition Workshop Series
Volume 28

POLYUNSATURATED FATTY ACIDS IN HUMAN NUTRITION

Editors

Umberto Bracco, Ph.D.
Deputy Director
Nestlé Research Center
Nestec Ltd.
Lausanne, Switzerland

Richard J. Deckelbaum, M.D.
Professor of Pediatrics
Director, Division of Gastroenterology
and Nutrition
Department of Pediatrics
College of Physicians and Surgeons
of Columbia University
New York, New York, USA

NESTLÉ NUTRITION SERVICES

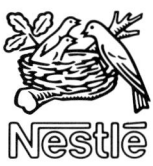

RAVEN PRESS ■ NEW YORK

Nestec Ltd., 55 Avenue Nestlé, CH-1800 Vevey, Switzerland
Raven Press, Ltd., 1185 Avenue of the Americas, New York,
New York 10036

© 1992 by Nestec Ltd. and Raven Press, Ltd. All rights reserved. This book is protected by copyright. No part of it may be reproduced, stored in a retrieval system, or transmitted, in any form or by any means, electronical, mechanical, photocopying, or recording, or otherwise, without the prior written permission of Nestec and Raven Press.

Made in the United States of America

Library of Congress Cataloging-in-Publication Data

Nestlé Nutrition Workshop (28th : 1990 : Mexico City, Mexico)
    Polyunsaturated fatty acids in human nutrition / editors, Umberto Bracco, Richard J. Deckelbaum.
        p.   cm.
    Proceedings of the 28th Nestlé Nutrition Workshop on "Polyunsaturated Fatty Acids in Human Nutrition," held in Mexico City Mexico, November 27–30th, 1990.
    Includes bibliographical references and index.
    ISBN 0-88167-933-X
    1. Unsaturated fatty acids in human nutrition—Congresses.
I. Bracco, Umberto. II. Deckelbaum, Richard J. III. Title.
    [DNLM: 1. Fatty Acids, Unsaturated—congresses. 2. Nutrition—congresses. W1 NE228 v.88 / QU 90 N468p 1990]
QP752.F35N47   1990
612.3'97—dc20
DNLM/DLC
for Library of Congress   92-11920

    The material contained in this volume was submitted as previously unpublished material, except in the instances in which credit has been given to the source from which some of the illustrative material was derived.
    Great care has been taken to maintain the accuracy of the information contained in the volume. However, neither Nestec nor Raven Press can be held responsible for errors or for any consequences arising from the use of the information contained herein.

9 8 7 6 5 4 3 2 1

Preface

Fatty acids in the diet undergo in the body various metabolic processes governing absorption and transport mechanisms, cell membrane activity modulation, and the pool of specific metabolites. The biochemical pathways possess high physiological significance at the tissue level, which has recently produced convincing evidence of the role of dietary fatty acids in human nutrition. In particular, long chain polyunsaturated fatty acids (LCPUFAs), major constituents of cell membrane phospholipids, represent extremely active substrates for metabolic processes mediating physiological activities.

This book presents the papers and discussions of the 28th Nestlé Nutrition Workshop held in Mexico City, November 27–30th, 1990. We address the new perspectives in human nutrition related to polyunsaturated fatty acids (PUFAs), focusing in particular on their biochemistry, metabolism, physiological role and nutritional impact.

We discuss PUFA transport and utilization, its role in phospholipid molecular species, extracellular and intracellular fate, and metabolism to oxidative derivatives. Then we consider the LCPUFAs as mediators—through eicosanoid-dependent and/or independent mechanisms—of physiological processes at the central nervous system level (brain and retinal development), in particular, of diseases such as cystic fibrosis and atopic eczema, as well as in relation to disturbances of lipoprotein metabolism and gynecological disorders. LCPUFAs are also precursors of eicosanoids, produced by a large variety of cells involved in immunoresponse, and they therefore intervene in problems related to immunomodulation.

Evidence of close relationships between dietary LCPUFAs and their structural-metabolic physiological role leads us to consider the problems and opportunities of LCPUFAs in the human diet, with particular emphasis on infant feeding.

The data presented in the chapters and discussion sections should contribute to a better understanding of the role of fatty acids in human biology, while pointing out existing gaps in the area and identifying research needs. The final aim is to contribute to a better knowledge of the role of lipids in human nutrition.

UMBERTO BRACCO, Ph.D. RICHARD J. DECKELBAUM, M.D.
Lausanne, Switzerland *New York, New York, USA*

Contents

Fatty Acids in Human Biology: Past and Future 1
Arthur A. Spector

Long Chain Fatty Acid Metabolism 13
Howard Sprecher

Physical Properties of Fatty Acids and their Extracellular and
　Intracellular Distribution 25
Donald M. Small

Long Chain Fatty Acids and Other Lipid Second Messengers   41
Alfred H. Merrill, Jr.

Long Chain Fatty Acids: Intake, Digestion, and Absorption
　in Newborn Infants 53
Olle Hernell and Lars Bläckberg

Long Chain Fatty Acids and Peroxisomal Disorders 65
Hugo W. Moser and Ann B. Moser

Long Chain Polyunsaturated Fatty Acid Metabolism and
　Cellular Utilization: Regulation and Interactions 81
Claudio Galli, Cristina Mosconi, and Franca Marangoni

Essential Fatty Acids in Early Development 93
Michael A. Crawford, K. Costeloe, W. Doyle, A. Leaf,
　M. J. Leighfield, N. Meadows, and A. Phylactos

Developmental Aspects of Long Chain Polyunsaturated Fatty
　Acid Metabolism: CNS Development 111
Michael Thomas Clandinin and Johny E. E. Van Aerde

Supply, Uptake, and Utilization of Docosahexaenoic Acid
　During Photoreceptor Cell Differentiation 121
Nicolas G. Bazan

CONTENTS

Long Chain Polyunsaturated Fatty Acids in the Diets of
  Premature Infants 135
Berthold Koletzko

Dietary Long Chain Polyunsaturated Fatty Acids: Sources,
  Problems, and Uses 147
Umberto Bracco

Long Chain Fatty Acid Metabolism and Essential Fatty Acid
  Deficiency with Special Emphasis on Cystic Fibrosis 159
Birgitta Strandvik

Effects of Dietary Essential Fatty Acid Balance on Behavior
  and Chronic Diseases 169
Harumi Okuyama

Long Chain Fatty Acids in Obstetrics, Gynecology, and
  Fertility: A Focus on Non-Eicosanoid-Mediated
  Mechanisms 179
Jamie Y. Jeremy

Thymus Eicosanoids Are Involved in Tolerance to Self 195
Norbert Gualde

Long Chain Fatty Acids and Atopic Dermatitis 211
Lennart Juhlin

Long Chain Fatty Acids and Cholesterol Metabolism 219
Richard J. Deckelbaum

Subject Index 233

Contributors

Nicolas G. Bazan
Department of Ophthalmology and
  Neuroscience Center
Louisiana State University Medical
  Center
2020 Gravier Street, Suite B
New Orleans, Louisiana 70112-2234,
  USA

Umberto Bracco
Nestlé Research Centre, Nestec Ltd.
Vers-chez-les-Blanc, P.O. Box 44
1000 Lausanne 26, Switzerland

Michael Thomas Clandinin
Nutrition and Metabolism Research
  Group
Departments of Foods and Nutrition
  and Medicine
University of Alberta
Edmonton, Alberta, Canada T6G 2C2

Michael A. Crawford
Institute of Brain Chemistry and Human
  Nutrition
Hackney Hospital
Homerton High Street
London E9 6BE, England

Richard J. Deckelbaum
Division of Gastroenterology and
  Nutrition
Department of Pediatrics
College of Physicians and Surgeons of
  Columbia University
630 West 168th Street
New York, New York 10032, USA

Claudio Galli
Institute of Pharmacological Sciences
School of Pharmacy
University of Milano
Via Balzaretti 9, 20133
Milano, Italy

Norbert Gualde
Université Bordeaux II
URA CNRS 1456 and Fondation
  Bergonié
180 Rue du Saint-Genès, 33076
Bordeaux Cédex, France

William C. Heird
Baylor College of Medicine
Children's Nutrition Research Center
1100 Bates Street
Houston, Texas 77030, USA

Olle Hernell
Department of Pediatrics
University of Umeå
S-90185 Umeå, Sweden

Jamie Y. Jeremy
Department of Chemical Pathology and
  Human Metabolism
Royal Free Hospital School of Medicine
University of London Pond Street
London NW3 2QG, England

Lennart Juhlin
Department of Dermatology
University Hospital
S-751 85 Uppsala, Sweden

Berthold Koletzko
Kinderpoliklinik der Ludwig-
  Maximilians-Universität
Universität, D-W-8000
Munich 2, Germany

Alfred H. Merrill, Jr.
Department of Biochemistry
Emory University School of Medicine
Atlanta, Georgia 30322, USA

CONTRIBUTORS

Hugo W. Moser
Johns Hopkins University
Kennedy Krieger Institute
707 North Broadway
Baltimore, Maryland 21210, USA

Harumi Okuyama
Faculty of Pharmaceutical Sciences
Nagoya City University
3-1 Tanabedori, Mizuhoku
Nagoya 467, Japan

Donald M. Small
Department of Biophysics
Boston University School of Medicine
80 East Concord Street
Boston, Massachusetts 02118-2394, USA

Arthur A. Spector
Department of Biochemistry
University of Iowa College of Medicine
Iowa City, Iowa 52242, USA

Howard Sprecher
Department of Medical Biochemistry
Ohio State University
1645 Neil Avenue
Columbus, Ohio 43210-1218, USA

Birgitta Strandvik
Department of Pediatrics
University of Göteborg
41685 Göteborg, Sweden

Kurt Widhalm
Department of Pediatrics
University of Vienna
Währinger Guntel 18-20
1090 Vienna, Austria

Invited Attendees

Narendra Singh Bhandari / *Bhopal, India*
Héctor Bourges Rodriguez / *Tlalpan, Mexico*
Daniel Brasseur / *Brussels, Belgium*
Margaret Cheney / *Ontario, Canada*
Stephen Cunnane / *Toronto, Canada*
Guy de Bethune / *Kortrijk, Belgium*
Baudouin de Bont / *Marche lez Ecaussines, Belgium*
Angel Lerdo de Tejada / *Coyoaca D. F., Mexico*
Bernard Duvivier / *Marche, Belgium*
Ephrem Eggermont / *Herent, Belgium*
Luc Emmery / *Opglabeek, Belgium*
Marilyn Escobedo / *San Antonio, Texas, USA*
Samuel Flores Huerta / *Mexico*
Pierre-Philippe Forget / *Embourg, Belgium*
Jose Alberto Garcia-Aranda / *Mexico*
Jean Gigot / *Brussels, Belgium*
Walter Glinsmann / *Washington, D.C., USA*
Tibor Heim / *Toronto, Canada*
Herwig Ingelaere / *Lembeke, Belgium*
Albert Jacob / *Agadir, Morocco*
Paul-Jacques Lamotte / *Embourg, Belgium*
William Laureys / *Halle, Belgium*
Denis Lauvau / *Binche, Belgium*
Paul Marien / *Edegem, Belgium*
Pierre Sarda / *Montpellier, France*
Phienvit Tantibhedhyankul / *Bangkok, Thailand*
Jan Taveirne / *Kortrijk, Belgium*
Jean Timmermans / *Bree, Belgium*
Victor Uzcànga Vicarte / *Monterrey, Mexico*

Jean-Pierre van Biervliet / *Brugge, Belgium*
Maurice van Eygen / *Roeselare, Belgium*

Bea Vanheule / *Roeselare, Belgium*
Gonde van Paemel / *Oostende, Belgium*
Marc Verghote / *Namur, Belgium*

Nestlé Participants

Karel de Block, *Brussels, Belgium*
Pierre R. Guesry, *Vevey, Switzerland*
Laila Khouri-Dufour, *Vevey, Switzerland*
Russell J. Merritt, *Glendale, California, USA*

Cedric de Prelle, *Brussels, Belgium*
Danièle Spielmann, *Lausanne, Switzerland*
Margaret Stedman, *Don Mills, Canada*

Nestlé Nutrition Workshop Series

Volume 29: Nutrition of the Elderly
*Hamish N. Munro and Günter Schlierf, Editors;
248 pp., 1992.*
Volume 28: Polyunsaturated Fatty Acids in Human Nutrition
*Umberto Bracco and Richard J. Deckelbaum, Editors;
256 pp., 1992.*
Volume 26: Perinatology
Erich Saling, Editor; 208 pp., 1992.
Volume 25: Sugars in Nutrition
*Michael Gracey, Norman Kretchmer, and Ettore Rossi, Editors;
304 pp., 1991.*
Volume 24: Inborn Errors of Metabolism
*Jürgen Schaub, François Van Hoof, and Henri L. Vis, Editors;
320 pp., 1991.*
Volume 23: Trace Elements in Nutrition of Children—II
Ranjit Kumar Chandra, Editor; 248 pp., 1991.
Volume 22: History of Pediatrics 1850–1950
*Buford L. Nichols, Jr., Angel Ballabriga, and Norman
Kretchmer, Editors; 320 pp., 1991.*
Volume 21: Rickets
Francis H. Glorieux, Editor; 304 pp., 1991.
Volume 20: Changing Needs in Pediatric Education
*Cipriano A. Canosa, Victor C. Vaughan III, and Hung-Chi Lue,
Editors; 336 pp., 1990.*
Volume 19: The Malnourished Child
*Robert M. Suskind and Leslie Lewinter-Suskind, Editors;
432 pp., 1990.*
Volume 18: Intrauterine Growth Retardation
Jacques Senterre, Editor; 336 pp., 1989.
Volume 17: Food Allergy
*Dietrich Reinhardt and Eberhard Schmidt, Editors;
320 pp., 1988.*
Volume 16: Vitamins and Minerals in Pregnancy and Lactation
Heribert Berger, Editor; 472 pp., 1988.
Volume 15: Biology of Human Milk
Lars Å. Hanson, Editor; 248 pp., 1988.

Fatty Acids in Human Biology: Past and Future

Arthur A. Spector

Department of Biochemistry, University of Iowa, College of Medicine, Iowa City, Iowa 52242, USA

This review is a brief summary of the nutritional, metabolic, and functional roles of fatty acids in mammalian systems, with emphasis on processes that play a role in human physiology and diseases. In this context I will point out existing gaps in our knowledge about fatty acids and suggest areas that appear to be most promising for further study.

Table 1 lists the long chain fatty acids that presently are known to have an important role in nutrition and metabolism. There are 20 to 30 additional fatty acids contained in the plasma and tissue lipids, many at a level of less than 1%. It seems likely that some of these also have important functional roles. A case in point is myristic acid (14:0).[1] Since the tissue contain only a very small amount of myristic acid, it was ignored in most studies. Recently, amino-terminal myristoyl groups have been found on several regulatory proteins, including the protein product of the ras oncogene and the catalytic subunit of protein kinase A, and myristic acid has become one of the most intensively studied fatty acids in biological research (1). Specific functions may be found for other fatty acids now classified as minor components, and the list in Table 1 is likely to expand in the future.

FATTY ACID UTILIZATION

Much of the fatty acid transported to the tissues is either in the form of free fatty acid (FFA) or triglycerides contained in very low density lipoproteins and chylomicrons. The lipoprotein triglycerides are hydrolyzed by lipoprotein lipase at the endothelial surface, and the released fatty acid passes into the tissues. As shown in Fig. 1, in both of these major transport systems, it is the fatty acid itself that is presented to the cells. In an attempt to model this physiologic situation, most studies of fatty acid utilization have been done by incubating tissues or cells directly with

---

[1] The fatty acids are abbreviated as number of carbon atoms: number of double bonds.

TABLE 1. *Biologically important long chain fatty acids*

Fatty acid	Carbons/double bonds	Unsaturated series	Functions
Myristic	14:0	—	Acylation of proteins
Palmitic	16:0	—	Energy storage
			Oxidative substrate
			Alkyl/alkenyl ethers
			Acylation of proteins
Stearic	18:0	—	Phospholipid structure
Oleic	18:1	ω-9	Regulation of bulk membrane fluidity
Linoleic	18:2	ω-6	Arachidonic acid precursor
Arachidonic	20:4	ω-6	Substrate for eicosanoid mediator synthesis
Eicosapentaenoic	20:5	ω-3	Competitor of arachidonic acid and the synthesis of arachidonate-derived eicosanoids
Docosahexaenoic	22:6	ω-3	Membrane structure

fatty acids (2,3). The fatty acid is usually in a physical complex with plasma albumin, the main fatty acid transport protein in the blood and extracellular fluid (4). Most of what we know about the mechanism of fatty acid utilization is based on studies using this experimental design.

Figure 2 summarizes what occurs when fatty acids are presented to cells as a complex with albumin. Although albumin contains multiple binding sites for fatty acid and the binding at several of these sites is strong, some of the fatty acid dissociates and passes to the cell surface in unbound form (4). The higher the molar ratio of fatty acid to albumin, the greater the unbound concentration. As the cells take up the unbound material more fatty acid dissociates from the albumin and

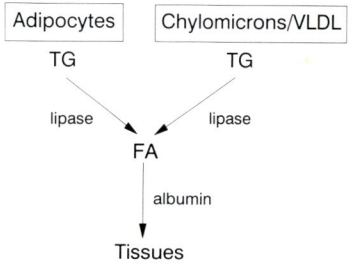

FIG. 1. Supply of circulating fatty acid to the tissues. Abbreviations used: VLDL, very low density lipoproteins; TG, triglycerides; FA, fatty acids. There are two major sources of fatty acid available to the tissues. There are plasma free fatty acid and triglycerides contained in chylomicrons and VLDL, which are large, triglyceride-rich plasma lipoproteins. The plasma-free fatty acid is derived from the hydrolysis of triglycerides stored in adipocytes, mediated by the hormone-sensitive lipase present in the adipocytes. After release into the plasma, the fatty acids bind to albumin, pass through the endothelium, and are transferred through the extracellular fluid to the cells. The circulating triglycerides contained in the chylomicrons and VLDL are hydrolyzed by lipoprotein lipase, an enzyme present on the endothelial surface of the capillaries. The released fatty acids cross the endothelium and pass through the extracellular fluid to the cells. In the extracellular fluid, the fatty acid associates transiently with albumin. Therefore, fatty acid derived from both of these major pathways becomes available to the tissues in the same final form, as free fatty acid bound to albumin.

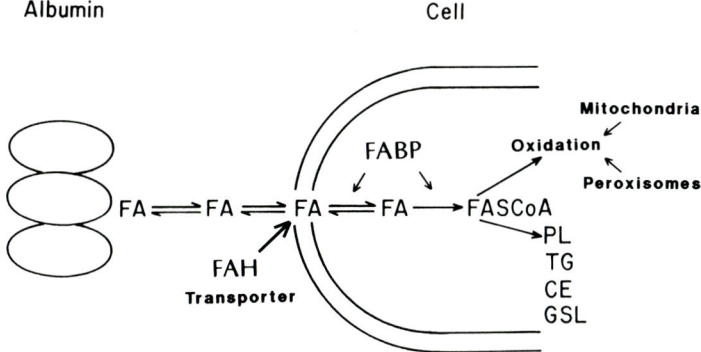

FIG. 2. Mechanism of fatty acid utilization by mammalian cells. Abbreviations used: FA, fatty acid anion; FAH, protonated form of fatty acid; FABP, fatty acid binding protein; FAS-CoA, fatty acyl coenzyme A; PL, phospholipids; TG, triglycerides; CE, cholesteryl esters; GSL, glycosphingolipids. Fatty acid dissociates from the albumin in the uptake process and initially enters a reversibly bound cellular pool. There is uncertainty as to whether the fatty acid crosses the membrane by diffusion of the protonated form, FAH, through the lipid bilayer, or in the anionic form (FA) through the action of a transporter. The cytosolic fatty acid binding protein, FABP, may facilitate uptake by desorbing fatty acid from the membrane, or by directing the fatty acid into specific metabolic pathways.

becomes available for uptake. The amount of fatty acid incorporated by the cells depends on the unbound concentration, which, in turn, depends on the molar ratio (2). Under physiologic conditions, the albumin concentration does not fluctuate much, so the main determinant of the molar ratio is the fatty acid concentration. This is governed by the entry of fatty acid from either the adipose tissue or the plasma lipoproteins.

The cells initially accumulate fatty acid in unesterified form and at this stage much of the uptake is reversible, as indicated by the double arrows in Fig. 2. Most of this fatty acid is probably associated with the plasma membrane, and its accumulation to excessive levels may alter the properties of the membrane and even produce cell injury. At a given molar ratio of fatty acid to albumin, stearic (18:0) and palmitic (16:0) acids accumulate to a greater extent than oleic acid (18:1), and to a much greater extent than linoleic acid (18:2) (5).

Two key questions involving the uptake mechanism remain unresolved. One is whether the fatty acid crosses the plasma membrane by diffusion, probably in the protonated form indicated as FAH (6), or in anionic form through the action of a membrane transporter (7,8). The other is whether the cytoplasmic fatty acid binding protein (FABP) plays a role in the transport process (9), such as by binding the fatty acid at the membrane-cytosol interface and thereby facilitating its desorption.

Oxidative Pathways

Following entry, the fatty acid is activated and the acylcoenzyme A thioester is channeled into the oxidation or esterification pathways. While most of the emphasis has been on mitochondrial β-oxidation, peroxisomes also are an important site of fatty acid oxidation, particularly for very long chain, highly polyunsaturated, hydroxylated, and branched chain fatty acids (10). As much as 30% of fatty acid oxidation in some cells occurs in the peroxisomes (10). The peroxisomal β-oxidation pathway generates H_2O_2, and this process will probably assume increasing importance as more becomes known about the role of peroxide tone and lipid peroxidation in cellular function and disease processes (11,12). The formation of the alkyl ether bond also occurs in the peroxisomes, and it seems likely that more emphasis will be placed on this organelle in the future because of the increasing number of functions that are becoming attributed to it.

Phospholipid Molecular Species

The incoming fatty acid also is incorporated into phospholipids and glycosphingolipids for membrane biogenesis or replacement, as well as into triglycerides and cholesteryl esters for storage. An aspect of these esterification pathways that is likely to assume increasing importance is the channeling of various fatty acids into different phospholipid molecular species. This is illustrated by the data in Table 2, obtained from human endothelial cultures (13). The diacyl form of phosphatidylcholine in the endothelial cell is composed of 37 different molecular species; those listed in Table 2 account for only 58% of the total in this fraction. The specific activity of labeled arachidonic acid (20:4) incorporated during a 24 hour incubation differs among the five fractions that contain 20:4. In particular, molecular species with two unsaturated fatty acids, the 20:4/20:4 and 16:1/20:4 + 18:2/20:4 fractions, have the highest specific activity. This suggests that they may act as acceptors for incoming arachidonic acid, be more active metabolically, or play a special role in intracellular channeling of arachidonic acid. Detailed information of this type ultimately will be needed for other fatty acids. The complexity of the problem becomes apparent when one considers that there are many different phospholipid classes in a cell besides diacyl

TABLE 2. *Endothelial cell diacyl phosphatidylcholine*

Molecular species[a]	Amount (mol %)	[^{3}H]Arachidonic acid (dpm × 10^{-5}/nmol)
16:0/16:0	11.7	
16:0/18:1	20.8	
18:0/18:1	5.8	
18:1/18:1	5.4	
16:0/20:4	5.0	1.7
18:0/20:4	5.2	1.7
18:1/20:4	3.9	2.3
16:1/20:4 + 18:2/20:4	0.9	4.5
20:4/20:4	0.3	3.1

[a] There are 37 molecular species; those listed total only 58.3 mol %.

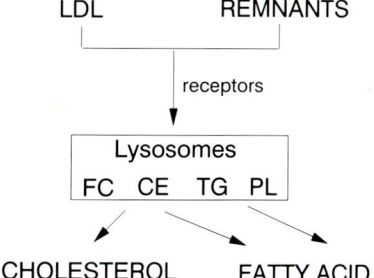

FIG. 3. Supply of fatty acid to the cells as a result of lipoprotein uptake by receptor-mediated endocytosis. Abbreviations used: LDL, low density lipoproteins; FC, cholesterol; CE, cholesteryl ester; TG, triglyceride; PL, phospholipids. In addition to cholesterol, fatty acid is released intracellularly when lipoproteins are degraded in the lysosomes. The processing and functional effects of fatty acids made available to cells in this way have not been adequately explored.

phosphatidylcholine and that the types of molecular species may differ in different subcellular compartments, or even in different domains within a single membrane.

Endocytosis of Plasma Lipoproteins

Cells also can obtain fatty acids through receptor-mediated endocytosis of lipoproteins, as illustrated in Fig. 3. The fatty acid aspect of this process has been almost completely ignored because work in this area has concentrated on cholesterol (14). However, when the phospholipids and cholesteryl esters of the low density lipoproteins are hydrolyzed in the lysosomes, fatty acids are released. Furthermore, the remnant lipoproteins taken up in the liver are rich in triglycerides and should provide even more fatty acid. The fundamental question of whether fatty acid released intracellularly during endocytosis is handled in the same way as fatty acid delivered as an albumin complex has not been addressed. Since arachidonic acid provided by low density lipoproteins is available for prostaglandin formation (15,16), the endocytosis route of fatty acid entry may be linked to important metabolic functions.

Phospholipid Fatty Acid Turnover

There is a continuous turnover of fatty acyl groups contained in the cell lipids, including the membrane phospholipids (17,18). This is illustrated schematically in Fig. 4. If fatty acid is present in the extracellular fluid, it will exchange with the intracellular fatty acid that is turning over as a result of mixing in the free fatty acid

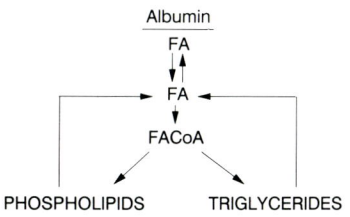

FIG. 4. Turnover of intracellular fatty acids. Abbreviations used: FA, fatty acid; FACoA, fatty acyl coenzyme A. The fatty acid contained in cell lipids, particularly the membrane phospholipids, undergoes continuous turnover. If fatty acids are available in the extracellular fluid, they will mix with the intracellular fatty acid undergoing turnover. Through this process, the intracellular fatty acid composition, including the fatty acid composition of the membrane phospholipids, can change somewhat to reflect the type of fatty acid available in the diet.

pool. This can lead to a change in the fatty acid composition of the intracellular lipids. The phospholipid storage pools that supply arachidonic acid for prostaglandin formation also turn over in this way, and their arachidonic acid content can increase or decrease fairly rapidly. Differences in cellular arachidonic acid that result from this turnover are sufficient to affect the amount of prostaglandin released in response to a stimulus (19,20). Therefore, the extent of certain cellular response mechanisms mediated by eicosanoids could be affected by dietary modification, a possibility that could have profound implications.

MEMBRANE FATTY ACID MODIFICATION

As predicted from the phospholipid turnover findings, it is possible to modify the fatty acid composition of cell membranes within certain limits (21). This can influence membrane fluidity and the properties of certain membrane transport systems. Substitution of large amounts of polyunsaturated fatty acid into experimental mouse leukemia cells has rendered them more sensitive to hyperthermia and chemotherapy with doxorubicin (22). Furthermore, liver membrane become more susceptible to lipid peroxidation when they are enriched with polyunsaturated fatty acids (23), raising the question of whether shifts to diets containing more polyunsaturation are universally desirable.

Ω-3 FATTY ACIDS

Eicosapentaenoic acid (20:5, EPA), an analog of arachidonic acid that competes for incorporation into the phospholipid substrate pools, reduces the amount of arachidonic acid available for eicosanoid formation when the cell is activated (24,25). EPA is also a poor substrate for cyclo-oxygenase and acts primarily as a competitive inhibitor of arachidonic acid conversion to the dienoic prostaglandins. While EPA is a good substrate for lipoxygenases, the lipoxygenase products formed from EPA are less active than those produced from arachidonic acid. These "anti-arachidonic acid" actions of EPA are probably responsible for many of the biological effects of the Ω-3 fatty acids.

The main Ω-3 fatty acid that accumulates in most tissue, especially the retina and brain, is docosahexaenoic acid (22:6, DHA), not EPA. It is crucial to determine whether DHA has a specific functional role. Although DHA can be retroconverted to EPA (26), it is most unlikely that DHA is simply a storage form for excess EPA. DHA could have special actions by producing unique structural effects in the membrane lipid bilayer (27). In this regard DHA is incorporated primarily into the ethanolamine and serine phosphoglycerides, especially the ethanolamine plasmalogens (28). The functions of these phospholipids are not fully understood, and the biologic role of DHA may be clarified as we learn more about the actions and effects of these phospholipid classes.

Another question that remains to be answered is how DHA is made available to the brain. One possibility is that DHA is formed in the liver and is then transported preformed across the blood-brain barrier (29). Alternatively, as suggested by work with mouse brain microvessel endothelial cultures (30), the endothelium of the blood-brain barrier may be a site of conversion of circulating ω-3 fatty acid precursors to docosapentaenoic acid (22:5). This intermediate may then be the form transported across the blood-brain barrier into the brain, where it is desaturated to DHA. The extent to which each of these mechanisms operates to supply the brain with DHA is an important area that requires clarification.

FATTY ACID ANALOGS

Most of the work to date deals with the straight chain fatty acids that are abundant in mammalian tissues. Recently, however, hydroxylated derivatives of linoleic acid (HODE) were found to be produced by a number of tissues, including endothelium (31,32). Furthermore, the lipoxygenase pathways produce hydroxylated forms of arachidonic acid (HETE). The HETEs can be incorporated into tissue phospholipids and oxidized in peroxisomes to chain-shortened metabolites (33,34). Epoxide derivatives of arachidonic acid, formed by the cytochrome P_{450} pathway, appear to act as mediators of certain cellular functions (35). Branched chain fatty acids can be incorporated into phospholipids and can perturb the packing of the membrane lipid bilayer (36). This may be one reason why phytanic acid accumulation produces neurologic defects. Finally, conjugated fatty acids such as cisparinaric acid can be incorporated into membranes and thereby serve as a fluorescent reporter group for functional studies (37). Further work with these and other analogs is likely to provide many new molecular insights into the effects that fatty acids can have in biological systems.

FUTURE DIRECTIONS

Table 3 lists the areas of fatty acid research which I believe hold the greatest promise for further study. This list is by no means complete. It is obvious that many

TABLE 3. *Promising areas for further study*

Protein acylation—myristic acid
Peroxisomes—function of β-oxidation, plasmalogens
Perodixation—fatty acid composition
Phospholipid molecular species
Docosahexaenoic acid—role in nervous system
FABP—role in fatty acid metabolism
HETE, HODE, eicosatrienoic acid epoxides—function
Membrane fatty acid modification—cell response mechanisms

FABP, fatty acid binding protein; HETE, hydroxyeicosatetraenoic acid; HODE, hydroxyoctadecadienoic acid.

vital questions remain to be explored, and new discoveries in the fatty acid field almost certainly will occur through the 1990s and beyond.

ACKNOWLEDGMENT

The studies from my group discussed in this review were supported by research grants HL14230, HL39308, and DK28516 from the National Institutes of Health.

REFERENCES

1. James G, Olson EN. Fatty acylated proteins as components of intracellular signaling pathways. *Biochemistry* 1990; 29: 2623–34.
2. Spector AA. The transport and utilization of free fatty acid. *Ann NY Acad Sci* 1968; 149: 768–83.
3. Spector AA, Mathur SN, Kaduce TL, Hyman BT. Lipid nutrition and metabolism of cultured mammalian cells. *Prog Lipid Res* 1981; 19: 155–86.
4. Spector AA. Fatty acid binding to plasma albumin. *J Lipid Res* 1975; 16:165–79.
5. Spector AA. The effect of fatty acid structure on utilization in Ehrlich ascites tumor cells. *Cancer Res* 1967; 27: 1587–94.
6. Cooper RB, Noy N, Zakim DA. Mechanism for binding of fatty acids to hepatocyte plasma membranes. *J Lipid Res* 1989; 30: 1719–26.
7. Stremmel W, Strohmeyer G, Berk PD. Hepatocellular uptake of oleate is energy dependent, sodium linked, and inhibited by an antibody to a hepatocyte plasma membrane fatty acid binding protein. *Proc Natl Acad Sci USA* 1986; 83: 3584–8.
8. Abumrad NA, Perkins RH, Park JH, Park CR. Mechanism of long chain fatty acid permeation in the isolated adipocyte. *J Biol Chem* 1981; 256: 9183–91.
9. Lowe JB, Sacchettini JC, Laposata M, McQuillan JJ, Gordon JI. Expression of rat intestinal fatty acid-binding protein in *Escherichia coli*. *J Biol Chem* 1987; 262: 5931–7.
10. Hiltunen JK, Karki T, Hassinene IE, Osmundsen H. β-Oxidation of polyunsaturated fatty acids by rat liver peroxisomes. *J Biol Chem* 1986; 261: 16484–93.
11. Lands WEM, Byrnes MJ. The influence of ambient peroxides on the conversion of 5,8,11,14,17-eicosapentaenoic acid to prostaglandins. *Prog Lipid Res* 1981; 20: 287–90.
12. Hempel SL, Haycraft DL, Hoak JC, Spector AA. Reduced prostacyclin formation following reoxygenation of anoxic endothelium. *Am J Physiol* 1990; 259: C738–45.
13. Blank ML, Spector AA, Kaduce TL, Snyder F. Composition and incorporation of [^{3}H]arachidonic acid into molecular species of phospholipid classes by cultured human endothelial cells. *Biochim Biophys Acta* 1986; 877: 211–5.
14. Brown MS, Goldstein JL. A receptor-mediated pathway for cholesterol hemeostasis. *Science* 1986; 232: 34–47.
15. Spector AA, Scanu AM, Kaduce TL, Figard PH, Fless GM, Czervionke RL. Effect of human plasma lipoproteins on prostacyclin production by cultured endothelial cells. *J Lipid Res* 1985; 26: 288–97.
16. Habenicht AJR, Salbach P, Goerig M, et al. The LDL receptor pathway delivers arachidonic acid for eicosanoid formation in cells stimulated by platelet-derived growth factor. *Nature* 1990; 345: 634–6.
17. Spector AA, Steinberg D. Release of free fatty acid from Ehrlich ascites tumor cells. *J Lipid Res* 1966; 7: 649–56.
18. Spector AA, Steinberg D. Turnover and utilization of esterified fatty acids in Ehrlich ascites tumor cells. *J Biol Chem* 1967; 242: 3057–62.
19. Lewis MG, Kaduce TL, Spector AA. Effect of essential polyunsaturated fatty acid modifications on prostaglandin production by MDCK canine kidney cells. *Prostaglandins* 1981; 22: 747–60.
20. Denning GM, Figard PH, Spector AA. Effect of fatty acid modification on prostaglandin production by cultured 3T3 cells. *J Lipid Res* 1982; 23: 585–96.
21. Lokesh BR, Mathur SN, Spector AA. Effect of fatty acid saturation on NADPH-dependent lipid peroxidation in rat liver microsomes. *J Lipid Res* 1981; 22: 905–15.

22. Spector AA, Yorek MA. Membrane lipid composition and cellular function. *J Lipid Res* 1985; 26: 1015–35.
23. Spector AA, Burns CP. Biological and therapeutic potential of membrane lipid modification in tumors. *Cancer Res* 1987; 47: 4529–37.
24. Kinsella JE, Lokesh B, Stone RA. Dietary n-3 polyunsaturated fatty acids and amelioration of cardiovascular disease: possible mechanisms. *Am J Clin Nutr* 1990; 52: 1–28.
25. Spector AA, Kaduce TL, Figard PH, Norton KC, Hoak JC, Czervionke RL. Eicosapentaenoic acid and prostacyclin production by cultured human endothelial cells. *J Lipid Res* 1983; 24: 1595–604.
26. Hadjiagapiou C, Spector AA. Docosahexaenoic acid metabolism and effect on prostacyclin production in endothelial cells. *Arch Biochem Biophys* 1987; 253: 1–12.
27. Applegate KR, Glomset JA. Computer-based modeling of the conformation and packing properties of docosahexaenoic acid. *J Lipid Res* 1986; 27: 658–80.
28. Yorek MA, Bohnker RR, Dudley DT, Spector AA. Comparative utilization of n-3 polyunsaturated fatty acids by cultured Y-79 retinoblastoma cells. *Biochim Biophys Acta* 1984; 795: 277–85.
29. Scott BL, Bazan NG. Membrane docosahexaenoate is supplied to the developing brain and retina by the liver. *Proc Natl Acad Sci USA* 1989; 86: 2903–7.
30. Moore SA, Yoder E, Spector AA. Role of the blood-brain barrier in the formation of long-chain ω-3 and ω-6 fatty acids from essential fatty acid precursors. *J Neurochem* 1990; 55: 391–402.
31. Buchanan MR, Haas TA, Lagarde M, Guichardant M. 13-Hydroxyoctadecadienoic acid is the vessel wall chemorepellant factor, LOX. *J Biol Chem* 1985; 260: 16056–9.
32. Kaduce TL, Figard PH, Leifur R, Spector AA. Formation of 9-hydroxyoctadecadienoic acid from linoleic acid in endothelial cells. *J Biol Chem* 1989; 264: 6823–30.
33. Spector AA, Gordon JA, Moore SA. Hydroxyeicosatetraenoic acid (HETEs). *Prog Lipid Res* 1988; 27: 271–323.
34. Gordon JA, Figard PH, Spector AA. Hydroxyeicosatetraenoic acid metabolism in cultured human skin fibroblasts. Evidence for peroxisomal β-oxidation. *J Clin Invest* 1990; 85: 1173–81.
35. Fitzpatrick FA, Murphy RC. Cytochrome P-450 metabolism of arachidonic acid. Formation and biological actions of "epoxygenase"-derived eicosanoids. *Pharmacol Rev* 1988; 40: 229–41.
36. King ME, Spector AA. Effect of specific fatty acyl enrichments on membrane physical properties detected with a spin label probe. *J Biol Chem* 1978; 253: 6493–501.
37. Rintoul DA, Simoni RD. Incorporation of a naturally occurring fluorescent fatty acid into lipids of cultured mammalian cells. *J Biol Chem* 1977; 252: 7916–8.

DISCUSSION

Dr. Glinsmann: In relation to the genetic changes that occur in lipoproteins, do you think there is also considerable genetic variation in the fatty acid pathways and that this may explain some of the differences observed?

Dr. Spector: I think there are probably mutations where the handling of fatty acids is not normal and this can lead to disease. I expect there are also genetic variations in fatty acid pathways. It will probably turn out that some people are better at elongating palmitic acid and at desaturating the resulting stearic acid, so they accumulate more monounsaturates. This is an area that needs to be explored.

Dr. Merrill: I found it interesting that the 22:6 fatty acids are incorporated in such large amounts into ethanolamine plasmalogens. What is the specificity for the addition of the alkyl ether group to the plasmalogens? Is it unusual for plasmalogens to be influenced by dietary fatty acids?

Dr. Spector: I am not sure whether the availability of certain fatty acids in the diet, such as 22:6, can affect the formation of ether lipids. Another possibility is that the genetic make-up may control the extent to which the ether bond is formed and the plasmalogens are produced.

Dr. Bracco: One interesting remark is that in the membrane you can change the phospholipid and the fatty acid composition; the membrane is changing, not only in terms of activity, but also in terms of polarity of the phospholipid. One should also consider what is called the flip flop mechanism which is one of the fields to be investigated again, how we can measure the change of the polarity of the membrane when we change the fatty acid composition and in particular the class of phospholipid. This is one of the techniques we need in order to explain the different effects of the kind of phospholipids in the membrane.

Dr. Spector: I agree completely. There will be some changes in the physical properties of the membrane as a result of these fatty acid substitutions. On the other hand, this probably will not be a very large effect in terms of the overall physical properties of the membrane. It is much more likely that localized domains, either localized phospholipid pools that feed into specific metabolic pathways or localized domains around certain membrane proteins, are where the functional changes will be observed. In terms of the measurement that we actually use to determine membrane fluidity, there is so much of the original fatty acid present that the change may not be very profound. Localized changes are probably going to be missed by fluidity measurements alone. Therefore, if we use physical probes, we may not see as much of a change as we would, if we were monitoring certain membrane proteins, or substrate pools that supply fatty acid to phospholipases.

Dr. Spielmann: Myristic acid is known to be one of the most important fatty acids in the induction of arteriosclerosis. Could you speculate on its possible role in this?

Dr. Spector: One possibility is that myristic acid is elongated to palmitic acid. The formation of monounsaturates like oleic acid from palmitic acid may not be as rapid as from stearic acid which comes directly from the diet. Apparently the step from stearic to oleic is much faster than the elongation step needed to convert palmitic to stearic acid. If the diet is rich in the tropical oils and a lot of medium chain saturates are absorbed, a build-up of the longer chain saturates may occur without corresponding conversion to monounsaturates. This could produce hypercholesterolemia.

Dr. Deckelbaum: You showed that hydroxy fatty acids can be part of the phospholipid molecule. We know that if you hydroxylate linoleic acid you produce ricinoleic acid, a major ingredient of castor oil which has important effects on the intestine. Do you think there is a mediatory role for nonphospholipid hydroxy fatty acids in the body outside the gut lumen?

Dr. Spector: Yes, I think hydroxy fatty acids have a role in the function of many tissues, in addition to the intestine. The hydroxylated arachidonic derivatives may be very important in transcytosis reactions and in signaling between cells. Other eicosanoids bind to receptors and induce a rapid response, whereas these substances could be taken up into membranes and produce slower, more prolonged changes in cell function.

Dr. Guesry: You make the point that cell membrane composition is highly dependent on the intake of specific fatty acids, and we know that breast milk long chain polyunsaturated fatty acid composition is also highly dependent on the maternal intake. This means that the cell composition of the baby is dependent on the intake of the mother. It is difficult for me to accept that there is no mechanism for defending the human body against variation in food composition.

Dr. Spector: This is a puzzling problem. I don't want to imply, however, that there is extreme variation in cell composition. In terms of the dietary fatty acids the human has protective mechanisms—the elongation and desaturation pathways. In spite of what is in the diet there is remarkable consistency in the membranes. On a scale of 0 to 1, 0 being the most fluid and 1 being the most rigid, the kinds of variations that can occur in membranes are somewhere between 0.40 and 0.46. We are talking about variations within a narrow range, so much of the structural consistency does not change. Some might say that a variation of 5% or so in a structural component is not important. I would say that overall there is the ability to compensate and to keep things within limits, but there is also an ability to vary membrane structure slightly. Local regions around key membrane proteins, or phospholipid pools that provide the prostaglandin substrates, may change to a much greater extent than the bulk membrane lipid.

Dr. Crawford: I should like to comment on the variability of human milk, as this is a particularly misconceived area. We have studied over 4,000 milk samples, a large proportion of which were collected over a 6 month lactation period from several different countries. The remarkable feature is that, while variability undoubtedly exists, the pattern of the fatty acids, and especially the composition of the long chain EFA derivatives, was remarkably constant. In particular the long chain essential fatty acid derivatives, which are the principal substrates for membrane growth, are strikingly similar. Shelia Innis compared Inuit Indian with Vancouver Canadian mothers' milks, which would be expected to be about as different as possible since the Inuits are fish eaters and therefore live on a diet rich in n-3 FA, while Vancouver mothers have a high proportion of lionelic acid in their diets. The remarkable feature was the similarity in the milk composition, the linoleic acid content being 11.5% and 12.7% in Inuit and Vancouver mothers, respectively (1).

Dr. Koletzko: We have found strong indications for a protective mechanism that regulates the content of long chain polyunsaturated fatty acids in human milk. Metabolic regulation in the maternal organism seems to keep the ratio between ω-6 and ω-3 long chain polyunsaturates relatively constant. It appears that the various essential fatty acids may have different physiological roles for the infant and are therefore subject to different regulatory mechanisms. Maybe linoleic acid intake does not matter that much for the infant at all, but it is the long chain metabolites that are important.

Dr. Crawford: I think that the confusion in the past has been that people thought that milk fat was just fat, whereas in fact it is provided for two purposes: providing energy and providing for cell growth and development. Fifty percent of the linoleic acid goes into the metabolic pools for oxidation, so a variability in the amount of linoleic acid supplied can be acceptable, the excess simply being burned as fuel. However there would probably be some low level at which there is an ultimate requirement to meet the needs for cell growth and function.

Dr. Heim: It is almost unbelievable that 50% of the linoleic acid is directed to oxidation. In our laboratory we found in formula-fed infants about 10% of the lipids are oxidized and the rest are deposited; in breast-fed infants up to 25% are oxidized at maximum. I think linoleic acid is largely deposited and not oxidized.

Dr. Crawford: In the very active phases of growth, such as in the premature infant, the situation may be different from the sort of experimental data I was referring to. What I was saying was that linoleic acid is compartmentalized into oxidative pools, with 50% going into triglycerides and 50% going into the phosphoglycerides. Under normal circumstances that 50% in the triglycerides would be available for oxidation, but not necessarily so, depending on the demands for growth which I assume would take priority.

Dr. Spielmann: Could you enlarge a little on the relationship between linoleic acid and the arachidonic acid content and PGE_2 production by endothelial cells?

Dr. Spector: The data I showed were from 3T3 cells, which predominantly synthesize PGE_2. A decrease in PGE_2 formation occurs at the highest linoleic acid concentrations and this is significant. As the linoleic acid content of the cell phospholipids increases, arachidonic acid goes down and less is available for prostaglandin formation. The same general effect occurs in the endothelium, which predominantly synthesizes PGI_2. In endothelium derived from large arteries this decrease occurs at much lower levels of linoleic acid. The endothelial cells are therefore especially sensitive to linoleic acid, and PGI_2 production is suppressed more than in 3T3 cells.

Dr. Jeremy: I should like to make a comment about low density lipoproteins (LDL) since I have done some experiments recently on human LDL. Others have shown that LDL stimulate prostacyclin synthesis in endothelial cells. We have repeated these experiments in human endothelial cells and isolated vessels and have found that the effect is probably due to release of arachidonic acid within the cell. We have not published this yet but the concept that LDL enter cell where they release fatty acids is absolutely right. Obviously other fatty acids may influence other functions, not just prostaglandin synthesis, depending on the relative fatty acid content of the LDL.

Dr. Cunnane: Do you believe there is a blood-brain barrier for long chain polyunsaturated fatty acids?

Dr. Spector: Our studies confirm the work of Bazan showing that polyunsaturates like 22:6 can pass right through the endothelium. However, I don't think the endothelium is passive. It plays an active role and can for a time trap these fatty acids in storage lipids and subsequently release them from the basolateral surface into the brain. Our studies indicate that the microvascular endothelium plays a critical role in processing the fatty acids that get into the nervous system.

REFERENCE

1. Innis S. Dietary ω3 and ω6 fatty acids. In: Galli C and Simopoulos AP, eds. *NATO ASI series.* 1989; 171: 142.

ABBREVIATIONS

EFA: essential fatty acids
PUFA: polyunsaturated fatty acids
LCPUFA: long-chain-polyunsaturated fatty acids
α-LNA: alpha-linolenic acid
γ-LNA, GLA: gamma-linolenic acid
EPA: eicosapentaenoic acid
DHA: docosahexaenoic acid
AA: arachidonic acid
n-3, ω-3, Ω-3:   omega 3 serie fatty acids
n-6, ω-6, Ω-6:   omega 6 serie fatty acids
CHOL: cholesterol
PGs: prostaglandins
LPs: lipoproteins

Long Chain Fatty Acid Metabolism

Howard Sprecher

Department of Medical Biochemistry, Ohio State University, Columbus, Ohio 43210-1218, USA

In recent years it has become ever more apparent that a variety of physiological processes are in part mediated by the types of unsaturated acids esterified in membrane lipids. These processes may broadly be categorized as being either eicosanoid-dependent or eicosanoid-independent. Eicosanoid-mediated events are frequently related to the amounts of esterified 20-carbon polyunsaturated fatty acid (PUFA) available for agonist-induced release followed by their metabolism via the cyclo-oxygenase or lipoxygenase pathways. For example, platelet aggregation (1) and neutrophil recruitment followed by degranulation (2) are both mediated in different ways by the types of prostaglandins, hydroxy acids, and leukotrienes produced from arachidonate *versus* those made from 20:5(n-3).

Membrane lipids from many cells and tissues also contain large amounts of 22-carbon (n-3) and (n-6) PUFA. Endothelial cells (3), kidney microsomes (4), and platelets (5) all metabolize exogenous 22-carbon (n-6) acids to eicosanoids and hydroxy acids. To date there is no evidence showing that exogenous 22-carbon (n-3) acids are metabolized by cyclo-oxygenase. Platelets metabolize both 22:5(n-3) and 22:6(n-3) into a isomeric pair of hydroxy fatty acids via the lipoxygenase pathway (5). *In vivo* the synthesis of cyclo-oxygenase and lipoxygenase products is coupled to the agonist-induced activation of phospholipases. There is, however, little evidence showing that 22-carbon acids are metabolized to eicosanoids *in vivo*. The reasons for this apparent lack of metabolism are not known but it may be due to the lack of release of 22-carbon acids from membrane lipids (6,7). There is, however, considerable evidence that processes such as visual acuity and learning ability correlate with the amount of 22:6(n-3) esterified in retina and brain phospholipids (8). It thus appears that 22-carbon (n-3) and (n-6) PUFA may exert their physiological roles primarily via eicosanoid-independent mechanisms.

Testes (9), retina (10), and brain (11) are examples of three tissues in which the phospholipids contain very long chain PUFA. These compounds have 24 to 38 carbons with 4, 5, or 6 double bonds. Little is known about the biological function of this interesting group of fatty acids.

The types of polyunsaturated fatty acids found in membrane lipids must be regulated by the coordinated control of the enzymes that synthesize and subsequently esterify acids into specific phospholipids. In addition, unique specificities must exist between cells to explain observed compositional differences. This review will summarize some of the factors regulating the metabolism and subsequent acylation of PUFA into membrane lipids.

FATTY ACID BIOSYNTHESIS

Desaturation

It is generally accepted that dietary 18:2(n-6) and 18:3(n-3) are metabolized, respectively, to 22:5(n-6) and 22:6(n-3) via an alternating sequence of position-specific desaturases and malonyl-coenzyme A (CoA)-dependent chain elongation steps (Fig. 1). Rate studies, using primarily rat liver microsomes (12), as well as experiments with hepatocytes (13) support the hypothesis that the 6-desaturase step is rate limiting in the synthesis of arachidonate. Although the 6-desaturase has been partially purified from rat liver microsomes (14) relatively little is known about what regulates the activity of this important enzyme *in vivo*. Some mutant cells lack the ability to desaturate fatty acids at position-6 even though they are able to introduce a double bond at the 5-position (15). These observations, along with altered rates of desaturation as induced by dietary or hormonal treatment of rats (16), support the hypothesis for separate 6- and 5-desaturases. Appropriate acyl-CoAs, as well as choline phosphoglycerides containing 8,11,14–20:3 at the *sn*-2 position, are both substrates for desaturation at position-5 (17). It remains to be determined whether a single protein can use both an acyl-CoA and an esterified fatty acid as substrates to introduce a double bond at position-5. It is generally accepted that 18:2(n-6) and 18:3(n-3) are metabolized, respectively, to 22:5(n-6) and 22:6(n-3). The last step in these reaction sequences requires a 4-desaturase (Fig. 1). However, the presence of a 4-desaturase has never really been established. For example, Ayala *et al.* (18) reported

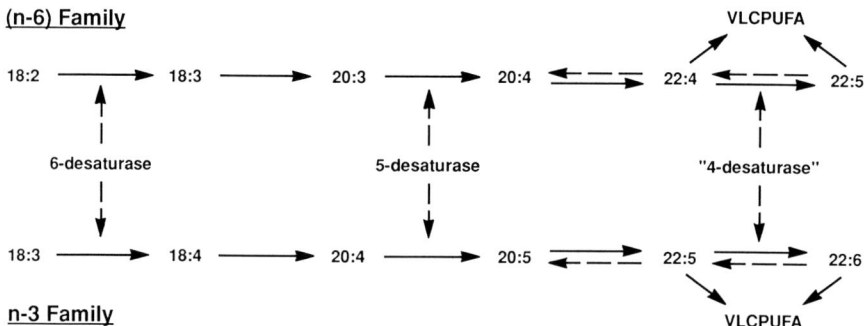

FIG. 1. Pathways for the microsomal desaturation and chain elongation of dietary linoleate and linolenate. The dashed arrows show that 22-carbon acids are in part metabolized to 20-carbon acids by retroconversion. In addition, 22-carbon acids serve as the precursors for the synthesis of very long chain polyunsaturated fatty acids (VLCPUFA).

that liver and testicular microsomes from chow-fed rats did not desaturate 22:4(n-6) to 22:5(n-6).

Chain Elongation and Retroconversion

Fatty acids are chain elongated via a malonyl-CoA-dependent process in which the substrates and products are the CoA derivatives (19) (Fig. 2). The condensation step is rate limiting for both saturated and 18-carbon unsaturated primers. Several studies now suggest that two separate condensing enzymes are used for saturated and unsaturated primers with the resulting β-ketoacyl-CoAs being channeled into a common set of enzymes to complete the chain elongation process (20,21). It is, however, not known if single or different condensing enzymes are used for chain-elongating 18- *versus* 20-carbon polyunsaturated fatty acids.

Rates of overall chain elongation are generally much more rapid than for desaturation. These observations suggest that chain elongation does not play a major role in regulating the synthesis of PUFA. The results in Table 1 show the unsaturated fatty acid composition of choline- and ethanolamine-containing phosphoglycerides from livers of chow-fed rats. These lipids contain large amounts of 20:4(n-6) but they have only low levels of 22:4(n-6) and 22:5(n-6). Conversely, they contain only trace amounts of 20:5(n-3), but 22:5(n-3) and particularly 22:6(n-3), are major components. Clearly *in vivo* different mechanisms must thus exist for regulating the

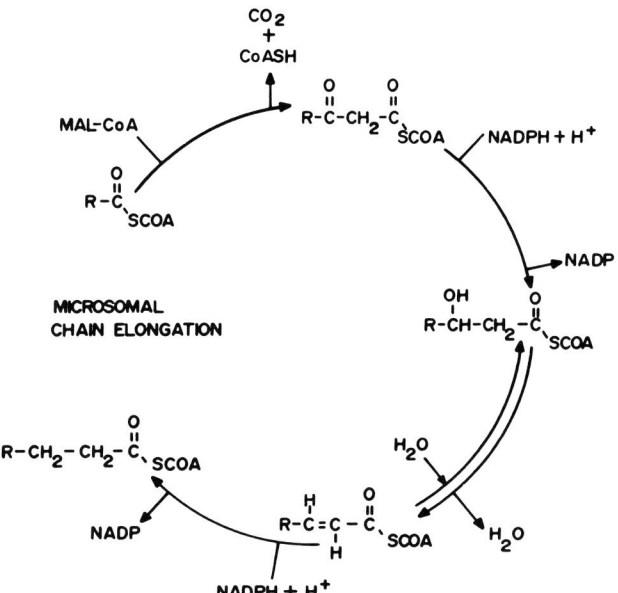

FIG. 2. The pathway for the malonyl-CoA-dependent chain elongation of fatty acids.

TABLE 1. *The unsaturated fatty acid composition of choline- and ethanolamine-containing phosphoglycerides from livers of rats maintained on a chow diet*

Fatty acid	Choline phosphoglycerides, weight	Ethanolamine phosphoglycerides, percent
18:2(n-6)	18.2	7.7
20:3(n-6)	1.2	0.5
20:4(n-6)	24.5	30.3
20:5(n-3)	0.7	1.1
22:4(n-6)	—	0.2
22:5(n-6)	0.3	—
22:5(n-3)	0.5	1.5
22:6(n-3)	4.1	10.3

conversion of 20:4(n-6) to 22:5(n-6) *versus* the metabolism of 20:5(n-3) to 22:6(n-3). These differences are not explained by enzymatic rate studies since both 20:4(n-6) and 20:5(n-3) are chain-elongated at about the same rate.

The amounts of 20- and 22-carbon PUFA available for acylation into membrane lipids *in vivo* is not totally dependent on anabolic specificities. It has long been recognized that membrane lipids accumulate 20-carbon PUFA when 22-carbon (n-6) and (n-3) PUFA are fed to rats (22). This catabolic process is frequently referred to as partial degradation or retroconversion. The pathway for retroconversion of 22:6(n-3), as elucidated by Shulz and Kunau (23), is shown in Fig. 3. This pathway requires the use of 2,4-dienoyl-CoA reductase and $\Delta 3$-*cis*-$\Delta 2$-*trans*-enoyl-CoA isomerase. Neither of these enzymes is required for the β-oxidation of saturated fatty acids. For reasons which are not yet understood a portion of the 22-carbon acids is metabolized to 20-carbon compounds followed by their removal from the β-oxidation process with subsequent acylation into membrane lipids. The intracellular location of this process remains to be more clearly defined. However, several studies suggest that it may be primarily peroxisomal (24,25). The amounts of 20- and 22-carbon PUFA available for acylation into lipids thus not only depend on the conversion of 20- to 22-carbon PUFA but, in addition, the composition of the intracellular fatty acid pool is in part regulated by the conversion of 22- to 20-carbon PUFA. However, it must be stressed that the mechanisms regulating retroconversion *versus* total β-oxidation are not elucidated. For example, both 22-carbon as well as 20-carbon

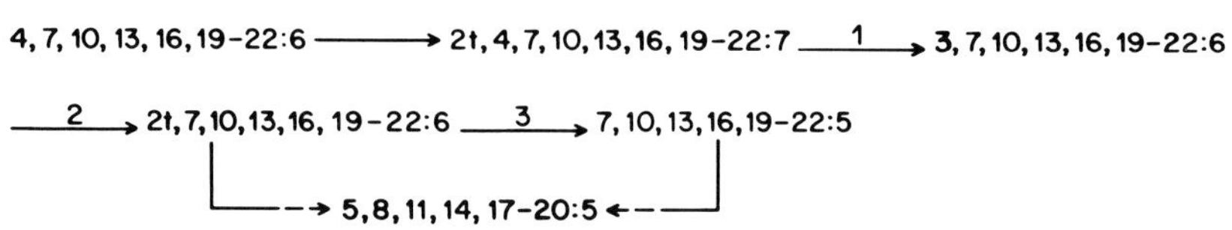

4, 7, 10, 13, 16, 19-22:6 ⟶ 2t, 4, 7, 10, 13, 16, 19-22:7 —1→ 3, 7, 10, 13, 16, 19-22:6

—2→ 2t, 7, 10, 13, 16, 19-22:6 —3→ 7, 10, 13, 16, 19-22:5

⟶ 5, 8, 11, 14, 17-20:5 ⟵

FIG. 3. The pathway for β-oxidation of polyunsaturated fatty acids. Reaction 1 is catalyzed by 2-*trans*-4-*cis*-dienoyl-CoA reductase; reaction 2 is catalyzed by $\Delta 3$-*cis*-$\Delta 2$-*trans*-enoyl-CoA isomerase; reaction 3 implies intramitochondrial nucleotide-dependent reduction.

PUFA are substrates for peroxisomal β-oxidation. Why then does 22-carbon β-oxidation, in part, stop when 20-carbon acids are produced and how are 20:4(n-6) and 20:5(n-3) transported out of peroxisomes or perhaps mitochondria to make these acids available for acylation into membrane lipids?

CELLULAR SPECIFICITIES FOR FATTY ACID BIOSYNTHESIS

Individual membrane lipids from various cells and tissues are characterized by differences in their unsaturated fatty acid composition. These compositional findings raise the following questions. Do various cells have unique capabilities to modify dietary fatty acids to specifically make those PUFA required for their own membrane lipid biosynthesis? Alternatively, is liver the primary site of PUFA biosynthesis and are specific PUFA then selectively taken up by various cells for subsequent acylation? In a recent review, Rosenthal (26) summarizes the evidence showing that extrahepatic cells have limited abilities to desaturate and chain-elongate fatty acids. Lefkowith *et al.* (27) reported there was a time-dependent movement of labeled 20:4(n-6) from liver lipids to those in heart and kidney, thus suggesting that dietary fatty acids were initially processed by the liver. Platelets and neutrophils are examples of two types of cells which contain large amounts of 20:4(n-6) but relatively small amounts of 22-carbon PUFA. Both cells are able to chain-elongate but not desaturate fatty acids (28–31). The physiological role of chain elongation in these cells is thus obscure. Conversely, heart lipids are characterized by their relatively high content of 22-carbon (n-3) PUFA. We, however, have been unable to show that cardiomyocytes or the perfused rat heart have the capacity to introduce a double bond at position-6 when either linoleate or linolenate was used as a substrate (32). In addition, neither 20:4(n-6) nor 20:5(n-3) was chain-elongated by cardiomyocytes. When cardiomyocytes were incubated with 3-^{14}C-labeled 22:4(n-6) or 22:5(n-3) it was not possible to detect any products of the 4-desaturase—i.e., 22:5(n-6) or 22:6(n-3) (33). Conversely, as shown in Table 2 both acids were substrates for retroconversion as measured by the acylation of radioactive arachidonate and 20:5(n-3) into myocyte phospholipids. Interestingly, the specificity for retroconversion followed by subsequent esterification was consistent with compositional data. More of the

TABLE 2. *Distribution of radioactivity in percent in phospholipid fatty acids after incubating rat cardiomyocytes with either 3-^{14}C-labeled 22:4(n-6) or 22:5(n-3)*

Component	Substrate	
	3-^{14}C-22:4(n-6)	3-^{14}C-22:5(n-3)
22:4(n-6)	52	—
20:4(n-6)	48	—
22:5(n-3)	—	88
20:5(n-3)	—	12

22:4(n-6) was retroconverted to 20:4(n-6) and esterified when compared to the amount of 20:5(n-3) that was made from 22:5(n-3) and subsequently acylated. The above examples suggest that liver plays a major role in supplying extrahepatic cells with the types of unsaturated acids required to make their membrane lipids. The physiological role of the retroconversion process in cells such as cardiomyocytes is, however, unclear.

The source of 22:6(n-3) for phospholipid synthesis in brain and retina has long been a matter of discussion. Scott and Bazan (34) recently presented evidence suggesting that 18:3(n-3) was metabolized to 22:6(n-3) in liver and transported to the brain. Another recent study by Moore et al. (35) showed that endothelial cells isolated from brain capillaries are able to metabolize 18:3(n-3) to potentially provide long chain (n-3) acids for brain phospholipid biosynthesis. A second important unresolved question is to define the site of synthesis for the very long chain PUFA that are found in brain and retina phospholipids. In essence, the horizontal pathways in Fig. 1 define how PUFA are produced in tissues such as liver. However, in brain the 20- and 22-carbon unsaturated acids can be viewed as the initial unsaturated precursors for additional families of polyunsaturated acids that are produced by repetitive chain elongation steps. Several lines of evidence now suggest that these enzyme activities may indeed reside in brain but it remains to be established whether they are absent in liver. Brain, but not liver, is able to chain elongate 18:0 to 20:0 (36,37). Robinson et al. (38) reported that when 1-^{14}C-26:4(n-6) was injected into brains of 1 and 16 day old rats it was chain-elongated to yield small amounts of 28:4, 30:4, 34:4, and 36:4. The above results document that brain has the capacity to chain-elongate both long chain saturated and long chain unsaturated fatty acids. However, it clearly raises the question as to whether brain contains unique chain-elongating or perhaps condensing enzymes that are absent in liver. This is indeed a distinct possibility since studies by Goldberg et al. (39) suggest that brain contains three separate chain-elongating enzymes. One uses 16:0-CoA as a primer, the second converts 18:0 to 20:0, while the third, which is absent in a demyelinating disease in quaking and jimpy mice, utilizes acyl-CoA derivatives of 20- and 22-carbons.

SPECIFICITIES IN PHOSPHOLIPID BIOSYNTHESIS

The types of PUFA found in membrane lipids depend not only on a readily available supply of PUFA but also on a myriad of specificities for acylating fatty acids into individual phospholipids. According to the Kennedy pathway, phosphatidic acid or the resulting diglyceride is a common intermediate for both phospholipid and triglyceride biosynthesis. However, the fatty acid composition of triglycerides and phospholipids differ. In part, this discrepancy was resolved by Lands when he described a deacylation-reacylation cycle. This pathway as shown in Fig. 4 is a remodeling pathway in which the fatty acid at the *sn*-2 position of an existing phospholipid is hydrolyzed by phospholipase A_2 followed by re-esterification with a second fatty acid. The discovery of this important pathway helped to clarify how

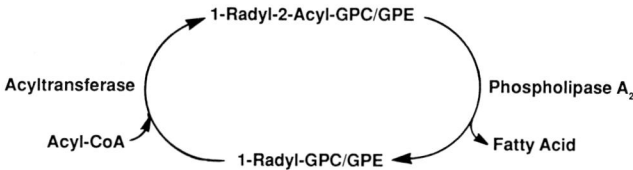

FIG. 4. The pathway for modifying phospholipid fatty acid composition by deacylation and subsequent reacylation.

phospholipids selectively obtain their highly unsaturated fatty acids. However, several important questions remain unresolved. For example, membrane lipids frequently contain large amounts of 18:2(n-6) and 20:4(n-6) but only low levels of 18:3(n-6) and 20:3(n-6), even though both of these latter acids are obligatory intermediates in the conversion of dietary 18:2(n-6) to 20:4(n-6). Table 3 compares the rate of desaturation and chain elongation for individual reactions required in converting 18:2(n-6) to 20:4(n-6). Rates of acylation using 1-acyl-*sn*-glycero-3-phosphocholine as an acceptor are also shown (40). Clearly, both 18:3(n-6) and 20:3(n-6) are removed more rapidly by acylation than by either chain elongation or desaturation. Reaction rates by themselves are thus poor predictors of the types of PUFA found in membrane lipids. Clearly, different mechanisms must operate *in vivo* to determine what regulates membrane lipid fatty acid composition. By using isolated hepatocytes we have presented evidence suggesting that some linoleate may be channeled directly to arachidonate in such a way that 18:3(n-6) and 20:3(n-6) are not made available for esterification (41). However, when 18:2(n-6) was incubated with hepatocytes some 18:3(n-6) was esterified (41). This 18:3(n-6), however, had a very rapid turnover rate, suggesting that it was part of a highly labile phospholipid pool (42). These findings suggest that a "ping-pong" mechanism may in part be involved in converting 18:2(n-6) to 20:4(n-6). Initially, 18:2(n-6) is desaturated to 18:3(n-6)

TABLE 3. *Rates of desaturation and chain elongation for individual reactions in (n-6) fatty acid biosynthesis and for acylation using 1-acyl-*sn*-glycero-3-phosphocholine as an acceptor*[a]

Reaction or substrate	Rate
Desaturation or chain elongation	
18:2(n-6) → 18:3(n-6)	0.2
18:3(n-6) → 20:3(n-6)	2.5
20:3(n-6) → 20:4(n-6)	0.4
20:4(n-6) → 22:4(n-6)	1.2
Acylation	
18:2(n-6)	56
18:3(n-6)	28
20:3(n-6)	79
20:4(n-6)	72

Adapted from Lands WEM, et al., ref. 40.
[a] All results are expressed as nmol/min/mg of rat liver microsomal protein.

which is then acylated into phospholipids followed by rapid release for conversion to 20:3(n-6). The 20:3(n-6) in turn may temporarily be trapped by esterification prior to its release for desaturation at position-5. This model suggests that PUFA and phospholipid biosynthesis, via the Lands pathway, may be coupled metabolic processes. It is, however, important to note that different mechanisms may control (n-6) *versus* (n-3) PUFA fatty acid metabolism. Membrane lipids of chow-fed animals generally contain low levels of both 18:3(n-3) and 20:5(n-3). Linolenate is an excellent substrate for both peroxisomal (25) and mitochondrial (43) β-oxidation. Its virtual absence from membrane lipids may thus, in part, be explained by its rapid catabolism. However, these findings do not explain why membrane lipids from chow-fed animals accumulate both 22:5(n-3) and 22:6(n-3) but not 20:5(n-3).

Inositol-containing phosphoglycerides play a unique role in the signal transduction process. This lipid, in chow-fed animals, contains primarily only stearic and arachidonic acids. When animals or humans are fed (n-3) acids only small amounts of 20:5(n-3) are acylated into phosphatidylinositol (44,45). Glomset and his colleagues have recently shown that Swiss 3T3 cells contain a diglyceride kinase that is highly specific for arachidonic-acid-containing diglycerides (46). The possibility thus exists that this specific diglyceride may selectively be used for phosphatidylinositol biosynthesis. These findings, however, do not explain why the fatty acid composition of phosphatidyl inositol, phosphatidylinositol 4-phosphate, and phosphatidylinositol-4,5-bisphosphate differ from cerebral cortical phosphoinositides of rats raised on a fat-free diet (47).

The mechanism dictating what fatty acids are found in membrane lipids is not only due to specificities for acyl transferases and selectivities for diglycerides but also by remodeling pathways between donor and acceptor phospholipids. Two general pathways have been described. One is adenosine triphosphate (ATP) and coenzyme (CoA) independent while the other is ATP independent but depends on a supply of CoASH (48). The former pathway has been extensively studied in circulating cells. It appears to function primarily to transfer fatty acids from diacyl phospholipids to alkyl and alkenyl phospholipids. The physiological role of the latter pathway is more uncertain. It is of minor importance in circulating cells but is very active in liver microsomes (48).

CONCLUSION

The objective of this brief review has been to outline some of the major pathways of PUFA and phospholipid biosynthesis. It is now clear that we can alter the long chain unsaturated fatty acid composition of membrane lipids by dietary fat change. It is also becoming ever more apparent that long chain unsaturated acids exert their biological effects in different ways. Arachidonate and 20:5(n-3) are both released from membrane lipids in response to agonists with subsequent metabolism via the cyclo-oxygenase and lipoxygenase pathways. Physiological processes such as thrombosis and inflammation can be down-regulated by replacing esterified arachidonate with 20:5(n-3).

Conversely, much less is known about the biological function of 22-carbon polyenoic acids. In this regard further studies are needed to elucidate what factors regulate the synthesis of 22-carbon (n-6) *versus* (n-3) acids. Membrane lipids from chow-fed animals as well as from humans who consume a typical diet contain large amounts of arachidonate but only low levels of 22:4(n-6) and 22:5(n-6). Arachidonate is the accepted biosynthetic precursor for 22:4(n-6) and 22:5(n-6). Membrane lipids generally contain little 18:3(n-3) and 20:5(n-3) but they accumulate large amounts of 22:6(n-3) and significant levels of 22:5(n-3). *In vivo* differences thus exist for regulating the synthesis and subsequent acylation of 22-carbon (n-6) *versus* (n-3) acids. It is, however, not known if these differences exist at the chain elongation step—i.e., 20:4(n-6) → 22:4(n-6) *versus* 20:5(n-3) → 22:5(n-3)—or for the 4-desaturase—i.e., 22:4(n-6) → 22:5(n-6) *versus* 22:5(n-3) → 22:6(n-3). Indeed it is not yet known if microsomes contain a 4-desaturase which is analogous to the well-characterized 9-desaturase. It is also now recognized that 22-carbon (n-6) and (n-3) acids are in part β-oxidized to arachidonate and 20:5(n-3) followed by their esterification into membrane lipids. The physiological role played by this pathway in maintaining a balance between 20- and 22-carbon acids is not known. Finally, it must be stressed that no physiological role has been ascribed to the very long chain polyunsaturated acids that accumulate in membrane lipids of brain and retina.

ACKNOWLEDGMENT

These studies were supported in part by NIH grants DK18844 and DK20387.

REFERENCES

1. Needleman P, Raz A, Minkes MSM, Ferrendelli JA, Sprecher H. Triene prostaglandins: prostacyclin and thromboxane biosynthesis and unique biological properties. *Proc Natl Acad Sci USA* 1979; 76: 944–8.
2. Lewis RA, Lee TH, Austen KF. Effects of omega-3 fatty acids on the generation of products of the 5-lipoxygenase pathways. In: Simopoulous AP, Kifer RR, Martin RE, eds. *Health effects of polyunsaturated fatty acids in seafoods.* New York: Academic Press, 1986: 227–38.
3. Campbell WB, Falck JR, Okida JR, Johnson AR, Callahan KS. Synthesis of dihomoprostaglandin from adrenic acid (7,10,13,16-docosatetraenoic acid) by human endothelial cells. *Biochim Biophys Acta* 1985; 837: 67–76.
4. Sprecher H, VanRollins M, Sun F, Wyche A, Needleman P. Dihomoprostaglandins and thromboxane: a novel prostaglandin family from adrenic acid that may be specifically synthesized in the kidney. *J Biol Chem* 1982; 257: 3912–8.
5. Sprecher H, Careaga MM. Metabolism of (n-6) and (n-3) polyunsaturated fatty acids by human platelets. *Prostaglandins Leukotrienes Med* 1986; 23: 129–34.
6. Rosenthal MD, Hill JR. Elongation of arachidonic and eicosapentaenoic acids limits their availability for thrombin-stimulated release from the glycerolipids of vascular endothelial cells. *Biochim Biophys Acta* 1986; 875: 382–91.
7. Rosenthal MD, Garcia MC, Sprecher H. Substrate specificity of the agonist-stimulated release of polyunsaturated fatty acids from vascular endothelial cells. *Arch Biochem Biophys* 1989; 274: 590–600.

8. Neuringer M, Connor WE. Omega-3 fatty acids in the retina. In: Galli C, Simopoulos A, eds. *Dietary ω3 and ω6 fatty acids biological effects and nutritional essentiality.* New York: Plenum Press, 1989: 179–90.
9. Grogan WM. Metabolism of arachidonate in rat testis: characterization of 26-30 carbon polyenoic acids. *Lipids* 1984; 19: 341–5.
10. Aveldano MI, Sprecher H. Very long chain (C_{24} to C_{36}) polyenoic fatty acids of the n-3 and n-6 series in dipolyunsaturated phosphatidylcholines from bovine brain retina. *J Biol Chem* 1987; 262: 1180–6.
11. Robinson BS, Johnson DW, Poulos A. Unique molecular species of phosphatidylcholine containing very-long-chain polyenoic fatty acids in rat brain. *Biochem J* 1990; 265: 763–7.
12. Brenner RR. The desaturation step in the animal biosynthesis of polyunsaturated fatty acids. *Lipids* 1971; 6: 567–75.
13. Christophersen BO, Hagve T-A, Norseth J. Studies on the regulation of arachidonic acid synthesis in isolated liver cells. *Biochim Biophys Acta* 1982; 712: 305–14.
14. Okayasu T, Nagao M, Ishibashi J, Imai Y. Purification and partial characterization of linoleoyl-CoA desaturase from rat liver microsomes. *Arch Biochem Biophys* 1981; 206: 21–8.
15. Dunbar LM, Bailey JM. Enzyme deletions and essential fatty acid metabolism in cultured cells. *J Biol Chem* 1975; 250: 1152–3.
16. Castuma JC, Catala A, Brenner RR. Oxidative desaturation of eicosa-8,11-dienoic acid to eicosa-5,8,11-trienoic acid: comparison of different diets on oxidative desaturation at the 5,6 and 6,7 positions. *J Lipid Res* 1972; 13: 783–9.
17. Pugh EL, Kates M. Direct desaturation of eicosatrienoyl lecithin to arachidonyl lecithin by rat liver microsomes. *J Biol Chem* 1977; 252: 68–72.
18. Ayala S, Gaspar G, Brenner RR, Kunau W. Fate of linoleic, arachidonic and docosa-7,10,13,16-tetraenoic acids in rat testicles. *J Lipid Res* 1973; 14: 296–305.
19. Bernert JT, Sprecher H. The isolation of acyl-CoA derivatives in partial reactions in the microsomal chain elongation of fatty acids. *Biochim Biophys Acta* 1979; 573: 436–42.
20. Bernert JT, Sprecher H. An analysis of partial reactions in the overall chain elongation of saturated and unsaturated acids by rat liver microsomes. *J Biol Chem* 1977; 252: 6736–44.
21. Prasad MR, Nagai MN, Ghesquier P, Cook L, Cinti D. Evidence for multiple condensing enzymes in rat hepatic microsomes catalyzing the condensation of saturated, monounsaturated and polyunsaturated acyl coenzyme A. *J Biol Chem* 1986; 261: 8213–7.
22. Sprecher H, James AT. Biosynthesis of long chain fatty acids in mammalian tissues. In: Emken EA, Dutton HJ, eds. *Geometrical and positional fatty acid isomers.* Champaign: American Oil Chemists Society, 1979: 303–38.
23. Schulz H, Kunau W-H. Beta-oxidation of unsaturated fatty acids: a revised pathway. *Trends Biochim Sci* 1987; 12: 403–6.
24. Hovik R, Osmundsen H. Peroxisomal β-oxidation of long-chain fatty acids possessing different extents of unsaturation. *Biochem J* 1987; 247: 531–5.
25. Hiltunen JK, Kärki T, Hassinen IE, Osmundsen H. β-oxidation of polyunsaturated fatty acids by rat liver peroxisomes. A role for 2,4-dienoyl-Coenzyme A reductase in peroxisomal β-oxidation. *J Biol Chem* 1986; 261: 16484–93.
26. Rosenthal MD. Fatty acid metabolism of isolated mammalian cells. *Prog Lipid Res* 1987; 26: 87–124.
27. Lefkowith JB, Flippo V, Sprecher H, Needleman P. Paradoxical conservation of cardiac and renal arachidonate content in essential fatty acid deficiency. *J Biol Chem* 1985; 260: 15736–44.
28. Needleman S, Spector AA, Hoak JL. Enrichment of human platelet phospholipids with linoleic acid diminishes thromboxane release. *Prostaglandins* 1982; 24: 607–22.
29. Weiner TW, Sprecher H. 22-carbon acids. Incorporation into platelet phospholipids and the synthesis of these acids from 20-carbon polyenoic acid precursors by intact platelets. *J Biol Chem* 1985; 260: 6032–8.
30. Cook HW, Clarke JTP, Spense MW. Inability of rabbit polymorphonuclear leukocytes to synthesize arachidonic acid from linoleic acid. *Prostaglandins Leukotrienes Med* 1983; 10: 39–52.
31. Kugi M, Yoshida S, Takeshita M. Characterization of fatty acid elongation system in porcine neutrophil microsomes. *Biochim Biophys Acta* 1990; 1043: 83–90.
32. Hagve T-A, Sprecher H. Metabolism of long-chain polyunsaturated fatty acids in isolated cardiac myocytes. *Biochim Biophys Acta* 1989; 1001: 338–44.
33. Mohammed BS, Hagve T-A, Sprecher H. The metabolism of 20- and 22-carbon unsaturated acids in rat heart and myocytes as mediated by feeding fish oil. *Lipids* 1990; 25: 854–8.

34. Scott BL, Bazan NG. Membrane docosahexaenoate is supplied to the developing brain and retina by the liver. *Proc Natl Acad Sci USA* 1989; 86:2903–7.
35. Moore SA, Yoder E, Spector AA. Role of the blood-brain barrier in the formation of long-chain ω3 and ω6 fatty acids from essential fatty acid precursors. *J Neurochem* 1990; 55: 391–402.
36. Bernert JT, Sprecher H. Factors regulating the elongation of palmitic and stearic acid by rat liver microsomes. *Biochim Biophys Acta* 1979; 574: 18–24.
37. Bernert JT, Bourre J-M, Baumann NA, Sprecher H. The activity of partial reactions in the chain elongation of palmitoyl-CoA and stearoyl-CoA by mouse brain microsomes. *J Neurochem* 1979; 32: 85–90.
38. Robinson BS, Johnson DW, Poulos A. Metabolism of hexacosatetaenoic acid ($C_{26:4,n-6}$) in immature rat brain. *Biochem J* 1990; 267: 561–4.
39. Goldberg I, Schechter I, Bloch K. Fatty acyl-coenzyme A elongation in brain of normal and quaking mice. *Science* 1973; 182: 497–9.
40. Lands WEM, Inoue M, Sugiura Y, Okuyama H. Selective incorporation of polyunsaturated fatty acids into phosphatidylcholine by rat liver microsomes. *J Biol Chem* 1982; 237: 14968–72.
41. Voss AC, Sprecher H. Regulation of the metabolism of linoleic acid to arachidonic acid in rat hepatocytes. *Lipids* 1988; 23: 660–5.
42. Voss AC, Sprecher H. Metabolism of 6,9,12-octadecatrienoic acid and 6,9,12,15-octadecatetraenoic acid by rat hepatocytes. *Biochim Biophys Acta* 1988; 958: 153–62.
43. Clouet P, Niot I, Bezard J. Pathway of α-linoleic acid through the mitochondrial outer membrane in the rat liver and influence on the rate of oxidation. *Biochem J* 1989; 263: 867–73.
44. Mahadevappa VG, Holub BJ. Quantitative loss of arachidonoyl-containing phospholipids in thrombin-stimulated platelets. *J Lipid Res* 1987; 28: 1275–80.
45. Weiner TW, Sprecher H. Arachidonic acid, 5,8,11-eicosatrienoic acid and 5,8,11,14,17-eicosapentaenoic acid. Dietary manipulation of the levels of these acids in rat liver and platelet phospholipids and their incorporation into human platelet phospholipids. *Biochim Biophys Acta* 1984; 792: 293–303.
46. MacDonald ML, Mack KF, Williams BW, King WC, Glomset UA. A membrane-bound diacylglycerol kinase that selectively phosphorylates arachidonoyl-diacylglycerol. *J Biol Chem* 1988; 263: 1584–92.
47. Haycock JC, Evers AJ. Altered phosphoinositide fatty acid composition mass and metabolism in brain essential fatty acid deficiency. *Biochim Biophys Acta* 1988; 960: 54–60.
48. Nakagawa Y, Waku K. The metabolism of glycerophospholipid and its regulation in monocytes and macrophages. *Prog Lipid Res* 1989; 28: 205–43.

DISCUSSION

Dr. Clandinin: What studies are you proposing to do as it relates to function and synthesis of long chain PUFA?

Dr. Sprecher: At the moment I want to primarily focus our efforts on describing how a double bond is introduced at position-4 during polyunsaturated fatty acid biosynthesis. Once we have synthesized 24-carbon polyunsaturated acids then we would like to determine whether liver has the capacity to chain-elongate these acids or whether these activities may be confined to brain and retina which is of course where these long chain acids are found.

Dr. Bracco: Do you think that this lack of δ-4 desaturase is also related to the steric hindrance of the enzyme? In other words is the double bond so close to carboxyl and the molecule so flexible that it is difficult for the enzyme to work on the C-20 fatty acid?

Dr. Sprecher: When we do microsomal incubations with linoleate it is readily desaturated at position 6 to 6,9,12–18:3. Conversely, we do not detect any conversion of 7,10,13,16,19–22:5 to 4,7,13,16,19–22:6 by the putative 4-desaturase. However there may be optimal ways to introduce a double bond into a fatty acid at position-4. Plasmalogen synthesis uses an ether as substrate, and Kates *et al.* have shown that esterified 8,11,14–20:3 is a substrate for the 5-desaturase. It is thus possible that phospholipids containing either 7,10,13,16–22:4 or 7,10,13,16,19–22:5 are the true substrates for a 4-desaturase.

Dr. Crawford: You mentioned two mechanisms for the effect of eicosapentaenoic acid in reducing arachidonic acid in the phosphoglycerides. The second was competition for incorporation. If that was the case wouldn't you be able to check by measuring the rate of arachidonic acid turnover, which should be increased, whereas an effect on the δ-6-desaturation would result in a decrease in turnover rate?

Dr. Sprecher: It would seem there are two general ways in which dietary eicosapentaenoic acid (EPA) could function to depress the amount of esterified arachidonate. It could function in some way to inhibit 6-desaturase, thus depressing the amount of arachidonate that is made for subsequent esterification. Alternatively it might have no effect on the conversion of linoleate to arachidonate. The arachidonate that is made from linoleate might simply mix with the preformed dietary EPA. Competition for acylation would then be the major site of regulation in defining membrane lipid fatty acid composition.

Dr. Crawford: You might expect the linoleic acid to compete with the 6-desaturase. I am not so sure if you would expect EPA to compete with it. Therefore if 6-desaturase is still functioning at the same rate in the presence of EPA it is producing the same amount of arachidonic acid, however much that is, but this is not getting into the cell membranes. It has to go somewhere, so it must be burned and there has to be a change in turnover.

Dr. Sprecher: That is correct. My hypothesis simply says that arachidonic acid is made and part of it is just burned. Whether that happens or not I do not know, but it is a possibility.

Dr. Bazan: We found that if we do *in vitro* incubations with very low concentrations of labeled fatty acids (50 nanomolar) we get different profiles of lipid labeling than we do at higher concentrations. One of the features in retina and brain is that phosphatidic acid is highly labeled with docosahexaenoic acid (DHA) at an early stage, and DHA is then incorporated into other phospholipids. So the question is whether we are missing some initial step in the cellular handling of PUFA if we offer the cells concentrations in the low nanomolar and micromolar range. The way we have done these experiments is with high specific activity labeled fatty acids. Is the issue of the activation, acylation, and subsequent metabolism an important event in the cellular uptake of PUFA?

Dr. Sprecher: In our studies we are indeed incubating hepatocytes with fairly high concentrations of a single fatty acid. Hepatocytes, unlike many other cells, have a high capacity to desaturate, chain-elongate, retroconvert, and acylate fatty acids. I do, however, certainly agree with you that no incubation with a single fatty acids mimics normal physiological conditions.

Physical Properties of Fatty Acids and their Extracellular and Intracellular Distribution

Donald M. Small

Department of Biophysics, Boston University School of Medicine, Boston, Massachusetts 02118-2394, USA

Fatty acids are ubiquitous biological molecules. They are esterified to many complex lipids such as triacylglycerols, phospholipids, and cholesterol esters, and as part of those molecules determine some of their physical properties. However, fatty acids *per se* exist in significant concentrations in extracellular compartments and within cells. For instance, fatty acids are liberated from complex fats and lipids during fat digestion, lipoprotein-lipase-catalysed lipolysis, hydrolysis of endocytosed lipoproteins in lysosomes, hydrolysis of stored fat in cells, and during phospholipid hydrolysis. In certain circumstances, for instance the hydrolysis of chylomicron triglyceride in capillaries, the local fatty acid concentration may be quite high. Furthermore, fatty acids may be exposed to a wide range of pH both in the intestinal lumen and in intracellular compartments such as lysosomes. This brief overview will cover three topics: 1) The physical properties of fatty acids in aqueous systems, 2) the interaction of fatty acids with key structures in the blood (albumin, lipoproteins, and cell membranes), and 3) the interaction of fatty acids with intracellular constituents, specifically fatty acid binding proteins and membranes. The work to be summarized was largely carried out in the Department of Biophysics at Boston University by Drs. David Cistola, John Parks, James Hamilton, and Paul Spooner.

PHYSICAL PROPERTIES OF FATTY ACIDS IN WATER

The short chain fatty acids such as acetic acid, propionic acid, and butyric acid are freely soluble in water and have a pKa of about 4.5 (1,2). These fatty acids are soluble both in the protonated form and in the ionized form and really should be considered as water-soluble molecules and not as typical lipids. As the aliphatic chain length of the fatty acid increases, lipid-like properties begin to appear. The protonated fatty acids become much less soluble as the chain length increases so that once the chain has reached 12 carbons the aqueous solubility is quite low (2.3×10^{-4} g/100 g solution, 11.5 μmolar, 25°C) (1). The solubility of palmitic acid (16 carbon atoms) at 25°C decreases to 3×10^{-6} g/100 g solution (0.12 μmolar) (1). On the other hand, at very high pH where these longer chained fatty acids are totally ionized, they have the possibility of forming micelles, that is, small thermodynamically stable aggregates of molecules in aqueous solution (1). This property gives the ionized fatty acids (i.e., soaps) their detergent properties. However to achieve a stable micellar solution most biologically active fatty acids must be present in a solution at a pH greater than 9, and this is generally unphysiologic. In fact the most probable state of fatty acids at physiological temperature and pH is a membrane-like bilayer structure.

Figure 1 summarizes in a very simple way the complex physical behavior of long-chain fatty acids in aqueous systems (see refs. 1,3–5). Besides the monomer concentration in solution (which is very low) the fatty acids form at least six different types of physical aggregates which depend on the temperature and the pH. Figure 2 gives the chain melting temperatures for the different physical states of fatty acids

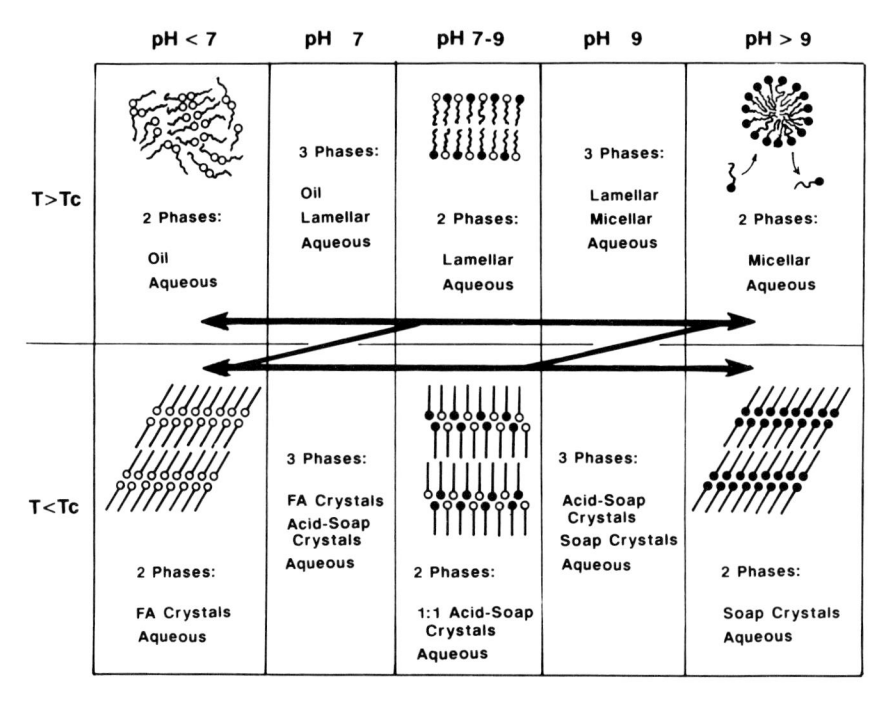

	pH < 7	pH 7	pH 7-9	pH 9	pH > 9
T>Tc	2 Phases: Oil Aqueous	3 Phases: Oil Lamellar Aqueous	2 Phases: Lamellar Aqueous	3 Phases: Lamellar Micellar Aqueous	2 Phases: Micellar Aqueous
T<Tc	2 Phases: FA Crystals Aqueous	3 Phases: FA Crystals Acid-Soap Crystals Aqueous	2 Phases: 1:1 Acid-Soap Crystals Aqueous	3 Phases: Acid-Soap Crystals Soap Crystals Aqueous	2 Phases: Soap Crystals Aqueous

FIG. 1. Schematic summary of the physical states formed by medium chain (≥10 carbons) and long chain fatty acids in excess water as a function of pH and temperature (T). Tc represents the hydrocarbon chain melting temperature in excess water. Tc increases with increasing chain length. In the hydrated state melting for fatty acids < 1:1 acid soaps < soaps (see Fig. 2). The aqueous phase is a saturated solution of fatty acid, acid soap, or soap, and the concentration of these molecules varies with ionization state and hydrocarbon chain length. The *solid circles* represent ionized (anionic) carboxylate groups (—COO⁻) and the *open circles* represent protonated carboxyl groups (COOH). The *straight lines* represent ordered hydrocarbon chains and the *curved lines* represent disordered (liquid) hydrocarbon chains. *Arrows* indicate possible isothermal titration paths. Adapted from Cistola DP, et al., ref. 3.

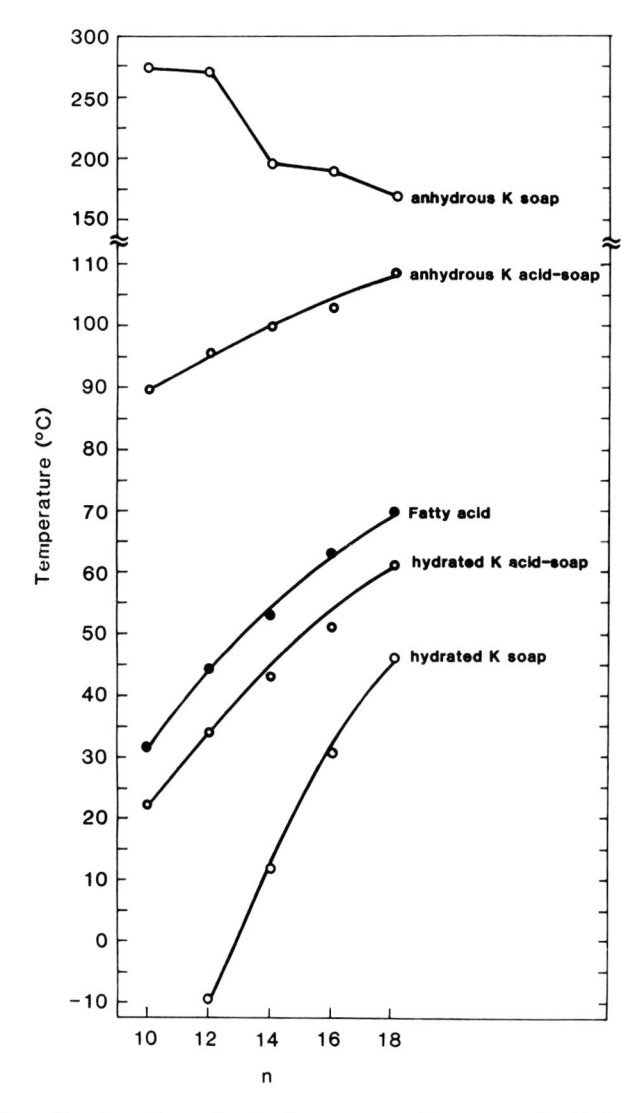

FIG. 2. Chain melting transitions of potassium soaps, acid soaps, and acids in anhydrous and hydrated states. The highest chain transitions are found in anhydrous K^+ soaps and the lowest in hydrated K^+ soaps. The decreasing order of chain melting is anhydrous soap > anhydrous acid soap > acid > hydrated acid soap > hydrated soap. n, number of carbons in the chain. From Small DM, ref. 1.

of different chain lengths (1). If the fatty acid is below its chain melting temperature, then, at low pH, it will crystallize and separate from an aqueous system as fatty acid crystals. These crystals will be in equilibrium with an extremely low concentration of fatty acid monomer. At high pHs (above 9) fatty acids form soaps. Below the melting temperature of the hydrated, crystalline soap, soap crystals will separate from an aqueous solution and be in equilibrium with a very low concentration of ionized soap molecules. At intermediate pHs between 7 and 9, below the melting temperature, the system will be partly ionized and partly unionized and will form a compound called an "acid soap." These crystalline solids are compounds of acid and soap with a 1:1 stoichiometry (e.g., potassium hydrogen dioleate) with extremely low solubility. Thus in all instances where the fatty acid chain remains unmelted, the fatty acid will crystallize in a specific form depending upon the pH (acid, acid soap, soap) and separate from the solution leaving a very low concentration of the monomer in slow equilibrium with the crystal. The actual monomer solubility increases as the chain length shortens, but in general it is below detection in biological systems.

Above the chain melting transition three new aggregated states occur. At low pH fatty acid exists as an oil which separates from the water; at intermediate pH it exists as a lamellar liquid crystalline phase which spontaneously forms vesicle-like bilayered membrane structures; and at high pH, where most of the fatty acid is fully ionized, it forms micelles. Thus, the most generally encountered forms of fatty acid in biological systems would not be micelles or soap crystals, but rather they would be acid soaps if the melting point is high, or lamellar liquid crystalline states or even oils if the pH is lower (for further details see refs. 1,3–5).

INTERACTIONS OF FATTY ACIDS WITH COMPONENTS OF THE BLOOD

As a general statement, fatty acids in the plasma compartment do not crystallize as acid soaps or form micelles; rather they partition into three different kinds of acceptors, proteins (specifically albumin), membrane-like structures such as plasma membranes of blood and endothelial cells, and lipoproteins. To model these three compartments (proteins, membranes, lipoproteins) we have utilized bovine serum albumin or human serum albumin, unilamellar vesicles, and triglyceride emulsion particles or isolated native lipoproteins. The emulsion particles mimic the triglyceride-rich particles such as chylomicrons and very low density lipoproteins. In most of the studies bovine serum albumin has been utilized (6–14) but human serum albumin has also been utilized and has been found to be quite similar in terms of its individual binding sites and capacity to bind fatty acids (15). While much work has been carried out on the binding of fatty acids to albumin [see reviews by Spector (16,17) and Brown and Shockley (18)], a noninvasive method using the signal from ^{13}C-enriched fatty acid was devised by us several years ago to monitor the binding of fatty acid to the different binding sites in albumin and to lipoproteins and membranes (6–15).

The natural abundance of ^{13}C is about 1%. Thus relatively concentrated solutions of fatty acids or other molecules are necessary to identify the ^{13}C spectra given by each of the carbons. However by utilizing fatty acids that are 90–99% ^{13}C enriched in the carboxyl carbon of the fatty acid a strong signal from the carboxyl fatty acid is produced at low fatty acid concentrations. Using these 1-^{13}C-enriched fatty acids in albumin (6,7,10,11,14) the different binding sites for long and short chain saturated fatty acids and oleic acid have been defined. Unfortunately ^{13}C-carboxyl-enriched polyunsaturates have not yet been studied. Each binding site which has a different chemical environment will absorb at a slightly different magnetic field (called chemical shift). When the exchange rate between different binding sites is slow, i.e., milliseconds or longer, the different sites will be resolved into separate peaks. Thus, the chemically different binding sites are defined by the chemical shift. About 10 years ago Parks et al. found that albumin had three different tight binding sites which filled with almost equal affinity (6). These three binding sites did not titrate normally and appeared to be bound not only hydrophobically around the chain (7) but also by ionic bonds to lysine groups in the albumin molecule (10,11). At least two weakly binding sites are present. Figure 3 illustrates the spectra of the different sites. The major weak site, called site C (6,11), can bind several moles of fatty acid per albumin and appears to have only hydrophobic bonding since the carboxyl group titrates like an acetic acid (pKa ~ 4.5). This suggests that the fatty acid carboxyl group is projecting into the aqueous phase where it can interact with hydrogen ions like a single free carboxyl.

Fatty acids can also bind to lipoproteins and cellular membranes. Figure 4 shows the different titration curves of the carboxyls in unilamellar vesicular membranes, chylomicrons, albumin (peak C), and as monomeric fatty acid plotted as chemical shift vs. pH of the medium. In each environment the titration curve and the apparent pKa are unique. Monomeric octanoic acid has a pKa of about 4.7. It is completely ionized by pH 6.5. The curves of membranes and lipoproteins are shifted to higher pH and have apparent pKa of 7.6–7.9 indicating that when the fatty acids are present in membranes or lipoproteins they are partly shielded from titration (8,9,11,12,15). Since at specific pHs, for instance pH 7.4 (see Fig. 4), the chemical shift for the fatty acid in each different compartment (e.g., in solution, on albumin, in lipoproteins, or in membranes) is different, by utilizing the appropriate NMR pulse sequences and calculating the area under each peak the mass of fatty acid associated with each compartment can be directly calculated (9,12,13,15).

Figure 5 shows the fraction of fatty acid bound to membranes or lipoproteins (in this case high density lipoproteins [HDL]) in the presence of human serum albumin (15). From these curves the approximate distribution ratios of fatty acid between albumin and membrane or lipoprotein can be estimated. These curves show that when the fatty acid to albumin ratio is 1 or less then virtually all the fatty acid binds to albumin. The normal physiologic range for plasma-free fatty acid give a mole ratio of fatty acids to albumin of 1 or less. As fatty acid to albumin ratios exceed 1, fatty acid begins to partition into both membranes and into lipoproteins. This is interesting since the three tight binding sites have nearly the same affinity and one would expect that they should fill first before fatty acid would partition to either membranes or lipoproteins. However, the very definite partitioning into lipoproteins and membranes below the 3:1 ratio indicates a negative cooperativity in the albumin at fatty acid-albumin ratios greater than 1 (15).

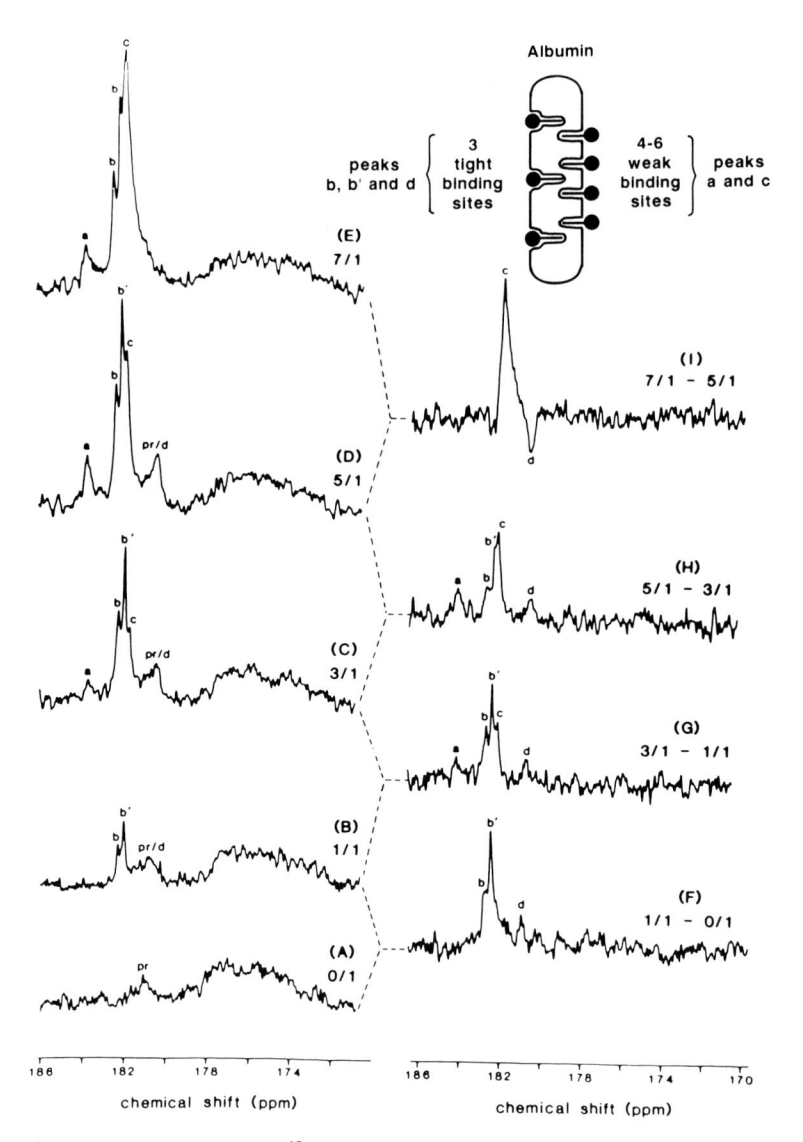

FIG. 3. Carboxyl/carbonyl region of ^{13}C NMR spectra **(A–E)** and difference spectra **(F–I)** for $C_{14.0}$ · bovine serum albumin (BSA) complexes with different $C_{14.0}$ · BSA mole ratios at pH 7.4 and 34°C. Difference spectra were obtained by digitally subtracting a spectrum at a given mole ratio from one at a higher mole ratio. This method removes BSA resonances from spectra and shows which fatty acid carboxyl resonances increased between two corresponding FA · BSA mole ratios. The pairs of spectra which are subtracted are indicated by the *dashed lines* in the middle of the figure. The *lower case letters* above each peak indicate specific FA carboxyl resonances (i.e., binding sites) with characteristic chemical shifts (see results in the text). For all samples, the BSA concentration was 7% (w/v). All spectra were recorded after 6000 accumulations with a pulse interval of 2.0 s, 16,384 time domain points, and a spectral width of 10,000 Hz. Line broadening (3 Hz) was used in all spectral processing. A: FA-free BSA spectrum. B: 1:1 $C_{14.0}$ · BSA spectrum. C: 3:1 $C_{14.0}$ · BSA spectrum. D: 5:1 $C_{14.0}$ · BSA spectrum. E: 7:1 $C_{14.0}$ · BSA spectrum. F: Difference spectrum, 1:1 $C_{14.0}$ · BSA minus FA-free BSA. G: Difference spectrum, 3:1 $C_{14.0}$ · BSA minus 1:1 $C_{14.0}$ · BSA. H: Difference spectrum, 5:1 $C_{14.0}$ · BSA minus 3:1 $C_{14.0}$ · BSA. I: Difference spectrum, 7:1 $C_{14.0}$ · BSA minus 5:1 $C_{14.0}$ · BSA. FA tightly bound to BSA contributes to peaks, b, b', and d; weakly bound FA contributes to peaks a and c. Adapted from Cistola DP, et al., ref. 10.

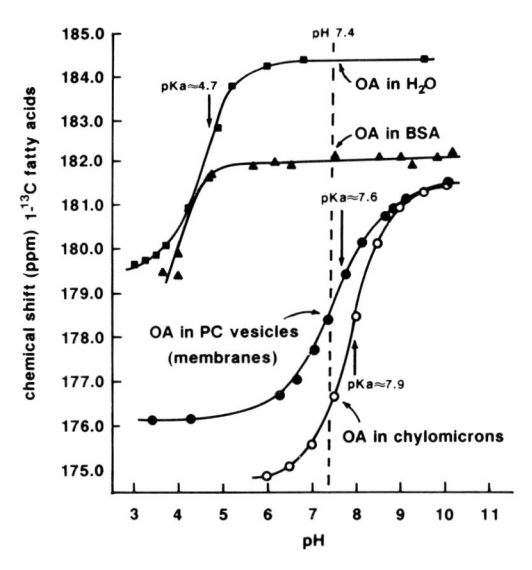

FIG. 4. Titration curves of fatty acid in different environments. Titration of 10^{-5} M 1-^{13}C-octanoic acid (■) in H_2O at concentrations when monomers are soluble. Titration of oleic acid in BSA (▲), in PC vesicles (●) (9,15), and in chylomicrons (○) (12).

While the physiological fatty acid to albumin ratio in plasma is 1 or less, under certain circumstances and in certain environments the ratio may be considerably higher. In uncontrolled diabetes mellitus (19–22) it often exceeds 2 and may be as high as 6. Nephrotic syndrome (23) and gram negative infection and sepsis (24) also increase the plasma ratio. Furthermore, in the capillary, where active lipolysis occurs, fatty acid to albumin ratio can be calculated to greatly exceed 1. Therefore, using the noninvasive ^{13}C NMR technique, the distribution coefficients of fatty acid at a mole ratio of 5 fatty acids to 1 albumin were determined between the three compartments, albumin, membranes, and triglyceride-rich lipoproteins, as a function of pH. Bovine serum albumin was used as a model for albumin, phospholipid unilamellar vesicles were used to model membranes, and emulsion particles resembling chylomicrons were used to model the chylomicrons and triglyceride-rich lipoproteins (10,11). Calculating the area under the peak corresponding to each individual compartment made it possible to estimate the distribution coefficients of fatty acids amongst these three intravascular compartments (Fig. 6). The distribution of fatty acid at pH 7.4 is as follows: albumin ~ 66%; membranes (phospholipid vesicles) ~ 16%; surface of chylomicrons (emulsion phospholipid surface) ~ 16%; lipoprotein triglyceride core 2%. Thus, only a small fraction of protonated fatty acids partition into the chylomicron core. The distribution coefficient of protonated fatty acid between surface and core is about 6:1 (12,25). No ionized fatty acid enters the core. As the pH falls fatty acid redistributes from albumin to the lipid acceptors so that at pH 5.5 the distribution is as follows: albumin 28%; membranes ~ 34%; chylomicron surface ~ 34%; and triglyceride core ~4%.

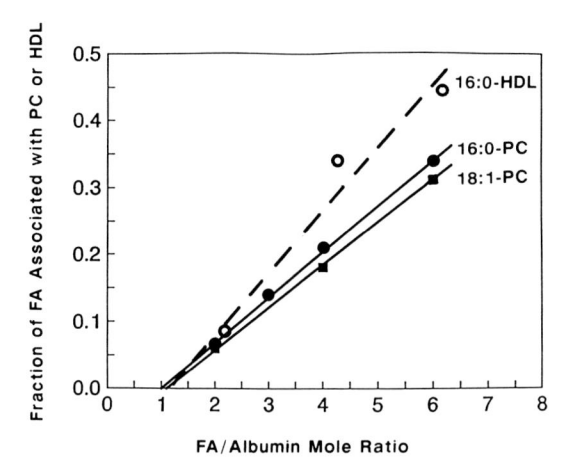

FIG. 5. Plots of the fraction of fatty acids (FA) molecules associated with phospholipid vesicles or human lipoproteins (HDL) in the presence of human serum albumin as a function of the total sample fatty acid/albumin mole ratio. All samples contained 47 mg/ml albumin. The fractions of fatty acids associated with each particle were calculated from the relative intensities of ^{13}C NMR carboxyl resonances corresponding to fatty acids bound to binding sites on particles and albumin. ○, Samples containing HDL at a concentration of 24 mg protein/ml (HDL) and increasing amounts of palmitic acid. ●, Samples containing EYPC vesicles (47 mg/ml) and increasing amounts of palmitic acid (16:0). ■, Samples containing EYPC vesicles (47 mg/ml) and increasing amounts of oleic acid (18:1). All NMR spectra were obtained at 37°C and pH 7.4. (Adapted from Cistola DP and Small DM, ref. 15.)

In theory these partition coefficients (Fig. 6) can be applied to the vascular compartment assuming that the partition into membranes will be reflected by the partitioning into vesicles and that the partitioning into lipoprotein surfaces will be reflected by the partitioning into emulsion phospholipid and emulsion triglyceride. I have estimated standard conditions (Fig. 7, top) as albumin being 3000 mg/dl, plasma lipoprotein phospholipid 300 mg/dl, triglyceride 100 mg/dl, and the membrane phospholipid of the blood elements at 350 mg/dl (26) and endothelium at 150 mg/dl for a total of 500 mg/dl. This last figure is arbitrary as it is difficult to calculate the membrane surface area of the endothelium since it will change with vessel size. With these "standard" or large vessel conditions and a fatty acid:albumin ratio of 5, about 93% of the fatty acid is partitioned into albumin, small amounts are in membranes and lipoprotein surfaces, and very little is in lipoprotein cores. As the pH is lowered there is a transfer of some fatty acid to membranes and lipoprotein surfaces, but 75% of the fatty acid remains partitioned with albumin even at pH 5.5. Three extremes that might be encountered physiologically are low albumin, hypertriglyceridemia, and high phospholipid membrane concentration such as might occur in a fine capillary bed. In low albumin (500 mg/dl) such as might occur in severe nephrosis, the albumin still carries 70% of the fatty acid. However at lower pHs this decreases sharply so that membranes and phospholipid surfaces of lipoproteins would carry a major fraction (Fig. 7). Increasing the concentration of membranes, as in a capillary bed, diminishes the albumin contribution and the membrane would carry the bulk

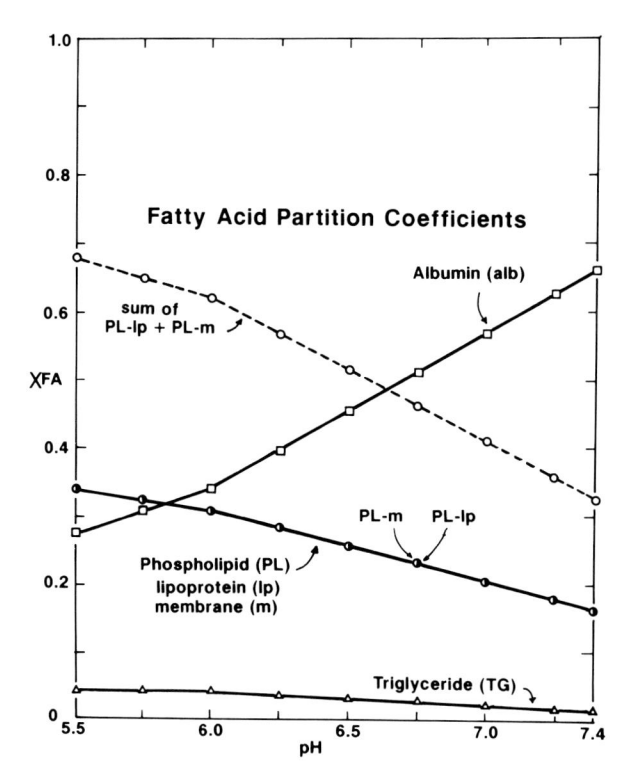

FIG. 6. Estimated distribution coefficients of fatty acid between equal masses of albumin, phospholipids in membranes, phospholipid surfaces in lipoproteins, and triglyceride cores of emulsions at an overall FA/albumin ratio of 5:1. The distribution coefficient is expressed as a fraction of the total fatty acid. Fatty acid distributes equally to phospholipid in lipoprotein surfaces (PL-lp) and in phospholipid membranes (PL-m). A very small fraction of fatty acid distributes to the core (TG). At pH 7.4 approximately 66% of the fatty acid distributes to albumin and approximately 34% to other compartments.

of the fatty acid particularly at low pH. When plasma triglycerides are greatly raised, such as in types I, IV, or V hyperlipidemias, the triglyceride cores of the lipoproteins become significant carriers of fatty acid, particularly at low pH. In a situation of hypertriglyceridemia, acidosis, and hypoalbuminemia (as could occur in a diabetic with nephrosis, acidosis, and type V hyperlipidemia), much of the fatty acid could be carried in capillary membranes and lipoproteins. This could have serious effects on capillary membranes and might alter the metabolic fate of lipoproteins.

DISTRIBUTION OF FATTY ACIDS WITHIN CELLS

Once fatty acids are delivered to cell membranes they become interdigitated between the phospholipid molecules with their aliphatic chains parallel to those of other

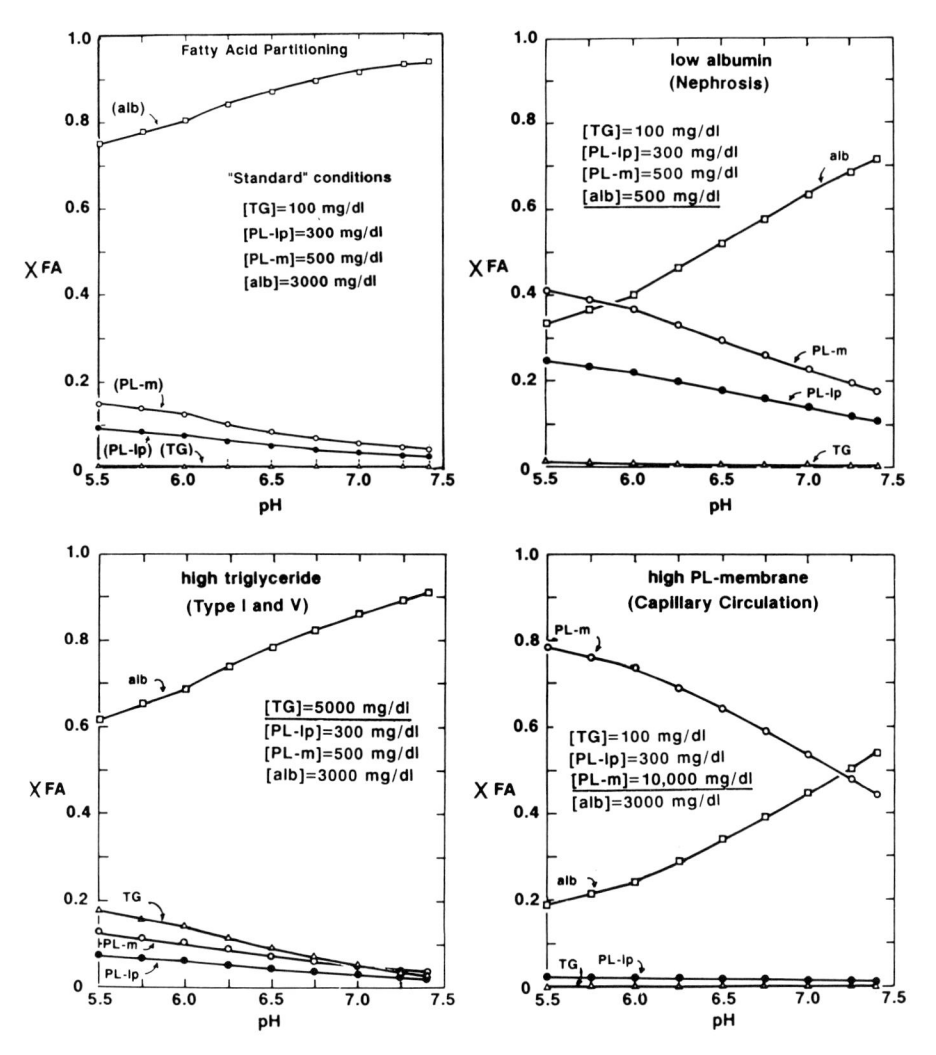

FIG. 7. The fraction of fatty acids associated with albumin (alb), lipoproteins surfaces (PL-IP), membranes (PL-m), and lipoprotein cores (TG) under standard conditions and under perturbed conditions. The effects of variations of pH (acidosis), low albumin (nephrosis), high membranes concentration (capillary bed), and high triglyceride (hypertriglyceridemia) at a 5:1 FA/albumin ratio are shown.

membrane lipids. Studies using radioactive fatty acids suggest that they can undergo transmembrane diffusion (flip flop) quite rapidly (27) and thus may translocate from the external surface of the plasma membrane to the internal surface. ^{13}C NMR has been used to attempt to locate slowly exchangeable pools of fatty acids present on the inside and outside of vesicles such as those seen for phospholipids (28), bile acids (29,30), and diacylglycerols (31). When the exchange rate between the internal and external leaflet pools is slow, two peaks corresponding to the slightly different chemical environments on the inside and outside of the vesicle can be seen (28–31). Attempts to find two pools for fatty acids have thus far failed, which suggests that the pools on the inside and the outside are in rapid equilibrium, i.e., rapidly flipping back and forth between the internal and external leaflet.

Once on the internal leaflet of the membrane the fatty acid may distribute to other compartments within the cell. Little is known of the specific components to which fatty acids distribute. However fatty acid binding proteins (FABP) are major potential carriers of fatty acids within the cytoplasm and may serve at least in part to shuttle fatty acids between membrane components or even to store excess fatty acids if they accumulate. FABPs are a family of proteins which bind hydrophobic molecules. They have a clamshell-like structure with a cleft into which the fatty acid or related hydrophobic molecules fit (32).

Several FABPs have been cloned and isolated in adequate quantities to carry out physical studies (33,34). Two of these proteins are present in the intestinal enterocyte, a cell which experiences a large fatty acid flux during fat absorption. These are intestinal fatty acid binding protein (I-FABP) and liver fatty acid binding protein (L-FABP) (34,35). Recently a third fatty acid binding protein called porcine intestinal peptide (PIP) was isolated from the ileum and found to bind not only fatty acid but chenodeoxycholic acid (36). It is possible that PIP is the ileal bile salt transporter. The liver cell (another cell which experiences large fluxes of fatty acid across its membrane (and within the cell)) also contains L-FABP in quite large quantities. Cistola *et al.*, utilizing 1-^{13}C-labeled fatty acids, have studied the binding and distribution of fatty acid among I-FABP, L-FABP, and membranes (phospholipid vesicles) (33–35). I-FABP can bind 1 mole of fatty acid per mole of protein. Excess fatty acid dissociates at pH 7.4 to form either a crystalline acid soap if below the chain melting point or a lamellar liquid crystalline phase if above. The binding site is both hydrophobic and ionic, binding the carboxyl to an arginine in the I-FABP molecule. I-FABP is stable at low pH and continues to bind the fatty acid in acidic conditions. L-FABP can accommodate 2 to 3 moles of fatty acids (33). Unlike I-FABP, L-FABP binding is mainly hydrophobic. Further at acid pH L-FABP is unstable and unfolds, dislodging its fatty acid (34,35). When the two proteins are mixed together in equal quantities and fatty acid is added they have a roughly equal affinity for the first mole of fatty acid, but when the mole ratio of fatty acid to total protein exceeds 1 then L-FABP takes up at least another mole at pH 7.4. When an equal mass of phospholipid membranes is added to L-FABP and increasing amounts of fatty acid are added, at ratios less than 1 mole of fatty acid to 1 mole of FABP, the fatty acid distributes between the membranes and the FABP indicating that the two acceptors in the cell (FABP and membranes) have similar affinity. After the first binding site is filled, that is when the mole ratio of fatty acid to the fatty acid binding protein exceeds 1, the excess fatty acid is partitioned into the membranes which can hold appreciably greater quantities of fatty acid per mass than fatty acid binding protein (33). As pH in the system is decreased, for instance toward lysosomal pH, more fatty acid partitions into membranes and less into fatty acid binding proteins.

SUMMARY AND CONCLUSION

In the vascular compartment, fatty acids are largely partitioned into albumin. However in capillaries, fatty acids may transfer from albumin to endothelial cell membranes. This shift is enhanced by acidosis and hypoalbuminemia. Within cells at least two general classes of acceptors are present for fatty acids: 1) FABPs, which appear to have a maximum binding stoichiometry in the presence of membranes of one fatty acid per FABP; and 2) the membranes, which appear to have a similar affinity and share fatty acids at low concentrations. At high concentrations of fatty acids they are the main acceptors. It is not known if this situation exists within living cells, but the use of ^{13}C NMR techniques may make it possible to study cell cultures by ^{13}C NMR and monitor the distribution of the fatty acids within cells actively turning over fatty acids.

REFERENCES

1. Small DM. The physical chemistry of lipids from alkanes to phospholipids. In: Hanahan D, ed. *Handbook of lipid research*, Vol 4. New York: Plenum Press, 1986: 1–672.
2. Cistola DP, Small DM, Hamilton JA. Ionization behavior of aqueous short-chain carboxylic acids: a carbon-13 NMR study. *J Lipid Res* 1982; 23: 795–9.
3. Cistola DP, Hamilton JA, Jackson D, Small DM. Ionization and phase behavior of fatty acids in water: application of the Gibbs phase rule. *Biochemistry* 1988; 27: 1881–8.
4. Cistola DP, Atkinson D, Hamilton JA, Small DM. Phase behavior and bilayer properties of fatty acids: hydrated 1:1 acid soaps. *Biochemistry* 1986; 25: 2804–12.
5. Cistola DP, Small DM. On micelle formation and phase separation. *J Am Chem Soc* 1990; 112: 3214–5.
6. Parks JS, Cistola DP, Small DM, Hamilton JA. Interactions of the carboxyl group of oleic acid with bovine serum albumin: a ^{13}C NMR study. *J Biol Chem* 1983; 258: 9262–9.
7. Hamilton, JA, Cistola DP, Morrisett JD, Small DM. Interactions of myristic acid with bovine serum albumin: a ^{13}C NMR study. *Proc Natl Acad Sci USA* 1984; 81: 3718–22.
8. Small DM, Cabral DJ, Cistola DP, Parks JS, Hamilton JA. The ionization behavior of fatty acids and bile acids in micelles and membranes. *Hepatology* 1984; 4: 77–9S.
9. Hamilton JA, Cistola DP. Transfer of oleic acid between albumin and phospholipid. *Proc Natl Acad Sci USA* 1986; 83: 82–6.
10. Cistola DP, Small DM, Hamilton JA. Carbon-13 NMR studies of saturated fatty acids bound to bovine serum albumin. I. The filling of individual fatty acid binding sites. *J Biol Chem* 1987; 262: 10971–9.
11. Cistola DP, Small DM, Hamilton JA. Carbon-13 NMR studies of saturated fatty acids bound to bovine serum albumin. II. Electrostatic interactions in individual fatty acid binding sites. *J Biol Chem* 1987; 262: 10980–5.
12. Spooner PJR, Bennett Clark S, Gantz DL, Hamilton JA, Small DM. The ionization and distribution behavior of oleic acid in chylomicrons and chylomicron-like emulsion particles and the influence of serum albumin. *J Biol Chem* 1988; 263: 1444–53.
13. Spooner PJR, Gantz DL, Hamilton JA, Small DM. The distribution of oleic acid between chylomicron-like emulsions, phospholipid bilayers and serum albumin. A model for fatty acid distribution between lipoproteins, membranes, and albumin. *J Biol Chem* 1990; 265: 12650–5.
14. Hamilton JA. Medium chain fatty acid binding to albumin and transfer to phospholipid bilayers. *Proc Natl Acad Sci USA* 1989; 86: 2663–7.

15. Cistola DP, Small DM. Fatty acid distributions in systems modeling the normal and diabetic human circulation: a ^{13}C NMR study. *J Clin Invest* 1991; 87: 1431.
16. Spector AA. Fatty acid binding to plasma albumin. *J Lipid Res* 1975; 16: 165–79.
17. Spector AA. Plasma albumin as a lipoprotein. In: Scann AM, Spector AA, eds. *Biochemistry and biology of plasma lipoproteins*. New York: Marcel Dekker, 1986: 247–79.
18. Brown JR, Shockley P. Serum albumin: structure and characterization of its ligand binding sites. In: Jost PC, Griffith OH, eds. *Lipid-protein interactions*, vol 1. New York: John Wiley, 1982: 26–8.
19. Laurell S. Plasma free fatty acids in diabetic ketoacidosis and starvation. *Scand J Clin Lab Invest* 1956: 8: 81–2.
20. Gerich JE, Martin MM, Recant L. Clinical and metabolic characteristics of hyperosmolar nonketotic coma. *Diabetes* 1971; 20: 228–38.
21. Reitsma WD. The relationship between serum free fatty acids and blood sugar in non-obese and obese diabetics. *Acta Med Scand* 1967; 182: 353–61.
22. Bierman EL, Dole VP, Roberts TN. An abnormality of non-esterified fatty acid metabolism in diabetes mellitus. *Diabetes* 1957; 6: 475–9.
23. Shaffir E. Partition of unesterified fatty acids in normal and nephrotic syndrome serum and its effect on serum electrophoretic pattern. *J Clin Invest* 1958; 37:1775–87.
24. Gallin JI, Kaye D, O'Leary WM. Serum lipids in infection. *N Engl J Med* 1969; 281: 1081–6.
25. Ekman S, Derksen A, Small DM. The partitioning of fatty acid and cholesterol between core and surfaces of phosphatidylcholine-triolein emulsions at pH 7.4. *Biochim Biophys Acta* 1988; 959: 343–8.
26. Nelson GJ, ed. *Blood lipids and lipoproteins: quantitation, composition, and metabolism*. Huntington, NY: Robert E. Krieger Publishing Co; 1979.
27. Brecher P, Saouaf R, Sugarman JM, Eisenberg D, LaRosa K. Fatty acid transfer between multilamellar liposomes and fatty acid-binding proteins. *J Biol Chem* 1984; 259: 13395–401.
28. Schmidt CF, Barenholz Y, Huang C, Thompson TE. Phosphatidylcholine ^{13}C-labeled carbonyls as a probe of bilayer structure. *Biochemistry* 1977; 16: 3948–54.
29. Cabral DJ, Hamilton JA, Small DM. The ionization behavior of bile acids in different aqueous environments. *J Lipid Res* 1986; 27: 334–43.
30. Cabral DJ, Small DM, Lilly HS, Hamilton JA. Transbilayer movement of bile acids in model membranes. *Biochemistry* 1987; 26: 1801–4.
31. Hamilton JA, Bhamidipati SP, Kodali DR, Small DM. The interfacial conformation and transbilayer movement of diacylglycerols in phospholipid bilayers. *J Biol Chem* 1991; 266: 1177–86.
32. Sacchettini JC, Gordon JI, Banaszak LB. Crystal structure of rat intestinal fatty acid-binding protein. Refinement and analysis of the *Escherichia coli*-derived protein with bound palmitate. *J Mol Biol* 1989; 208: 327–39.
33. Cistola DP, Walsh MT, Corey RP, Hamilton JA, Brecher P. Interactions of oleic acid with liver fatty acid binding protein: a carbon-13 NMR study. *Biochemistry* 1988; 27: 711–7.
34. Cistola DP, Sacchettini JC, Banaszak LJ, Walsh MT, Gordon JI. Fatty acid interactions with *E. coli*. Expressed rat intestinal and liver fatty acid binding protein(s): a comparative ^{13}C NMR study. *J Biol Chem* 1988; 264: 2700–10.
35. Cistola DP, Sacchettini JC, Gordon JI. ^{13}C NMR studies of fatty acid-protein interactions: comparison of homologous fatty-acid-binding proteins produced in the intestinal epithelium. *Mol Cell Biochem* 1990; 98: 101–10.
36. Sacchettini JC, Hauft SM, Van Camp SL, Cistola DP, Gordon JI. Developmental and structural studies of an intracellular lipid binding protein expressed in the ileal epithelium. *J Biol Chem* 1990; 265: 19199–207.

DISCUSSION

Dr. Guesry: What about competition between the different fatty acids with regard to acceptors?

Dr. Small: We have studied oleic and saturated fatty acids such as stearic, palmitic, and myristic acid which compete pretty much equally for albumin sites but have not studied polyunsaturates. It will be particularly important to synthesize some of the polyunsaturated fatty acids (PUFA) labeled with 13C. So far we have not been able to obtain those kinds of labels in adequate purity. So our studies are still limited to saturated and monounsaturated fatty acids.

Dr. Bazan: The competition studies should perhaps include other fatty acids such as lysophospholipids that can bind physiologically to albumin. The complexity of the biological setting should be kept in mind, since there are interstitial lipoproteins and other factors, such as the possible role of the endothelial cell. Have you looked at how the fatty acid composition of phosphatidylcholine from HDL affects the fatty acid partition? Dietary modifications are likely to have an important impact on the fatty acid composition of HDL; therefore one would expect that when they get together physiologically with albumin they might distribute in different ways according to fatty acid composition.

Dr. Small: What we are able to do now is to add ^{13}C-labeled fatty acid to a patient's plasma and by recording the ^{13}C NMR spectrum of the plasma we can determine the partitioning to albumin and lipoprotein species within the plasma, without separating the plasma (see ref. 15, above). Thus we shall be able to tell how oleic acid or palmitic acid distributes in plasmas of different composition.

Dr. Bracco: Do we know if this partition between the membrane and serum albumin is related to the polarity of the fatty acid itself?

Dr. Small: Yes. By polarity I mean the degree of ionization of the carboxyl group. As you lower the pH and protonate some of the fatty acids they come off albumin and go into the membranes. Interestingly, protonated fatty acids partition rather poorly to the core of the lipoproteins. We have determined that the partition coefficient of protonated fatty acids between the core and the surface of a lipoprotein is 1 to 6 (see refs. 12 and 25, above).

Dr. Galli: In your studies on the partition of fatty acids in the plasma is it possible that the uptake in lipoproteins might be dependent upon esterification processes, and that these enzyme activities may thus affect their partition?

Dr. Small: Using fluorescent probes it can be shown that the movement of fatty acids between albumin and lipoproteins is quite rapid. Where you have a rapid enzymatic reaction like lipolysis occurring in the capillary bed and where albumin concentration is limited by the flow through the capillary, then one can calculate that you can produce quite an excess of fatty acids under these circumstances and that the distribution into membranes must be quite large.

Dr. Merrill: Could you elaborate on the effect of the charge of the phospholipid? You described the effects of zwitterionic, neutral phosphatidylcholine, but if you have phosphatidylserine or any other phospholipids with a net charge, would this affect the partitioning?

Dr. Small: We have not done those experiments yet, but that is a good question. The other question which has not been asked is what is the effect of cholesterol, because cholesterol is in most membranes. We know that the partitioning of fatty acid into artificial membranes is not influenced by the amount of cholesterol in the membrane (see ref. 25 above) unlike the partitioning of cholesterol ester or triacylglyercol which is pushed out by high cholesterol (1,2).

Dr. Crawford: The fatty acids must behave very differently depending on the pKa. If you have a fatty acid with pKa around 8.4, at pH 7.4 only about 10% is in the ionized state, so the distribution of that fatty acid within the albumin would favor the loose binding site. But if you have fatty acid with pKA around 6.4 it will be the other way around.

Dr. Small: You are correct; what we report is apparent pKa in each system. The real pKa of fatty acids is around 4.5. However a fatty acid in a membrane or micelle is shielded by other components. Thus the effective H+ concentration in the interface is lower and the PKa appears higher. When you look at a mixed system with albumin and a membrane in which the fatty acid has an apparent pKa of 7.6 at pH 7.4, about half the fatty acid in the membrane is ionized but at that pH all the fatty acid in site C in the albumin is ionized.

REFERENCES

1. Spooner PJR, Hamilton JA, Gantz D, Small DM. The effects of free cholesterol on the solubilization of cholesteryl oleate in phosphatidylcholine bilayers: a ^{13}C-NMR study. *Biochim Biophys Acta* 1986; 860: 345–53.
2. Spooner PJR, Small DM. Effect of free cholesterol on incorporation of triolein in phospholipid bilayers. *Biochemistry* 1987; 26: 5820–25.

Long Chain Fatty Acids and Other Lipid Second Messengers

Alfred H. Merrill, Jr.

Department of Biochemistry, Emory University School of Medicine, Atlanta, Georgia 30322, USA

The ability of long chain fatty acids and complex lipids to control cell behavior was once thought to reside solely in their function as sources of energy and as structural elements for cells and tissues. There is no question that they serve these functions, and that dietary long chain fatty acids can influence cell behavior by governing membrane "fluidity" (1,2). However, the discovery that some long chain fatty acids (i.e., the eicosanoids) are converted to prostaglandins, leukotrienes, thromboxanes, and other compounds presented a new and exciting paradigm—that is, that membrane lipids are dynamic participants in the regulation of cell behavior through their turnover to highly bioactive metabolites.

This paradigm has now been extended to many types of lipids (e.g., other unsaturated fatty acids, diacylglycerols, lysophospholipids) which are generally referred to as lipid second messengers (3) (Fig. 1). Most of these compounds are obtained by the cleavage of a more complex lipid by various lipases (e.g., phospholipases A_2, C, and D) followed by metabolism to generate (or remove) the regulatory molecule(s). This article will given an overview of some of the different ways in which long chain fatty acids participate in signal transduction and will describe another, even more recently discovered, class of bioactive lipids, the long chain (sphingoid) bases.

LONG CHAIN FATTY ACIDS AND LIPOXYGENASE/CYCLO-OXYGENASE PRODUCTS

Arachidonic acid is the precursor for a large number of products that are best known for their regulation of the immune system and inflammation (via vasodilatation and vasoconstriction, platelet aggregation, leukocyte chemotaxis, etc.), although they also have effects on other cell types (4–6). The formation of these compounds begins after arachidonic acid is cleaved from the 2-position of phospholipids by phospholipase A_2. Arachidonic acid is then metabolized via several enzymatic and non-enzymatic pathways initiated by either cyclo-oxygenase (to form 15-hydroperoxy-9,11-endoperoxide PGG_2) or by lipoxygenase, which forms 5-hydroperoxy-6,8-*trans*-

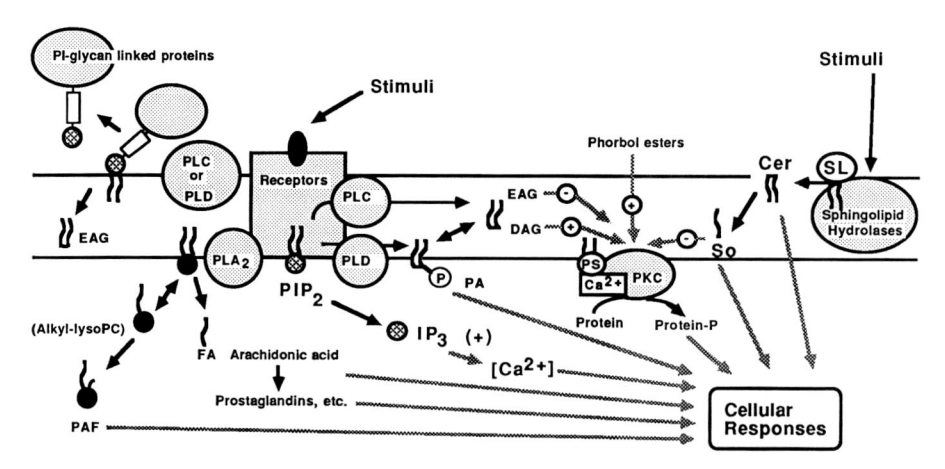

FIG. 1. Signal transduction pathways involving lipid biomodulators. Binding of stimuli (hormones, growth and differentiation factors, etc.) to membrane receptors causes cleavage of membrane lipids to bioactive products. Examples of the relevant lipases are phospholipase C (PLC), which yields diacylglycerols (DAG) and 1-alkyl-2-acylglycerols (EAG); phospholipase D (PLD), which releases phosphatidic acid (PA), which is interconvertable with diacylglycerol via PA phosphatase and DAG kinase; and phospholipase A_2 (PLA$_2$), which produces arachidonic acid and other (typically unsaturated) fatty acids as well as lysophospholipids. Phospholipases of both C and D type also cleave phosphatidylinositol-glycan-linked proteins to release them from the membrane, with EAG or PA as byproducts. The lipid products participate in multiple intracellular signal transduction pathways. For example, DAG and EAG affect protein kinase C (PKC); when PLC acts on phosphatidylinositol diphosphate (PIP$_2$), release of IP$_3$ stimulates the release of calcium, which activates calcium and calcium/calmodulin-dependent protein kinases. PLA$_2$ yields precursors for prostaglandins, leukotrienes, etc. as well as products (unsaturated fatty acids and lysophospholipids) that can affect PKC. In some cells, the product of PLA$_2$ is a 1-alkyl-2-acyl phosphatidylcholine that undergoes reacylation to produce platelet-activating factor (PAF). Recent studies indicate that sphingolipid turnover may constitute another type of lipid signaling pathway. For example, PKC is inhibited by sphingosine (So), which can be formed by the turnover of sphingolipids (SL) via ceramides (Cer) in plasma membranes and intracellular compartments (not shown). So affects other cellular systems, such as the epidermal growth factor receptor. Cer has been implicated in the action of 1-α-25-dihydroxyvitamin D$_3$.

11,14-*cis*-eicosatetraenoic acid (5-HPETE). These products are converted to other prostaglandins (i.e., D, E, and F series), prostacyclin, thromboxanes, 5-hydroxyeicosatetraenoic acid 5-HETE, and leukotrienes (4–6).

It is well established that the fatty acid composition of dietary fats can alter arachidonic acid metabolism (6–12). There has been considerable recent interest in interactions between eicosanoid production and the so-called n-3 fatty acids (e.g., α-linolenic acid) that are prevalent in fish oils *versus* n-6 fatty acids (γ-linolenic acid) (13–16). For example, the n-3 fatty acids of fish oils reduce the levels of thromboxane B_2 (TXB$_2$), prostaglandin E_2 (PGE$_2$), and 12-HETE formed by activated platelets, but increase tissue amounts of 5- and 12-HETE (10). This is of evident clinical concern because the composition of dietary oils affects bleeding times (17), thrombosis (18), and immune function (19,20), and is probably important in various disease including cancer (21).

LONG CHAIN FATTY ACIDS AND PROTEIN KINASE C

The hydrolysis of membrane phosphoglycerolipids by phospholipases A_2, C, and D releases several compounds that are able to activate the Ca^{2+}, phospholipid-dependent protein kinase termed protein kinase C (22–25). Whereas most investigations have focused on the phospholipase C-type hydrolysis of phosphoinositol (IP)-containing lipids (which liberates IP_3 as an additional second messenger), other phospholipids are also cleaved (26,27) and other products (e.g., phosphatidic acid and unsaturated fatty acids) appear to be involved in the regulation of this protein kinase C (25,28,29). This provides the potential for generation of second messengers in multiple sites and of different types and combinations. Furthermore, some phospholipids yield 1-alkyl-2-acylglycerols, which can be inactive or inhibitory for protein kinase C (30).

Protein kinase C is actually a family of enzymes that appear to translocate to the membrane in response to activation (25). Protein kinase C contains both catalytic and membrane-binding regulatory domains and is activated by the binding of natural activators such as DAG or by phorbol esters to the regulatory domain (25). Unsaturated fatty acids (sodium oleate) appear to activate "soluble" protein kinase C *in vitro* at a site distinct from that of DAG or phorbol esters, however (29).

The activation of protein kinase C by unsaturated fatty acids may have both physiological and pathophysiological implications. Protein kinase C is sensitive to changes in its lipid environment; hence, modulation of the composition of cell membranes by dietary lipids could provide a mechanistic link between diet and disease. For example, Donnelly *et al.* (31) have found that basal epidermal cells isolated from mice receiving high dietary fat had an increased proportion of protein kinase C in the particulate *versus* soluble fractions. High fat diets have been correlated with neoplasia, and instillation of arachidonic acid (but not palmitic acid) into colonic loops has been shown to increase the particulate protein kinase C, thymidine incorporation into DNA, and ornithine decarboxylase (a marker of tumor promotion) (32). Caution should be observed in linking protein kinase C to carcinogenesis because this process is complex (33); however, this remains an interesting and promising hypothesis for some of the biological effects of fatty acids.

Aberrant activation of protein kinase C has a reasonable probability of contributing to other disorders. For example, protein kinase C controls superoxide generation and secretion of some of the hydrolytic granules of human neutrophils (34). These events can be damaging to host tissues, and activation of leukocytes has been associated with cancer (35), atherosclerosis (36), reperfusion injury (37), arthritis (38), and other inflammatory disease (39). In fact, one wonders if there is frequent "accidental" activation of protein kinase C by cellular fatty acids or diacylglycerols, as well as by release of fatty acids from lipoproteins via the action of lipoprotein lipase. Perhaps this is not more prevalent because there are also a number of naturally occurring and synthetic compounds that inhibit protein kinase C, one of which (sphingosine) will be discussed in a later section.

LONG CHAIN FATTY ACIDS AND OTHER SIGNALING PATHWAYS

Relatively little is known about possible interactions between the availability of long chain fatty acids and other lipid signaling pathways. Nonetheless, fatty acyl-coenzyme A's (CoAs) and fatty acyl-carnitines have long been known to have fairly potent effects on various cellular enzymes. Fatty acyl-CoAs are activators and inhibitors of soluble and membrane-bound enzymes, receptors, and carriers (40–43), and as such may play a role in cell regulation. Fatty acyl-carnitines can also affect protein kinase C (44).

Lysophospholipids are another type of bioactive lipid encountered in cells and in circulation under various physiological conditions (45). One of the more recent proposals for lysophospholipids has been as activators and inhibitors of protein kinase C (46). One of the best characterized lysophospholipids is an acetylated derivative of lysophosphatidylcholine (1-alkyl-2-acetyl-sn-glycerol-3-phosphocholine) called platelet-activating factor (PAF), which induces aggregation of platelets at picomolar concentrations and is antihypertensive when injected into rats (47). There are several pathways for PAF formation (47,48), and once formed PAF appears to remain cell-associated, which could enhance the spacial localization of the agonist and the responding cells (49). PAF acetylhydrolase is found in plasma, where it is associated with lipoprotein particles (50).

Long chain fatty acids and other lipids also participate in the covalent attachment of proteins to membranes, and this is becoming a widespread occurrence among membrane receptors and other proteins associated with plasma membranes. A variety of proteins contain long chain fatty acids (such as myristic acid or palmitic acid) (51) or isoprenyl groups (52), and as perhaps the most complex example among mammalian proteins, a number have been discovered recently to be attached at membranes via phosphatidylinositol-glycan linkages (53,54) and to participate in hormone action (55). Cleavage of the membrane anchor of phosphatidylinositol-glycan linked proteins by phospholipase C (53) and D (54,55) releases not only the protein but also alkylacylglycerols, which may affect protein kinase C, or phosphatidic acid, another bioactive lipid.

LONG CHAIN (SPHINGOID) BASES AS A NEW CLASS OF PUTATIVE LIPID SECOND MESSENGERS

Sphingosine and other long chain bases are surfacing as another class of second messenger that can arise by cleavage of more complex precursors: in this case, sphingomyelins, gangliosides, and other ceramide derivatives (Fig. 2). These compounds are major constituents of tissues, lipoproteins (especially low density lipoproteins), milk, and other structures. Complex sphingolipids are associated with the maintenance of membrane and lipoprotein structure, cell-cell communication, modulation of cell surface receptors, differentiation, and neoplastic transformation, *inter alia* (56,57).

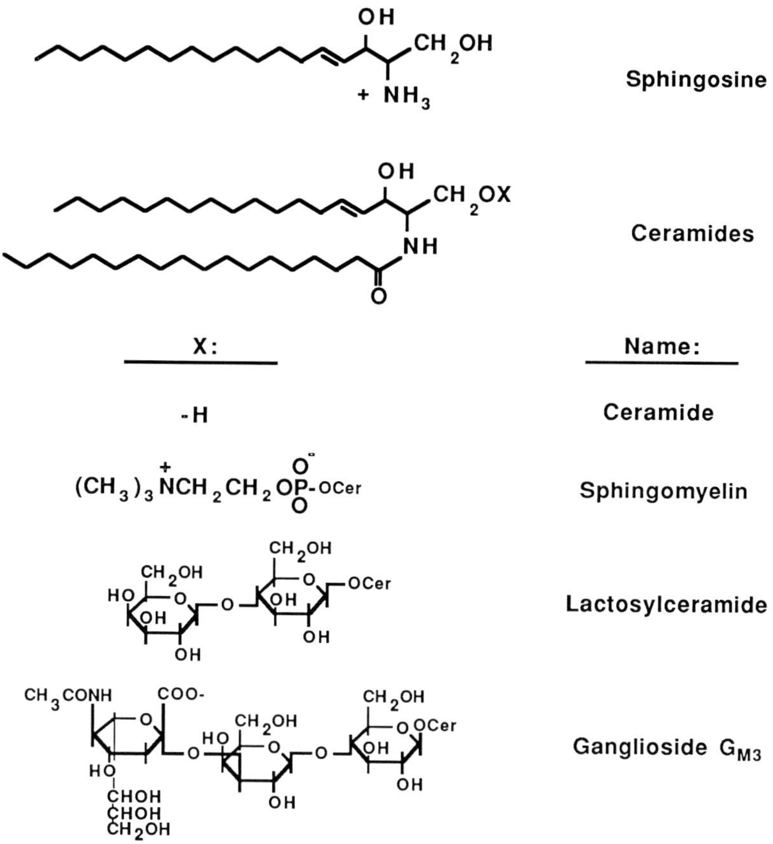

FIG. 2. Structure of sphingosine and representative sphingolipids. Shown are the structures of the major long chain (sphingoid) base (sphingosine). There are also smaller amounts of dihydrosphingosine (sphinganine), which lacks the 4,5-trans double bond, phytosphingosine (4-D-hydroxysphinganine), which has a hydroxylgroup at the 4-position instead of the double bond, as well as trace amounts of various chain length homologs of these three compounds. Ceramide has a long chain fatty acid in amide linkage at position 2, and more complex sphingolipids (shown for lactosylceramide and gangliosides) are modified at position 1.

One hypothesis for the mechanism of action of these compounds is that they are hydrolyzed to free sphingosine, which is a potent inhibitor of protein kinase C *in vitro* (58) and of cellular events dependent on this enzyme (57–60). Among the systems that have been found to be affected by adding sphingosine exogenously are the host defense system (activation of platelets, neutrophils, and natural killer cells); the cytolytic activity of pathogens and expression of viral genes; cell growth and differentiation in several cell types (including leukemic and neuronal cells); the control of insulin-stimulated hexose transport and metabolism in adipocytes and ion-transport systems in various models; the response of neuronal cells to excitatory compounds; and receptor desensitization (57,59,60). Sphingosine blocks ornithine decarboxylase induction by phorbol esters in mouse skin (61); hence these compounds may be able to interfere with tumor promotion as predicted for an inhibitor of protein kinase C (58). In addition to affecting protein kinase C, sphingosine activates the epidermal growth factor receptor and has a number of effects on various other cell regulatory systems (57). Furthermore, other products of sphingolipid turnover appear to be bioactive, such as ceramide, which has been associated with the action of 1-α,25-dihydroxyvitamin D_3 (62).

Ongoing research is evaluating how cells form free sphingosine and the effects of endogenous sphingosine on cell behavior. Free sphingosine has been found to be a constituent of all cells examined to date (57) and, in liver, is primarily localized in the plasma membrane (63) where it might affect protein kinase C, growth factor receptor(s), or other cell regulatory systems. Little is known about factors that can alter cellular levels of sphingosine. Various agonists and lipoproteins decrease and increase, respectively, the free sphingosine levels of human neutrophils (64); furthermore, dexamethasone increases sphingosine in 3T3-L1 fibroblasts (65).

Since sphingolipids have long been associated with cell-cell and cell-substratum contact (56,57), we have recently examined sphingosine formation by J774A.1 cells, a mouse macrophage-like cell line. The questions that we wanted to ask are the following: 1) do the cells contain sphingosine, 2) does the level change as the cells adhere to a surface (as a model for the movement of macrophages from circulation to tissues), and 3) what is the source of the sphingosine? Our findings have been that suspended J774 cells contain from 10 to 30 pmol of free sphingosine/10^6 cells, which is similar to our analyses of other systems (57). To determine the effect of adherence, the cells were grown in a spinner flask then recovered by centrifugation, resuspended in new medium (DMEM), and transferred to glass tubes or to another spinner bottle. As shown in Fig. 3, the amount of free sphingosine in J774 cells increases by four- to tenfold when the cells are allowed to adhere, whereas there is a lesser increase when the cells are returned to a spinner flask. The cause of the

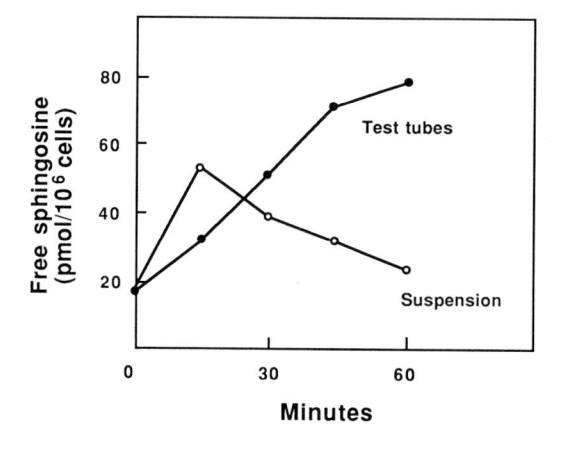

FIG. 3. Time course of sphingosine formation by J774 cells. The cells were grown in spinner flasks in DMEM supplemented with 10% fetal calf serum until a density of 0.5 to 1 × 10^6 cells/ml was reached. They were removed, centrifuged, then resuspended in DMEM and either returned to a spinner bottle (*open circles*) or placed in glass test tubes (*solid circles*) and incubated for the times shown. After incubation, the amount of sphingosine was assayed by HPLC.

temporary increase is not known, but may reflect partial activation during the cell surface contact that occurred during centrifugation of the cells.

We have seen increases in sphingosine as high as 200 pmol/10^6 cells in this model, which is the highest level ever reported (57). In studies of human neutrophils, this level of sphingosine (achieved by adding sphingosine exogenously) is able to inhibit protein kinase C and cell events dependent on this enzyme (66). While a direct effect of this endogenous sphingosine on protein kinase C is purely speculative at this point, preliminary studies have indicated that ^{3}H-phorbol dibutyrate binding by these cells is reduced, as would have been predicted by the fact that sphingosine is a competitive inhibitor of phorbol ester binding by protein kinase C (58).

Sphingosine might be formed by turnover of more complex sphingolipids in the plasma membrane (as we have seen in liver) (63) or in an acidic compartment, because lysosomes are well known to contain acidic sphingolipid hydrolases (55,57). To test the latter possibility, J774 cells were incubated with 10 mM ammonium ion or 25 µM chloroquine, both of which raise the pH of acidic compartments as lyso-osmotrophic agents. In each case, there was >95% inhibition of the increase in sphingosine (the NH$_4$Cl concentration for 50% inhibition was 2 mM); hence the source of free sphingosine in J774 cells appears to be an endosomal or lysosomal compartment. These findings establish that cells have multiple mechanisms for forming free sphingosine, as illustrated in Fig. 4, which lends additional support for the hypothesis that this bioactive molecule can be formed by cells as part of normal cell function or, perhaps, under pathological conditions.

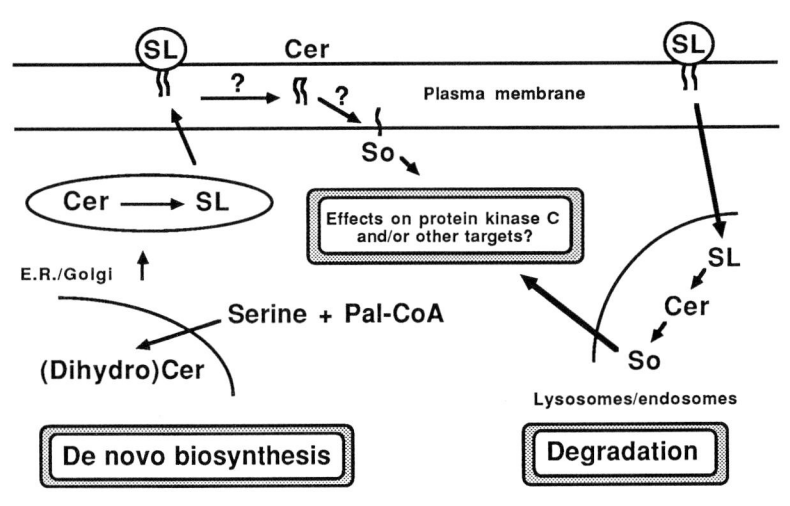

FIG. 4. Possible sources and fates of sphingosine formed by J774A.1 cells. Sphingosine is formed by *de novo* biosynthesis by the reactions shown, which do not appear to involve free sphingosine *per se*. The likely routes for formation of free sphingosine are at the plasma membrane or via lysosomal/endosomal compartments, the latter of which appear to predominate in this study. Once formed, sphingosine will exit these compartments and either undergo further metabolism or, possibly, interact with protein kinase C and other targets.

CONCLUSION

It has been estimated that mammalian cells contain approximately 3,000 different molecular species of lipids, considering the variation in lipid classes and alkyl chain composition. The functions of very few of these molecules have been established, and even fewer have been compared in animals fed different types and amounts of fat. The existence of diverse mechanisms whereby lipids participate in cell regulation, and the likelihood that even more will be found, presents exciting opportunities for understanding how dietary fats can be positive and negative factors in the etiology of disease.

ACKNOWLEDGMENTS

The new research from our laboratory presented in this report was conducted with the assistance of Lisa Warden and Elizabeth Smith and was supported by grants from the NIH (GM33369) and the Office of Naval Research (N0001489J1027).

REFERENCES

1. Cullis PR, Hope MJ, de Kruijff B, Verkleij AJ, Tilcock CPS. Structural properties and functional roles of phospholipids in biological membranes. In: Kuo JF, ed. *Phospholipids and cellular regulation*, Vol. I. Boca Raton, FL: CRC Press, 1985: 1–59.
2. Berdanier C. Role of membrane lipids and metabolic regulation. *Nutr Rev* 1988; 46: 145–52.
3. Merrill AH Jr. Lipid modulators of cell function. *Nutr Rev* 1989; 47: 161–9.
4. Needleman P, Turk J, Jakschik BA, Morrison AR, Lefkowith JB. Arachidonic acid metabolism. *Annu Rev Biochem* 1986; 55: 69–102.
5. Parker CW. Lipid mediators produced through the lipoxygenase pathway. *Annu Rev Immunol* 1987; 5: 65–84.
6. Lewis RA, Austen KF, Soberman RJ. Leukotrienes and other products of the 5-lipoxygenase pathway. *N Engl J Med* 1990; 323: 645–55.
7. Willis AL. Nutritional and pharmacological factors in eicosanoid biology. *Nutr Rev* 1961; 39: 289–301.
8. Terano T, Salmon JA, Moncada S. Effect of orally administered eicosapentaenoic acid (EPA) on the formation of leukotriene B_4 and leukotriene B_5 by rat leukocytes. *Biochem Pharmacol* 1984; 33: 3071–6.
9. Mathias KM, DuPont J. Quantitative relationships between dietary linoleate and prostaglandin (eicosanoid) biosynthesis. *Lipids* 1985; 20: 791–801.
10. Lee TH, Austen KF. Arachidonic acid metabolism by the 5-lipoxygenase pathway and the effects of alternative dietary fatty acids. *Adv Immunol* 1986; 39: 145–75.
11. Hwang DH, Boudreau M, Chanmugan P. Dietary linolenic acid and long-chain n-3 fatty acids: comparison of effects on arachidonic acid metabolism in rats. *J Nutr* 1988; 118: 427–37.
12. Lokesh BR, Black JM, German JB, Kinsella JE. Docosahexaenoic acid and other dietary polyunsaturated fatty acids suppress leukotriene synthesis by mouse peritoneal macrophages. *Lipids* 1988; 23: 968–72.
13. Kunkel SL, Ogawa H, Ward PA, Zurier RB. Suppression of chronic inflammation by evening primrose oil. *Prog Lipid Res* 1981; 20: 885–9.
14. Magrum LJ, Johnston PV. Modulation of prostaglandin synthesis in rat peritoneal macrophages with omega-3 fatty acids. *Lipids* 1983; 18: 514–21.
15. Miller CC, Ziboh VA. Gammalinolenic acid-enriched diet alters cutaneous eicosanoids. *Biochem Biophys Res Commun* 1988; 154: 967–74.
16. Miller CC, Ziboh VA, Wong T, Fletcher MP. Dietary supplementation with oils rich in (n-3) and

(n-6) fatty acids influences in vivo levels of epidermal lipoxygenase products in guinea pigs. *J Nutr* 1990; 120: 36–44.
17. Band HO, Dyerberg J, Hjorne W. The composition of foods consumed by Greenland Eskimos. *Acta Med Scand* 1976; 200: 69–73.
18. Whitaker MO, Wyche A, Fitzpatrick F, Sprecher H, Needleman P. Triene prostaglandins: prostaglandin D$_3$ and icosapentaenoic acid as potential antithrombotic substances. *Proc Natl Acad Sci USA* 1979; 76: 5919–23.
19. Somers SD, Chapkin RS, Erickson KL. Alteration of in vitro murine peritoneal macrophage function by dietary enrichment with eicosapentaenoic and docohexaenoic acids in menhaden oil. *Cell Immunol* 1989; 123: 201–11.
20. Meydani SN. Dietary modulation of cytokine production and biologic functions. *Nutr Rev* 1990; 48: 361–9.
21. Erickson KL, Hubbard NE. Dietary fat and tumor metastasis. *Nutr Rev* 1990; 48: 6–14.
22. Nishizuka Y. Studies and perspectives of protein kinase C. *Science* 1986; 233:305–12.
23. Berridge MJ. Inositol triphosphate and diacylglycerol: two interacting second messengers. *Annu Rev Biochem* 1987; 56: 159–93.
24. Bishop WR, Bell RM. Functions of diacylglycerol in glycerolipid metabolism, signal transduction, and cellular transformation. *Oncogene Res* 1988; 2: 205–18.
25. Nishizuka Y. Studies and perspectives of the protein kinase C family for cellular regulation. *Cancer* 1989; 63: 1892–903.
26. Slivka SR, Meier KE, Insel PA. Alpha 1-adenergic receptors promote phosphatidylcholine hydrolysis in MDCK-D1 cells. A mechanism for rapid activation of protein kinase C. *J Biol Chem* 1988; 263: 12242–6.
27. Billah MM, Anthes JC. The regulation and cellular functions of phosphatidylcholine hydrolysis. *Biochem J* 1990; 269: 281–91.
28. Ganong BR, Loomis CR, Hannun YA, Bell RM. Specificity and mechanism of protein kinase C activation by sn-1,2-diacylglycerols. *Proc Natl Acad Sci USA* 1986; 83: 1184–8.
29. El Touny S, Khan W, Hannun YA. Regulation of platelet protein kinase C by oleic acid. *J Biol Chem* 1990; 265: 16437–3.
30. Daniel LW, Small GW, Schmitt JD, Marasco CJ, Ishaq K, Piantadosi C. Alkyl-linked diglycerides inhibit protein kinase C activation by diacylglycerols. *Biochem Biophys Res Commun* 1988; 151: 291–7.
31. Donnelly TE Jr, Birt DF, Sittler R, Anderson CA, Choe M, Julius A. Dietary fat regulation of the association of protein kinase C activity with epidermal cell membranes. *Carcinogenesis* 1987; 8: 1867–70.
32. Craven PA, De Rubertis FR. Role of activation of protein kinase C in the stimulation of colonic epithelial proliferation by unsaturated fatty acids. *Gastroenterology* 1988; 95: 676–85.
33. Hansen LA, Monteiro-Riviere NA, Smart RC. Differential down-regulation of epidermal protein kinase C by 12-O-tetradecanoylphorbol-13-acetate and diacylglycerol: association with epidermal hyperplasia and tumor promotion. *Cancer Res* 1990; 50: 5740–5.
34. Wilson E, Rice WG, Kinkade JE Jr, Merrill AH Jr, Arnold RR, Lambeth JD. Protein kinase C inhibition by sphingoid long-chain bases: effects of secretion in human neutrophils. *Arch Biochem Biophys* 1987; 259: 204–14.
35. Weitzman SA, Weitberg AB, Clark EP, Stossel TP. Phagocytes as carcinogens: malignant transformation produced by human neutrophils. *Science* 1985; 227: 1231–3.
36. Quinn MT, Parthasarathy S, Fong LG, Steinberg D. Oxidatively modified low density lipoproteins: a potential role in recruitment and retention of monocyte/macrophages during atherogenesis. *Proc Natl Acad Sci USA* 1987; 84: 2995–8.
37. Simpson PJ, Lucchesi BR. Free radicals and myocardial ischemia and reprofusion injury. *J Lab Clin Med* 1987; 110: 13–30.
38. Terkeltaub R, Curtiss LK, Tenner AJ, Ginsberg MH. Lipoproteins containing apoprotein B as a major regulator of neutrophil responses to monosodium urate crystals. *J Clin Invest* 1984; 73: 1719–30.
39. Babior BM. Oxidants from phagocytes: agents of defense and destruction. *Blood* 1984; 64: 959–66.
40. Block K, Vance DE. Control mechanisms in the synthesis of fatty acids. *Annu Rev Biochem* 1977; 46: 263–98.
41. Brecher P. The interaction of long-chain fatty acyl-CoA with membranes. *Mol Cell Biochem* 1983; 57: 3–15.
42. Shoyab M. Long-chain fatty acyl-Coenzyme A's activate both the ligand-binding and protein kinase activities of phorboid and ingenoid receptor. *Arch Biochem Biophys* 1985; 236: 435–40.

43. Kakar SS, Huang W-H, Askari A. Control of cardiac sodium pump by long-chain acyl coenzymes A. *J Biol Chem* 1987; 262: 42–5.
44. Nakadate T, Blumberg PM. Modulation by palmitoylcarnitine of protein kinase C activation. *Cancer Res* 1987; 47: 6537–42.
45. Graham A, Bennett AJ, McLean AAM, Zammit VA, Brindley DN. Factors regulating the secretion of lysophosphatidylcholine by rat hepatocytes compared with the synthesis and secretion of phosphatidylcholine and triacylglycerol. *Biochem J* 1988; 253: 687–92.
46. Oishi K, Raynor RL, Charp PA, Kuo JF. Regulation of protein kinase C by lysophospholipids. Potential role in signal transduction. *J Biol Chem* 1988; 263: 6865–71.
47. Hanahan DJ. Platelet activating factor: a biologically active phosphoglyceride. *Annu Rev Biochem* 1986; 55: 483–509.
48. Blank ML, Lee YJ, Cress EA, Snyder F. Stimulation of the de novo pathway for the biosynthesis of platelet-activating factor (PAF) via cytidylyltransferase activation in cells with minimal endogenous PAF production. *J Biol Chem* 1988; 263: 5656–61.
49. McIntyre TM, Zimmerman GA, Satoh K, Prescott SM. Cultured endothelial cells synthesize both platelet-activating factor and prostacyclin in response to histamine, bradykinin, and adenosine triphosphate. *J Clin Invest* 1985; 76: 271–80.
50. Stafforini DM, McIntyre TM, Carter ME, Prescott SM. Human plasma platelet-activating factor acetylhydrolase. Association with lipoprotein particles and role in the degradation of platelet-activating factor. *J Biol Chem* 1987; 262: 4215–22.
51. James G, Olson EN. Identification of a novel fatty acylated protein that partitions between the plasma membrane and cytosol and is deacylated in response to serum and growth factor stimulation. *J Biol Chem* 1989; 264: 20997–1006.
52. Repko EM, Maltese WA. Post-translational isoprenylation of cellular proteins is altered in response to mevalonate availability. *J Biol Chem* 1989; 264: 9945–52.
53. Low MG, Prasad ARS. A phospholipase D specific for the phosphatidylinositol anchor of cell-surface proteins is abundant in plasma. *Proc Natl Acad Sci USA* 1988; 85: 980–4.
54. Low MG. Biochemistry of the glycosyl-phosphatidylinositol membrane protein anchors. *Biochem J* 1987; 244: 1–13.
55. Saltiel AR, Osterman DG, Darnell JC, Sorbara-Cazan LR, Chan BL, Low MG, Cuatrecasas P. The function of glycosyl phosphoinositides in hormone action. *Philos Trans R Soc Lond [Biol]* 1988; 26: 345–58.
56. Hakomori S-I. Glycosphingolipids in cellular interaction, differentiation, and oncogenesis. *Annu Rev Biochem* 1981; 50: 733–64.
57. Merrill AH Jr. Cell regulation by sphingosine and more complex sphingolipids. *J Bioenerg Biomembr* 1991; 23: 83–104.
58. Hannun YA, Loomis CR, Merrill A, Bell RM. Mechanism of sphingosine inhibition of protein kinase C activity and of phorbol-dibutyrate binding. *J Biol Chem* 1986; 261: 12604–9.
59. Hannun YA, Bell RM. Functions of sphingolipids and sphingolipid breakdown products in cellular regulation. *Science* 1989; 243: 500–7.
60. Merrill AH Jr, Stevens VL. Modulation of protein kinase C and diverse cell functions by sphingosine—a pharmacologically interesting compound linking sphingolipids and signal transduction. *Biochim Biophys Act* 1989; 1010: 131–9.
61. Enkvetchakul B, Merrill AH Jr, Birt DF. Inhibition of ornithine decarboxylase activity in mouse epidermis by sphingosine sulfate. *Carcinogenesis* 1989; 10: 379–81.
62. Okasaki T, Bielawska A, Bell RM, Hannun YA. Role of ceramide as a lipid mediator of 1-alpha,25-dihydroxyvitamin D_3-induced HL-60 cell differentiation. *J Biol Chem* 1990; 265: 15823–31.
63. Slife CW, Wang E, Hunter R, *et al.* Free sphingosine formation from endogenous substrates by a liver plasma membrane system with a divalent cation dependence and a neutral pH optimum. *J Biol Chem* 1989; 264: 10371–7.
64. Wilson E, Wang E, Mullins RE, *et al.* Modulation of free sphingosine levels in human neutrophils by phorbol esters and other factors. *J Biol Chem* 1988; 263: 9304–9.
65. Ramachandran CK, Murray DK, Nelson DH. Dexamethasone increases neutral sphingomyelinase activity and sphingosine levels in 3T3-L1 fibroblasts. *Biochim Biophys Res Commun* 1990; 167: 607–13.
66. Wilson E, Olcott MC, Bell RM, Merrill AH Jr, Lambeth JD. Inhibition of the oxidative burst in

human neutrophils by sphingoid long-chain bases: role of protein kinase C in activation of the burst. *J Biol Chem* 1986; 261: 12616–23.

DISCUSSION

Dr. Jeremy: Does the alteration of the acyl moiety on diacylglycerol change its biological activity?

Dr. Merrill: There are various reports claiming that you can see small changes if you alter the structure of the diacylglycerol moiety. It is hard to interpret the available data because of the difficulty in creating a model system that presents diacylglycerols, phospholipids, calcium, and protein kinase C in the *in vivo* conformation. Donnelly *et al.* (1) found that feeding animals high levels of fat increased the portion of membrane-associated protein kinase C in epidermal cells. Since protein kinase C is translocated to membranes during activation it may be that high fat diets increase the membrane association of protein kinase C and thereby affect cell behavior.

Dr. Bazan: Do you know of any specific agonists for the formation of free sphingosine?

Dr. Merrill: We have looked very hard for agonists that change cellular levels of sphingosine, but the effects we have seen are not adequate as proof that this compound is a second messenger. We originally showed that lipoproteins increase the level of sphingosine in neutrophils by about 50% and that was one of the factors that led us to continue studies on leukocytes, such as the J774 macrophage. This cell has shown the largest increases and the cleanest data indicating that by altering the sphingosine level you can see an effect on protein kinase C.

Dr. Juhlin: Have you used sphingosine in any clinical conditions? The reason for my question is that protein kinase C is supposed to be involved in the development of psoriatic lesions. However, when we applied a 2% sphingosine cream on the psoriatic plaques for 2 weeks we could not see any effect.

Dr. Merrill: A couple of groups have tried sphingosine unsuccessfully, but I still think it is an excellent idea because of the apparent association of protein kinase C with psoriasis. The reason it has not worked may be that the system is much more complicated than has been thought, and it is possible that the sphingosine has been removed by metabolism.

Dr. Bracco: Sphingosine comes from the hydrolytic splitting of ceramide, the skin being very rich in ceramide. We don't know exactly what kinds of fatty acid are bound to ceramide that could influence sphingosine production. We know from the work of Wertz that in a particular case of acne the ceramide contained less linoleic acid than in normal individuals. I believe that sphingosine in the skin is dependent on the ceramide level, which itself depends on the fatty acid bound to the ceramide.

Dr. Merrill: I agree entirely. We have recently synthesized a family of fluorescent ceramides so that we can watch them become internalized and see what their intracellular location is. I think the intracellular distribution of these molecules will be very critical.

Dr. Forget: You showed that sphingosine had a negative influence on tissue growth and differentiation and that ammonium chloride decreases sphingosine levels. Do you think that polyamines could have a negative influence on sphingosine levels in the same way as ammonium chloride?

Dr. Merrill: We know that in several transformed cell lines addition of sphingosine is growth-inhibitory. Since the original discovery of sphingosine it has been shown by four independent groups that it is also an activator of tyrosine kinase on the epidermal growth factor receptor. So sphingosine has the potential to be either growth inhibitory or growth stimulatory.

REFERENCE

1. Donnelly TE, Jr, Birt DF, Sittler R, Anderson CA, Choe M, Julius A. Dietary fat regulation of the association of protein kinase C activity with epidermal cell membranes. *Carcinogenesis* 1987; 8: 1867–70.

Long Chain Fatty Acids: Intake, Digestion, and Absorption in Newborn Infants

Olle Hernell and Lars Bläckberg

Department of Pediatrics, University of Umeå, S-90185 Umeå, Sweden

Triglyceride (triacylglycerol) constitutes more than 98% of the dietary fat and provides about half the energy intake for breast-fed as well as formula-fed infants. Each triglyceride molecule consists of three fatty acids esterified to one molecule of glycerol. In human milk these fatty acids are almost exclusively long chain fatty acids (LCFA), which thus become the major energy substrate during early life (1). Therefore, with only few exceptions, the milk fatty acids have been regarded merely as a source of exchangeable energy. This is evident from current guidelines on infant feeding and composition of infant formulas. Except for the amount of fat, specific recommendations on intakes are given only for the so-called essential fatty acids (2,3).

ESSENTIAL FATTY ACIDS

Because humans are devoid of enzyme systems that introduce double bonds into the n-6 and n-3 positions, linoleic acid (18:2 n-6) and α-linolenic acid (18:3 n-3) must be supplied with the food to prevent deficiency symptoms. Hence these two are classified as essential fatty acids. While it is accepted that linoleic acid should account for at least 1% of the energy intake, the minimum amount of α-linolenic acid required to avoid deficiency symptoms is not known. Present recommendations for newborn infants are therefore based on the average content of human milk, i.e., 0.5% of the energy content, or 1% of the fatty acids (1,2). Generally, the concentration of 18:2 n-6 in human milk is 5–15 times higher than that of 18:3 n-3 (1,4).

Long Chain Polyunsaturated Fatty Acids

At present there are reasons to believe that, at least for preterm infants, derivatives of linoleic and α-linolenic acids should also be classified as essential nutrients. These are the parent fatty acids from which, by a series of chain elongation and desaturation

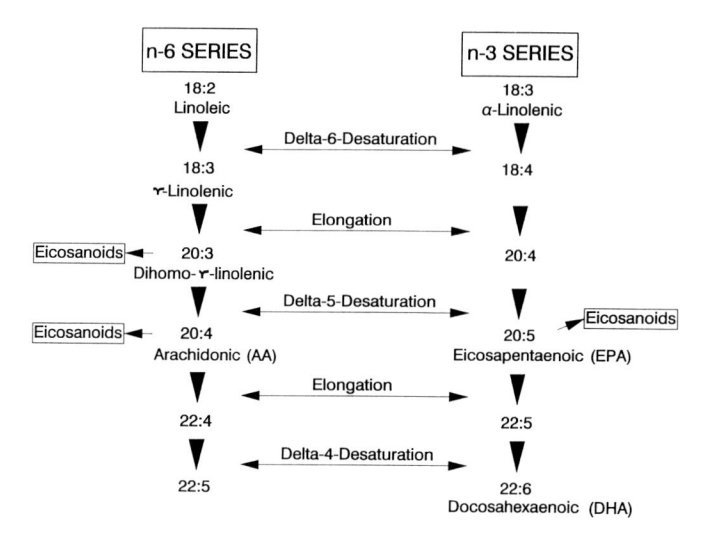

```
           n-6 SERIES                                n-3 SERIES
              18:2                                      18:3
            Linoleic                                 α-Linolenic
              ▼        ◄── Delta-6-Desaturation ──►    ▼
              18:3                                      18:4
           γ-Linolenic
              ▼        ◄──── Elongation ────►           ▼
Eicosanoids ◄─ 20:3                                     20:4
            Dihomo-γ-linolenic
              ▼        ◄── Delta-5-Desaturation ──►    ▼
Eicosanoids ◄─ 20:4                                     20:5      ─► Eicosanoids
            Arachidonic (AA)                        Eicosapentaenoic (EPA)
              ▼        ◄──── Elongation ────►           ▼
              22:4                                      22:5
              ▼        ◄── Delta-4-Desaturation ──►    ▼
              22:5                                      22:6
                                                  Docosahexaenoic (DHA)
```

FIG. 1. Synthesis of long chain fatty acids of the n-6 and n-3 series by chain elongation and desaturation of linoleic and α-linolenic acids, respectively.

reactions, long chain polyunsaturated fatty acids (LCPUFA) of the n-6 and n-3 series, respectively, are synthesized. Although, the same enzyme systems are shared by the two series there is no interconversion between the series (Fig. 1).

As indicated (Fig. 1), certain of these LCPUFA are precursors of the biologically potent eicosanoids. Others, e.g., arachidonic acid (20:4 n-6) and docosahexaenoic acid (22:6 n-3), are important constituents of membrane phospholipids. As such they are particularly enriched in the membrane phospholipids of retina and brain grey matter, whereas these tissues contain only minor concentrations of the parent linoleic and α-linolenic acids (5,6). Thus, during the rapid phase of brain growth, i.e., the last trimester of pregnancy and early extrauterine life, significant amounts of n-6 and n-3 LCPUFA are incorporated into brain lipids. The development of visual acuity in preterm infants was recently found to correlate to the n-3 LCPUFA concentration of erythrocyte membrane phospholipids (7,8). After birth this concentration is influenced by type of feeding. Compared to breast-fed infants, the erythrocyte membrane phospholipids of formula-fed infants become depleted of n-3 LCPUFA (9,10), the likely explanation being that in contrast to human milk conventional infant formulas do not contain LCPUFA (11). The conclusion has therefore been drawn that the enzyme systems required for chain elongation and desaturation of 18:2 n-6 and 18:3 n-3 (Fig. 1) are not fully developed at birth in preterm infants (12). If so, then not only the parent acids but also their LCPUFA derivatives should be considered essential nutrients, at least for a certain, as yet not defined, period of early life.

DIGESTION OF HUMAN MILK TRIGLYCERIDES

Milk lipids are secreted as fat globules composed of a core of mainly triglyceride which when secreted becomes enveloped by the apical part of the phospholipid-rich plasma membrane of the synthesizing mammary gland epithelial cell. Although in human milk LCPUFA are also enriched in the phospholipid fraction, since this fraction accounts for less than 1% of total lipids the bulk of the LCPUFA are constituents of the triglyceride fraction (1). Hence utilization of LCPUFA is dependent on milk triglyceride digestion and subsequent product absorption (13).

Gastric Lipolysis

Before absorption from the aqueous portion of small intestinal contents dietary triglycerides must be hydrolyzed into absorbable products, i.e., a mixture of monoglycerides, free fatty acids and glycerol. We have recently studied the sequential steps of human milk triglyceride hydrolysis *in vitro* by use of purified human enzymes (14). The first step in this digestive process is accomplished by gastric lipase secreted from the chief cells of the gastric mucosa. Not only is this enzyme particularly well suited to function in the environment of gastric contents (15) but it also has the unique property that its activity is not hampered by the milk fat globule membrane (16). This first step of triglyceride digestion is important even under circumstances when the contribution of gastric lipolysis to overall triglyceride digestion is minor.

Intestinal Lipolysis

The reason behind this effect of gastric lipase is that native milk fat globules, in contrast to globules partially digested by gastric lipase, are resistant to hydrolysis by colipase-dependent pancreatic lipase. This lipase, together with its cofactor colipase, is secreted from the pancreas into the duodenal contents where it catalyzes the subsequent triglyceride digestion in the upper small intestinal contents (14). Long chain fatty acids released by gastric lipase enforce binding between the colipase-lipase complex and the globules and by this mechanism the inhibition is abolished (16).

Because it is a constituent of human milk the bile salt-stimulated lipase (BSSL) contributes to milk fat digestion in breast-fed but not in formula-fed infants. After activation by bile salts in duodenal contents, BSSL, being a non-specific lipase, will not only support colipase-dependent lipase in hydrolysis of tri- and diglyceride but it will also hydrolyze *sn*-2 monoglyceride. Thus, at least *in vitro*, BSSL causes a shift in final products of triglyceride digestion from one *sn*-2 monoglyceride and two free fatty acids to one glycerol and three fatty acids for each triglyceride (14,17). As discussed below, BSSL may therefore be beneficial not only to milk fat digestion but also to product absorption.

Release of LCPUFA From Triglyceride

Although many reports suggest that infant formulas should contain certain concentrations of LCPUFA there are virtually no studies that have focused on how well

LCPUFA are utilized from human milk or from infant formulas. There are however some indications that they may be less efficiently utilized than fatty acids containing 16–18 carbons, including the parent n-6 and n-3 precursors. For instance, when whale oil triglycerides were hydrolyzed by colipase-dependent lipase, eicosapentaenoic acid (EPA, 20:5 n-3) and docosahexaenoic acid (DHA, 22:6, n-3) (Fig. 1) were relatively resistant to hydrolysis (18). Heimermann *et al.* (19) used 15 sets of synthetic triglycerides containing 12:0, 14:0, 16:0, 18:2 and one positional isomer of cis-18:1 (the position of the double bond varying from carbon 2 to carbon 16, the carboxyl carbon being number 1) to study the effect of the double bond position on hydrolysis. After a systematic exposure of these triglycerides to colipase-dependent lipase and subsequent analysis of reaction products, they concluded that ester bonds containing the isomers of 18:1 with the double bond in the second through the seventh position from the carboxyl group were relatively resistant to hydrolysis, the most hindered being the isomer with the double bond between carbons 5 and 6, while no discrimination could be seen beyond carbon 7. In this context it should be noted that position-5 coincides with the position of the nearest double bond in EPA and arachidonic acid, while it is 4 for DHA, 9 for linoleic acid and α-linolenic acid.

Relevance of these *in vitro* studies may gain support from a recent observation of LCPUFA absorption in adults. Relative to α-linolenic acid (free acid or linseed oil), when given as fish oil triglycerides EPA and DHA were absorbed to only 68% and 57%, respectively, as compared to greater than 95% when given as free acids. After stereospecific analysis it was concluded that the results obtained were best explained by EPA and DHA being relatively resistant to hydrolysis by colipase-dependent lipase, which seemed to be independent of the *sn* position of the fatty acid (20).

Does BSSL Augment Utilization of Milk Triglyceride LCPUFA?

We have recently initiated studies addressing the question whether or not also human milk triglyceride LCPUFA are less well utilized than their precursor fatty acids. In a first series of *in vitro* experiments we used double labeled rat chylomicron triglyceride as substrate. These chylomicrons were incubated with purified human colipase-dependent lipase alone, with purified BSSL alone, or with the two lipases operating simultaneously to resemble the situation in breast-fed infants (21). When colipase-dependent lipase was incubated with 18:2 n-6 and 20:4 n-6 double labeled chylomicrons the release of 20:4 was clearly retarded relative to 18:2 (Fig. 2). After 60 min incubation the mol% 20:4 released was only 60% that of 18:2. When the two lipases were operating together this difference was almost abolished (Fig. 2A, left panel), the mol% released as free fatty acid being about 70 for both fatty acids (Fig. 2A, middle panel). As expected, the explanation was that BSSL, in contrast to colipase-dependent lipase, does not discriminate between the two fatty acids (Fig. 2A, right panel).

The reason why 20:4 was released at a slower rate by colipase-dependent lipase was that this acid, but not 18:2, accumulated in the diglyceride fraction; more than

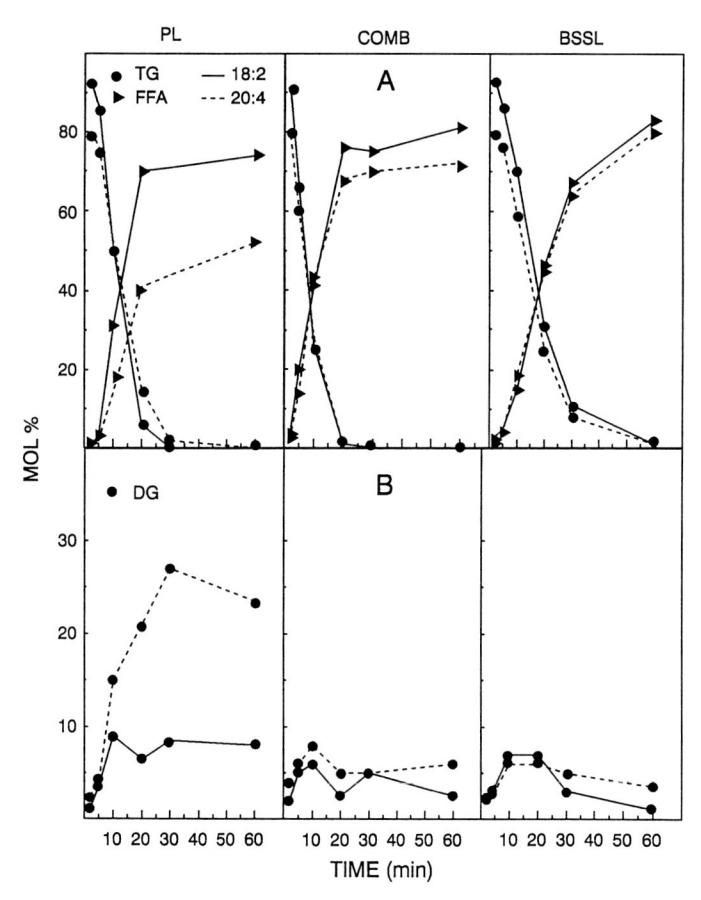

FIG. 2. Mesenteric lymph duct cannulated rats were fed, via a gastric fistula, ^{14}C-labeled linoleic acid (18:2 n-6) and ^{3}H-labeled arachidonic acid (20:4 n-6) dispersed in a parenteral fat emulsion. Chyle was collected and chylomicrons were isolated by ultracentrifugation. The chylomicrons were used as lipase substrate *in vitro* as previously described (22). Final bile salt concentration was 10.5 mM (sodium taurocholate:sodium taurodeoxycholate, 4.5:6). Incubations were done with purified human colipase-dependent lipase and colipase (PL, *left panels*) alone, with purified bile salt-stimulated lipase (BSSL, *right panels*) alone, or with the two in combination (COMB, *middle panels*). During the 60 min of incubation, aliquots were withdrawn at various time intervals, the lipids were extracted, lipid fractions were separated by thin-layer chromatography, and the different lipid fractions were transferred to counting vials and the radioactivity determined (22). The amount of the respective labeled fatty acid present in triglycerides (TG) and free fatty acids (FFA) is shown in the *upper panels* (A) and amount present in diglyceride (DG) is shown in the *lower panels* (B). Data are presented as percentage of the total lipid radioactivity (^{14}C and ^{3}H, respectively) present in each lipid class.

25 mol% as compared to less than 10 mol% after 60 min (Fig. 2B, left panel). This is in accord with previous observations (17,18,21), and with the resistance to hydrolysis being dependent on the fatty acid itself rather than on its *sn* position on the acylglycerol. No such accumulation was seen with BSSL alone or with the two lipases in combination (Fig. 2B, right and middle panels). This further illustrates the nonspecific nature of BSSL as a lipase; its activity has previously been shown to be relatively independent of the physical state as well as of the chemical structure of the lipid substrate (23). This may well be explained by the fact that BSSL is structurally clearly different from colipase-dependent lipase. In fact, the N-terminal half of BSSL shows striking homology to acetylcholine esterase, while the C-terminal part is unique (24).

To compare LCPUFA from the n-6 and n-3 series we carried out identical experiments, but with chylomicrons labeled with 20:4 n-6 and 20:5 n-3. There was no obvious difference in rate of release between the two when incubated with colipase-dependent lipase alone, with BSSL alone, or with the two lipases in combination. However, when hydrolysis by colipase-dependent lipase on one hand and BSSL on the other were compared, both fatty acids were released slower by the former lipase. Thus, when the two lipases acted simultaneously, in this case the release of both fatty acids was augmented. It is interesting to note that for both 20:4 n-6 and 20:5 n-3 the double bond nearest to the carboxyl group is positioned between carbons 5 and 6, which coincides with the most unfavorable position for hydrolysis by colipase-dependent lipase (19).

PHYSICAL-CHEMICAL BEHAVIOR AND ABSORPTION OF LIPOLYSIS PRODUCTS

Efficient utilization of dietary triglycerides depends on sufficient capacity for gastrointestinal lipolysis, and on subsequent efficient solubilization of the water-insoluble lipolysis products in the aqueous portion of upper small intestinal contents. Such solubilization is achieved by bile salt micelles (25), and, after transport as mixed micelles to the mucosal surface, absorption of the products occurs, presumably in monomolecular state. Not only is the newborn infant's endogenous capacity for fat digestion limited because of low intraluminal concentrations of colipase-dependent lipase (26), but due to low intraluminal bile salt concentrations the capacity for micellar solubilization and transport is also comparatively low (27). The compensatory role of BSSL makes fat digestion an efficient process in breast-fed infants. The relatively unimpaired fat absorption in breast-fed infants, together with the observation in adult patients with bile fistulas (28) that even in the almost complete absence of bile salts in the intestinal contents more than 50% of dietary triglyceride is digested and absorbed, suggests that a micellar phase is not indispensable for substantial fat absorption.

The Physical-Chemical Phases of Lipids in Intestinal Contents

We have recently studied the physical-chemical state of lipolysis products during established fat digestion and absorption, first by the use of model experiments *in*

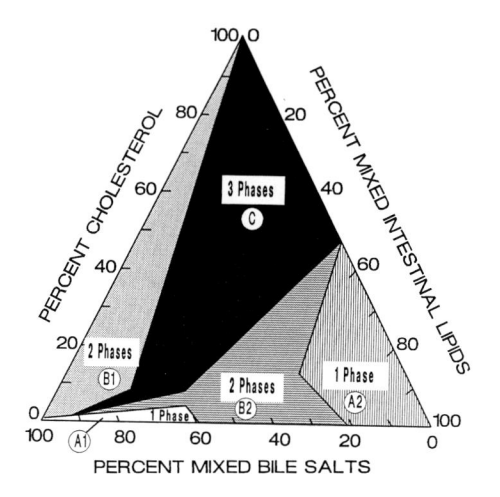

FIG. 3. Equilibrium phase diagram plotted on triangular coordinates. Ternary lipid system composed of a physiological mixture of mixed bile salts, mixed lipolysis products (partially ionized fatty acid, monoglyceride, and diglyceride), phospholipid, and cholesterol, all at fixed aqueous (99%) and electrolyte (0.15 M Na$^+$) concentrations, pH (6.5), temperature (37°C), and pressure. The total lipid concentration was 1 g/dl, with the following molar ratio; FA:MG:DG:PL, 5:1:0.2:1. The compositions of the respective zones (A1-C) are discussed in the text. The physiologically relevant zones are the micellar zone (A1) and the B2 zone composed of coexisting mixed micelles and unilamellar vesicles. Reproduced from Staggers JE, et al., ref. 29.

vitro (29) and then by chemical and physical-chemical *ex vivo* analyses of aspirated duodenal contents after triglyceride-rich meals given to healthy human adults (30). Equilibrium phase diagrams corresponding to the aqueous lipid compositions of upper small intestinal contents were developed. We identified (Fig. 3) two one-phase zones composed of mixed micelles (A1) and lamellar liquid crystals (A2), respectively, and two two-phase zones, one composed of cholesterol crystals and cholesterol-saturated micelles (B1) and the other of physiologic relevance (B2) composed of coexisting cholesterol- and mixed lipids (ML)-saturated mixed micelles and unilamellar vesicles, as judged by size and freeze-fracture technique. A single large three-phase zone in the system (C), was composed of cholesterol-saturated micelles, cholesterol crystals, and liquid crystals (29).

Micellar phase boundaries (A1) for typical physiological conditions were expanded by increase in total lipid concentration (0.25–5 g/dl), pH (5.5–7.5), and FA-to-MG molar ratio (5–20:1), resulting in reduction of the size of the physiologic two-phase (B2) zone (Fig. 3). Mean particle size (hydrodynamic radii, R_h), measured by quasielastic light scattering (QLS), demonstrated an abrupt increase from micellar (<40 Å) to micelle plus vesicle sizes (400–700 Å) as the B2 zone was entered. By phase separation and analysis, tie lines for the constituent phases of this zone demonstrated that the mixed micelles were saturated with mixed lipids and cholesterol, whereas the coexisting vesicles were saturated with bile salts but not with cholesterol (Fig. 3).

Analyses *ex vivo* of aspirated duodenal contents, in which lipolysis was immediately inhibited (30), confirmed the principal observations made in the model experiments. Relative lipid compositions of the so-called micellar phase, collected after ultracentrifugation, generally fell within the physiologic two-phase (B2) zone of the condensed ternary phase diagram (Fig. 3). As judged by QLS, *ex vivo* micellar sizes were similar (R_h < 40 Å), whereas unilamellar vesicle sizes (R_h = 200–600 Å) were smaller. When followed as functions of time, vesicles frequently dissolved spontaneously into mixed micelles, indicating that under the nonequilibrium *in vivo* conditions the constituent micellar phase was often unsaturated with lipids.

These two studies (29,30) support a model of intestinal fat digestion and absorption by which biliary lipids, mainly BS, phospholipid, and cholesterol, first mix with colipase-dependent lipase/colipase complex, and together adsorb to the crude tri- and diglyceride emulsion surfaces resulting from gastric lipolysis, entering from the stomach. The emulsion particles are thus further stabilized and inhibition of colipase-dependent lipase relieved, initially by FA released by gastric lipase and then continuously as lipolysis products are formed. Any surplus of biliary lipids will remain as a coexisting micellar phase in aqueous duodenal contents. During lipolysis, products formed will locate mainly at the emulsion surface, presumably as multilamellar, liquid-crystalline bilayers (31). As the core of the emulsion droplet shrinks, parts of the surface coat pinch off as large liquid-crystalline structures. Provided sufficient bile salts are present, they will catalyze formation of small unilamellar vesicles from these multilamellar liposomes, and, in healthy adults via the continued presence of bile, a two-phase system of mixed micelles and unilamellar vesicles (zone B2, Fig. 3) will form.

Provided that dissolution of vesicles into unsaturated micelles is faster than mucosal product absorption the micellar phase will become more and more saturated with products of lipolysis. Most of the products will be carried by micelles prior to absorption. However, absorption could also take place from unilamellar, and perhaps also multilamellar, vesicles. Under conditions of low intraluminal bile salt concentrations, the normal state for newborn infants, the abundance of multi- and unilamellar vesicles could explain the relatively unimpaired fat absorption. If so, one would expect hydrolysis of MG to glycerol and FA by BSSL in breast-fed infants to improve overall fat absorption for two reasons. The first is that the micellar phase is expanded by increase in the FA:MG molar ratio (29), and the second is that it is likely, even in the complete absence of bile salts, that spontaneous vesiculation will occur in the presence of high dilution, physiological ionic strength, and multilayers of partially ionized fatty acids.

DIRECTIONS FOR FUTURE RESEARCH

Research by many groups in the last 25 years has provided much information concerning the lipases involved in gastrointestinal fat digestion and absorption. The structure of gastric lipase, colipase-dependent lipase, and bile salt-stimulated milk lipase has been revealed from amino acid sequencing or cloning and sequencing of isolated cDNAs, and many of the physiologically relevant properties and other characteristics of these enzymes are known from studies *in vitro*. With accessibility to relevant probes it will now be possible to study how the levels and activities of these lipases are regulated on a molecular level and what effects dietary components, hormones, and gut peptides have on these enzymes.

During the last decade we have gained further insight into the physical-chemical behavior of dietary lipids during established fat digestion. It now seems that lipolysis products are dissolved in the aqueous portion of duodenal contents not only by the previously recognized mixed micelles. Moreover, absorption may occur directly from these other particles, e.g., unilamellar vesicles. Better definition of the occurrence and function of such "new" product phases in health and disease may have considerable impact on our understanding of intestinal absorption of lipids as well as of other nutrients, antibiotics, carcinogens, etc.

Of particular interest to this workshop have been the LCPUFA of the n-6 and n-3 series. Triglycerides rich in such fatty acids are presently fed to many patients for various purposes. For instance, there are indications that LCPUFA should be added to infant formulas in a concentration approximating that of human milk. Data presented at this meeting suggest that some LCPUFAs are more resistant than others to hydrolysis from triglycerides by colipase-dependent pancreatic lipase. However, such differences are abolished when bile salt-stimulated lipase acts together with colipase-dependent lipase. These data may favor a view that LCPUFAs are more efficiently utilized in breast-fed than in formula-fed infants. If so, this must be an important factor to consider when decisions are made about which LCPUFAs, and in what proportions, should be added to formulas. This, and the general mechanisms of LCPUFA utilization, are important questions to address within the near future.

ACKNOWLEDGMENTS

Financial support from the Swedish Medical Research Council (19X-05708) and the Medical Faculty, University of Umeå is gratefully acknowledged.

REFERENCES

1. RG Jensen, ed. *The lipids of human milk*. Boca Raton: CRC Press; 1989.
2. ESPGAN: Committee on Nutrition. Committee report. Nutrition and feeding of preterm infants. *Acta Paediatr Scand* [Suppl] 1987; 336: 1–14.
3. American Academy of Pediatrics. Committee on nutrition. Nutritional needs for low-birth weight infants. *Pediatrics* 1985; 75: 976–86.
4. Carrol KK. Upper limits of nutrients in infant formulas: polyunsaturated and *trans* fatty acids. *J Nutr* 1989; 119: 1810–3.
5. Svennerholm L. Distribution and fatty acid composition of phosphoglycerides in normal human brain. *J Lipid Res* 1968; 9: 570–9.
6. Martinez MM, Ballabriga A, Gil-Gibernau JJ. Lipids of the developing human retina: 1. Total fatty acids, plasmalogens and fatty acid composition of ethanolamine and choline phosphoglycerides. *J Neurosci Res* 1988; 20: 484–90.
7. Uauy R. Are n-3 fatty acids required for normal eye and brain development in the human? *J Pediatr Gastroenterol Nutr* 1990; 11: 296–302.
8. Carlson SE, Cooke RJ, Peeples JM, Werkman SH, Tolley EA. Docosahexaenoate and eicosapentaenoate status of preterm infants: relationship to visual acuity in n-3 supplemented and unsupplemented infants. *Pediatr Res* 1989; 25: 285A, 1696(abst).
9. Carlson SE, Rhodes PG, Fergusson MG. Docosahexaenoic acid status of preterm infants at birth and following feeding with human milk or formula. *Am J Clin Nutr* 1986; 44: 798–804.
10. Koletzko B, Schmidt E, Bremer HJ, Haug M, Harzer G. Effect of dietary long-chain polyunsaturated fatty acids on the essential fatty acid status of premature infants. *Eur J Pediatr* 1989; 148: 669–75.

11. Koletzko B, Bremer HJ. Fat content and fatty acid composition of infant formulae. *Acta Paediatr Scand* 1989; 78: 513–21.
12. Clandinin MT, Chapell JE, Van Aerde JEE. Requirements of newborn infants for long-chain polyunsaturated fatty acids. *Acta Paediatr Scand* [Suppl] 1989; 351: 63–71.
13. Hernell O. The requirements and utilization of dietary fatty acids in the newborn infant. *Acta Paediatr Scand* [Suppl] 1990; 365: 20–7.
14. Bernbäck S, Bläckberg L, Hernell O. The complete digestion of milk triacylglycerol *in vitro* requires gastric lipase, pancreatic colipase-dependent lipase, and bile salt-stimulated lipase. *J Clin Invest* 1990; 85: 1221–6.
15. Bernbäck S, Hernell O, Bläckberg L. Bovine pregastric lipase: a model for the human enzyme with respect to properties relevant to its site of action. *Biochim Biophys Acta* 1987; 922: 206–13.
16. Bernbäck S, Bläckberg L, Hernell O. Fatty acids generated by gastric lipase promote human milk triacylglycerol digestion by pancreatic colipase-dependent lipase. *Biochim Biophys Acta* 1989; 1001: 286–93.
17. Hernell O, Bläckberg L. Digestion of human milk lipids: physiologic significance of sn-2 monoacylglycerol hydrolysis by bile salt-stimulated lipase. *Pediatr Res* 1982; 16: 882–5.
18. Bottino NR, Vandenburg GA, Reiser R. Resistance of certain long-chain polyunsaturated fatty acids of marine oils to pancreatic lipase hydrolysis. *Lipids* 1967; 2: 489–93.
19. Heimermann WH, Holman RT, Gordon DT, Kowalyshyn DE, Jensen RG. Effect of double bond position in octadecanoates upon hydrolysis by pancreatic lipase. *Lipids* 1973; 8: 45–7.
20. Lawson LD, Hughes BG. Human absorption of fish oil fatty acids as triacylglycerols, free acids, or ethyl esters. *Biochem Biophys Res Commun* 1988; 152: 328–35.
21. Hernell O, Bläckberg L, Chen Q, Nilsson Å. Utilization of human milk long-chain polyunsaturated fatty acids. In: Van Biervielt JP, *et al.*, eds. *Recent advances in infant feeding*. Stuttgart: Thieme Verlag; 1991 [in press].
22. Chen Q, Sternby B, Nilsson Å. Hydrolysis of triacylglycerol arachidonic and linoleic acid ester bonds by human pancreatic lipase and carboxyl ester lipase. *Biochim Biophys Acta* 1989; 1004: 372–86.
23. Bläckberg L, Hernell O. Further characterization of the bile salt-stimulated lipase in human milk. *FEBS Lett* 1983; 157: 337–41.
24. Nilsson J, Bläckberg L, Carlsson P, Enerbäck S, Hernell O, Bjursell G. cDNA cloning of human milk bile salt-stimulated lipase and evidence for its identity to pancreatic carboxylic ester hydrolase. *Eur J Biochem* 1990; 192:543–50.
25. Hoffman AF, Borgström B. The intraluminal phase of fat digestion in man: the lipid content of the micellar and oil phase of intestinal content obtained during fat digestion and absorption. *J Clin Invest* 1964; 43: 247–57.
26. Fredrikzon B, Olivecrona T. Decrease of lipase and esterase activities in intestinal contents of newborn infants during test meals. *Pediatr Res* 1978; 12: 631–4.
27. Brueton MJ, Berger HM, Brown GA, Ablitt L, Iyangkaran N, Wharton BA. Duodenal bile acid conjugation patterns and dietary sulphur amino acids in the newborn. *Gut* 1978; 19: 95–8.
28. Porter HP, Saunders DR, Tytgat G, Brunser O, Rubin CE. Fat absorption in bile fistula man. *Gastroenterology* 1971; 60: 1008–19.
29. Staggers JE, Hernell O, Stafford RJ, Carey MC. Physical-chemical behavior of dietary and biliary lipids during intestinal digestion and absorption. 1. Phase behavior and aggregation states of model lipid systems patterned after aqueous duodenal contents of healthy adult human beings. *Biochemistry* 1990; 29: 2028–40.
30. Hernell O, Staggers JE, Carey MC. Physical-chemical behavior of dietary and biliary lipids during intestinal digestion and absorption. 2. Phase analysis and aggregation states of luminal lipids during duodenal fat digestion in healthy adult human beings. *Biochemistry* 1990; 29: 2041–56.
31. Rigler MW, Honkanen RE, Patton JS. Visualisation by freeze fracture, *in vitro* and *in vivo*, of the products of fat digestion. *J Lipid Res* 1986; 27: 836–57.

DISCUSSION

Dr. Small: In the two-phase region, even if you are very close to single phase on the right hand side (which is actually a mixed, probably multilamellar, phase at that concentration) you still have micelles in equilibrium with vesicles. Over a long stretch of the intestine those micelles might be adequate to carry all the lipid molecules for absorption.

Dr. Hernell: I agree, but it is very difficult to establish that you are not completely devoid of micelles. In our *in vitro* system we could separate vesicles from micelles by centrifugation, but this is not possible with intestinal contents. Thus it is difficult to give a definite answer to your question.

Dr. Small: Since the pH precludes the formation of micelles by fatty acids, you can rule out the presence of micelles by measuring bile salt concentration and showing that it is clearly well below the mixed micelle concentration.

Dr. Bazan: Your work indicates the future directions in nutrition. The cDNA cloning that you have described for colipase-dependent lipase and the BSSL opens up the opportunity to develop probes to see how dietary intake would modify messenger abundance for these lipases. I wonder whether you have done any such studies.

Dr. Hernell: The data that I presented was on the milk lipase, on the BSSL, but the colipase-dependent lipase has also been cloned. No, we have not yet done such experiments but we certainly intend to do so.

Dr. Spector: How much modification is there in the dietary fat in the intestinal mucosa? In other words is the mucosa an active site for elongation and desaturation of different fatty acids?

Dr. Hernell: I don't know but I believe Dr. Clandinin may be able to answer.

Dr. Clandinin: We have done some recent work on this with Alan Thompson's group. The enterocyte does contain Δ-9 and Δ-6 desaturase activities. Both respond fairly quickly to a number of physiological changes such as overnight fasting and change in fatty acid intake.

Dr. Spector: What about the phospholipids in the chylomicrons? It would seem that the phospholipid fatty acid composition would have to be somewhat more regulated than would be the case if it simply reflected whatever is available in the diet.

Dr. Clandinin: The composition of the chylomicrons reflects the triglyceride composition of the fat fed. The aspect that has been of interest to us is how the membrane in the enterocyte is altered by diet. This involves both the absorptive membrane and the membrane that is coated on the chylomicrons.

Dr. Crawford: When considering these phosphoglycerides one is not just thinking about the coating of the chylomicrons but also about the synthesis of lipoprotein by the small intestine, which involves picking up a lot of phosphoglyceride en route; this phosphoglyceride would go preferentially down the portal system. The early experiments of Borgstrom show that significant amounts of the phosphoglyceride fatty acids were indeed going via that route rather than via the lymphatics. What is known about what happens to these phosphoglycerides? Do they provide the lipoprotein in human milk?

Dr. Hernell: To my knowledge no one has looked at the milk phospholipids and the fate of the phospholipid fraction.

Dr. Crawford: It is relevant that there is a small proportion of the fatty-acid-rich pool which is dominated by the phosphoglyceride pattern. This is destined for some different purpose than being dumped in adipose tissue for energy, and this may have a quite disproportionately interesting biological significance because its destination would be for cell membrane growth, differentiation, and regulatory processes.

Dr. Hernell: Dr. Åke Nilsson has pursued this problem by studying the hydrolysis of similarly labeled chylomicrons by lipoprotein lipase—that is, what happens when the chylomicrons enter the blood stream. It appears that lipoprotein lipase discriminates between fatty acids. Those with the first double bond close to the carboxyl carbon are not so readily hydrolyzed. Thus such fatty acids remain in the diglycerides, and perhaps this is a way to channel these fatty acids to the liver as chylomicron remnants. This would fit a hypothesis of a specific route to spare certain fatty acids for a particular purpose.

Long Chain Fatty Acids and Peroxisomal Disorders

Hugo W. Moser and Ann B. Moser

Johns Hopkins University, Kennedy Krieger Institute, Baltimore, Maryland 21210, USA

INITIAL DEMONSTRATION THAT PEROXISOMES OXIDIZE FATTY ACIDS

A connection between peroxisomes and fatty acid metabolism was established first by Lazarow and deDuve in 1976, who demonstrated a fatty acid coenzyme A (CoA) oxidizing system in rat liver that is enhanced by peroxisome proliferators (1). The system is most active toward saturated acyl-CoAs with chain lengths of C12–C16 and long chain unsaturated fatty acids (2,3). The enzymes involved in peroxisomal fatty acid oxidation are totally distinct from those in the mitochondria (4). The physiological contribution of peroxisomes to long chain fatty acid oxidation has been estimated to vary from 5% to 30% (5,6) depending upon physiological conditions.

PEROXISOMES AND VERY LONG CHAIN FATTY ACIDS

That peroxisomes have a major role in the oxidation of very long chain fatty acids (VLCFA) was discovered serendipitously through the study of disease states that only subsequently were shown to be peroxisomal disorders. In 1976 Igarashi *et al.* demonstrated abnormally high levels of saturated VLCFA, particularly hexacosanoic acid (C26:0), in the postmortem brain and adrenal glands of patients who had died of X-linked adrenoleukodystrophy (ALD) (7). Similar accumulations were also present in patients with the neonatal form of this disease (8), which resembles the Zellweger cerebro-hepato-renal syndrome (9). Because of this resemblance, VLCFA levels were measured in patients with Zellweger syndrome and found to be elevated consistently and to such an extent that this is now the most frequently used diagnostic assay (10). It had been shown previously that patients with Zellweger syndrome lack demonstrable peroxisomes (11). Singh *et al.* then showed that VLCFA are metabolized mainly, and possibly exclusively, in the peroxisome (12). Increased VLCFA

TABLE 1. *Classification of peroxisome disorders*

Group 1	Group 2	Group 3
Abnormalities		
Peroxisomes reduced or absent; multiple enzyme defects	Peroxisomes look normal; single enzyme defect	Peroxisomes present; more than one enzyme defective
Diagnosis		
Zellweger syndrome	X-linked ALD	Rhizomelic chondrodysplasia punctata
Neonatal ALD	Acatalasemia	
Infantile Refsum	Hyperoxaluria type 1	
Hyperpipecolic acidemia	3-Oxoacyl thiolase deficiency	
	Thiolase deficiency	
	Bifunctional enzyme deficiency	
	Acyl-CoA oxidase deficiency	

ALD, adrenoleukodystrophy.

levels serve as diagnostic markers for 8 of the 12 disorders that are now assigned to the peroxisome disease category (Table 1).

DISORDERS OF PEROXISOME BIOGENESIS

The disorders of peroxisome biogenesis comprise a group of genetic diseases in which peroxisomes are deficient in number or lacking altogether. The peroxisome is a subcellular organelle which normally is present in all cells other than the mature erythrocyte (13,14). There is increasing evidence that all of the dysfunction in this group of disorders is attributable to the peroxisome defect. Study of these disorders thus can contribute to the understanding of the normal role of this subcellular organelle. That the peroxisome has a significant role in humans is evidenced by the fact that patients with the Zellweger syndrome, the most severe phenotype, show abnormalities in nearly all organs and tissues and rarely survive beyond the 4th month. An analogous peroxisome defect has recently been described in a Chinese hamster ovary cell mutant (15).

Structural Organelle Defect

In tissue sections peroxisomes appear as round or oval structures that are bounded by a single membrane and have a diameter that varies from 0.1 to 0.5 μm. At least 40 enzymes have been localized to the peroxisome (16), and additional functions continue to be assigned. Catalase has long been known to be located in the peroxisome, and cytochemical evidence (17) that an organelle contains this enzyme has long been used as a criterion for its identification as a peroxisome. It was with the use of this technique that the deficiency of peroxisomes was first demonstrated in the liver and kidney of patients with the Zellweger syndrome (11). More recently it was shown that cultured skin fibroblasts of Zellweger disease patients do have membranous structures that contain the proteins characteristic of peroxisomal membranes, but that they lack proteins that are normally found in the matrix. These empty or partially empty membranous structures are referred to as peroxisome ghosts (18).

The Biogenesis Defect

Peroxisome proteins are encoded by nuclear genes and synthesized on free polyribosomes in the cytosol (19). The newly synthesized proteins diffuse through the cytosol and are imported post-translationally into pre-existing peroxisomes. Peroxisomal integral membrane proteins are not deficient in the liver (20) or cultured skin fibroblasts of Zellweger disease patients (18). Furthermore chase studies in cultured skin fibroblasts of Zellweger disease patients have shown that matrix enzymes are synthesized, but that they are degraded with abnormal rapidity (21). These observations have led to the hypothesis that the basic defect in the disorders of peroxisome biogenesis involves the mechanisms that target to the peroxisome the proteins that are normally destined to enter that organelle.

Except for 3-oxoacyl-CoA thiolase, peroxisomal enzymes are synthesized in the mature form (19). A carboxy terminal serine-lysine-leucine sequence (22) appears to be involved in the targeting or 40% of more of peroxisomal proteins (23). Other targeting sequences have been identified (24). As will be discussed, complementation analysis indicates that the disorders of peroxisome biogenesis can be subdivided into at least six groups. It is hypothesized that some or all of these mutants involve abnormalities of these targeting or import mechanisms.

Biochemical Consequences of Peroxisome Deficiency

The disorders of peroxisome biogenesis have in common a panel of morphological and biochemical abnormalities that are listed in Table 2. All can be traced to the defect in peroxisome structure. Ultrastructural and immunocytochemical studies of liver biopsy or cultured skin fibroblasts have revealed a deficiency or absence of catalase-containing particles (11). Unlike many other peroxisomal enzymes, catalase

TABLE 2. *Diagnostically significant abnormalities in disorders of peroxisome biogenesis*

Peroxisomes absent or reduced in number
Catalase in cytosol
Defective oxidation and abnormal accumulation of very long chain fatty acids
Deficient synthesis and reduced tissue levels of plasmalogens
Deficient oxidation and age-dependent accumulation of phytanic acid
Defects in certain steps of bile acid formation and accumulation of bile acids
Defects in oxidation and accumulation of L-pipecolic acid

is not degraded rapidly in the cytosol. Total catalase activity is not diminished, and may even be increased, but it is located in the cytosol rather than the particulate fraction (25).

Immunoblot studies have shown that livers and cultured skin fibroblasts of Zellweger or neonatal ALD patients lack or are deficient in one or more of the peroxisomal β-oxidation enzymes (26). Since these enzymes are synthesized in Zellweger fibroblasts (21) but are mislocated, their absence or low concentration is attributable to their rapid degradation in the cytosol. The deficiency of these enzymes can account for the abnormally high levels of VLCFA that are characteristic for this group of disorders. The pattern of VLCFA accumulation is complex. Unlike X-linked ALD, where only saturated VLCFA accumulate, unsaturated VLCFA also accumulate in the Zellweger syndrome (10,27), including polyenic fatty acids with a chain length up to C38 (28).

The other biochemical abnormalities can also be traced to peroxisomal dysfunction. The low tissue levels of plasmalogens (29) are due to defective function of the first three steps of plasmalogen synthesis which are known to take place in the peroxisome (30). The accumulation of dihydroxy- and trihydroxycholestanoic acid (31) results from a deficiency in the peroxisomal steps of bile acid formation (32). The moderate accumulation and impaired oxidation of phytanic acid (33) appears to be due to impaired oxidation of pristanic acid (34,35), which is the product of α-oxidation of phytanic acid, and thus differs from the defect in classical Refsum disease, where the defect involves the α-oxidation of phytanic acid itself (36). The increased levels of pipecolic acid (37) are attributable to the deficiency of peroxisomal L-pipecolic acid oxidase (38).

Phenotype-Genotype Correlations

The names assigned to the disorders of peroxisome biogenesis are historically based. The Zellweger syndrome was first described in 1963 (39), long before the peroxisomal defect was recognized. Neonatal ALD (40), infantile Refsum disease (41), and hyperpipecolic acidemia (42) were so named because initial metabolic studies pointed to a single abnormality. It was only years later that all of these disorders were found to display the panel of abnormalities listed in Table 2. The disorders differ in respect to severity, the Zellweger syndrome being the most severe, followed by neonatal ALD, with infantile Refsum relatively milder, but still severely disabling. Hyperpipecolic acidemia is not considered to be a distinct entity (14). The clinical features of these disorders have been reviewed (14). The main characteristics of the Zellweger syndrome are profound hypotonia, virtual absence of psychomotor development, neonatal seizures, multiple malformations, eye abnormalities, renal cysts, and cirrhosis of the liver. The children rarely survive beyond the 4th month. The neurological abnormalities appear to be due to a striking and characteristic defect of neuronal migration (43). Patients with neonatal ALD or infantile Refsum disease may survive to the third decade and possibly even longer. Nevertheless they are severely disabled. All are mentally retarded, usually in the severe or profound range; they have impaired hearing, retinal degeneration, liver disease, and often have seizures. Dysmorphic features are usually present.

Definition of the genotype has been aided by complementation analysis. To perform such analyses cultured skin fibroblast cell lines from two patients are fused with polyethylene glycol and a Ficoll gradient is used to separate multinucleate from mononuclear cells. Complementation is present when fused cell lines acquire capacities that the individual cell lines lack. The following properties have been used to assess complementation: acquisition of the capacity to synthesize plasmalogens (44,45), to oxidize phytanic acid (46), to oxidize VLCFA (47), or to assemble peroxisomes based upon the appearance of organelles that contain catalase (48). Results with these assays have been congruous for the most part. In this way cell lines from patients with disorders of peroxisome biogenesis have been subdivided into at least six complementation groups (45), one large and five smaller groups that so far include only one or two patients. It is presumed that each of these groups represents a distinct genotype, each of which possibly involves a different defect in the previously mentioned targeting-import mechanisms. Current research is aimed to define these defects by cell and molecular biology techniques. So far it has not been possible to establish correlations between genotype and phenotypes as they are currently defined. The large complementation group includes cell lines from patients with Zellweger syndrome, neonatal ALD, infantile Refsum disease, and hyperpipecolic acidemia, while the most common phenotype (Zellweger syndrome) was represented in four of the five small groups (45).

GROUP 2: DEFECTS THAT INVOLVE A SINGLE PEROXISOMAL ENZYME

These disorders differ fundamentally from the disorders of peroxisome biogenesis. Peroxisome structure is normal, and there is a mutation that involves a single enzyme. Table 1 lists the disorders that have been identified so far.

X-Linked Adrenoleukodystrophy

X-linked ALD is characterized by the abnormal accumulation of saturated VLCFA, particularly hexacosanoic acid (C26:0), but also tetracosanoic (C24:0), pentacosanoic (C25:0), and those with still longer chain lengths (7,49). The accumulation is due to impaired capacity to oxidize VLCFA, a reaction that normally takes place in the peroxisome (12). While ALD patients have an impaired capacity to oxidize free VLCFA, they metabolize their coenzyme derivative at a normal rate. This led to the hypothesis that the defect involves the coenzyme ligase for VLCFA, and experimental support for a defective function of this enzyme has been provided by two research groups (50,51). The ligase for VLCFA appears to be distinct from that for palmitic acid (52). Palmitoyl-CoA ligase is located in mitochondria, while that for VLCFA (lignoceroyl-CoA ligase) is present in microsomes and peroxisomes. The activity of peroxisomal lignoceroyl-CoA ligase is reduced in X-linked ALD cells, but the microsomal lignoceroyl-CoA activity is normal (50,51). The difference between the microsomal and peroxisomal enzyme activity is unexplained; possibly there are two distinct VLCFA CoA ligases, or the defect involves the import of the enzyme or the substrate to the organelle. The VLCFA CoA ligases have not yet been purified. The X-linked ALD gene has been mapped to Xq28, the terminal segment of the long arm of the X-chromosome (53).

X-linked ALD must be differentiated sharply from neonatal ALD. Neonatal ALD has an autosomal recessive mode of inheritance and is one of the disorders of peroxisome biogenesis. The two disorders have never occurred in the same family. X-linked ALD has several phenotypes, which do often occur in the same family. Approximately 50% of patients have the childhood cerebral form, a serious disease which presents most commonly between 4 and 8 years of age as a learning disability or dementing illness. It often progresses rapidly so that the child is left in an apparently vegetative state within 1 to 4 years, and dies within a few years thereafter. The neurological disturbance is due to a cerebral demyelination which begins in the parieto-occipital region and resembles multiple sclerosis because of intense perivascular lymphocyte infiltration in the actively demyelinating regions (49). In approximately 25% of patients there is slowly progressive involvement of the long tracts in the spinal cord, referred to as adrenomyeloneuropathy. These patients present with progressive paraparesis and sphincter and sexual disturbances beginning in the third or fourth decade which are slowly progressive over decades. The remainder of the patients may have adrenocortical insufficiency with little or no nervous system involvement and thus are diagnosed as having Addison disease. Still others have brain or cerebellar involvement in adulthood, and may be misdiagnosed as Alzheimer disease or brain tumor. A small proportion of men with the biochemical defect of X-linked ALD remain asymptomatic even in middle age or later. Approximately 15% of female heterozygotes develop neurological disability that resembles adrenomyeloneuropathy, but usually of later onset and milder.

OTHER DEFECTS OF PEROXISOMAL FATTY ACID OXIDATION

Figure 1 shows the pathways of peroxisomal β-oxidation and their interrelation with certain steps of bile acid synthesis. The genes for acyl-Co oxidase (54), bifunctional enzyme (54), and 3-oxo-acyl CoA thiolase (55) have been cloned. The bifunctional enzyme has recently been shown to be trifunctional. In addition to enoyl-CoA hydratase and 3-hydroxy-acyl CoA dehydrogenase it also has δ-3, δ-2 enoyl-CoA isomerase activity (56).

Disease states have now been identified for each of these enzymatic steps. They are acyl-CoA deficiency, also referred to as pseudo-neonatal ALD (57), bifunctional enzyme deficiency (58), and 3-oxo-coenzyme A thiolase deficiency (59), also referred to as pseudo-Zellweger syndrome (60). An unexplained and interesting feature is that

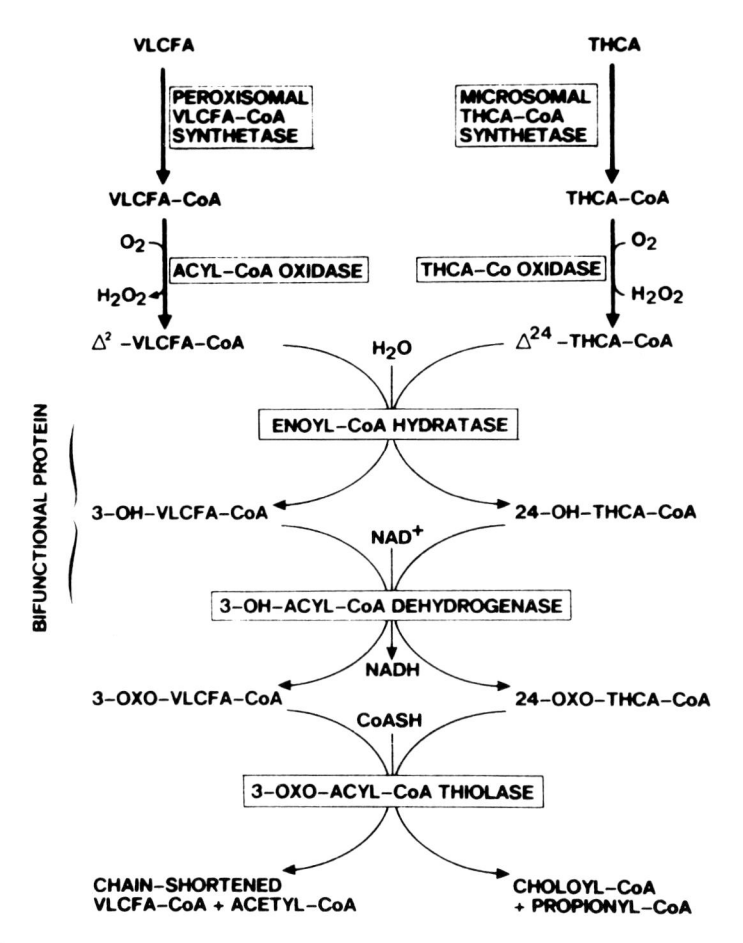

```
              VLCFA                                    THCA
                │                                        │
                ▼                                        ▼
          ┌─────────────┐                         ┌─────────────┐
          │PEROXISOMAL  │                         │MICROSOMAL   │
          │VLCFA-CoA    │                         │THCA-CoA     │
          │SYNTHETASE   │                         │SYNTHETASE   │
          └─────────────┘                         └─────────────┘
                │                                        │
                ▼                                        ▼
          VLCFA-CoA                                  THCA-CoA
         O₂ ┐                                           ┌ O₂
            │  ┌──────────────────┐   ┌─────────────────┐│
            │  │ ACYL-CoA OXIDASE │   │ THCA-Co OXIDASE ││
        H₂O₂┘  └──────────────────┘   └─────────────────┘└ H₂O₂
                │                                        │
                ▼                                        ▼
          Δ²-VLCFA-CoA          H₂O            Δ²⁴-THCA-CoA
```
```
                         ┌──────────────────────┐
                         │ ENOYL-CoA HYDRATASE  │
                         └──────────────────────┘
```

FIG. 1. Pathway of peroxisomal fatty acid and bile acid degradation. Note that for the CoA ligase and oxidase reactions the fatty acids and bile acids are processed by separate enzymes, while for the last two steps the two substrates are processed by the same enzymes.

the phenotype of patients with these single enzyme defects resembles that of the disorders of peroxisome biogenesis (as evidenced even by the names assigned). The patients have profound neurological defects at birth, including defects of neuronal migration. In the oxidase deficiency patients, LCFA accumulation is the only substrate abnormality. In the two other disorders there is also accumulation of bile acid intermediates. It appears that the accumulation of VLCFA and of bile acid intermediates may have serious deleterious effects on nervous system development.

OTHER PEROXISOMAL DISORDERS

The other peroxisomal disorders do not affect fatty acid metabolism, and will only be discussed briefly. In hyperoxaluria type 1 there is a deficiency of hepatic peroxisomal alanine:glyoxalate aminotransferase. The main complications are oxalate renal stones and renal failure. Neurological function is not impaired. Most patients with acatalasemia are asymptomatic. Rhizomelic chondrodysplasia punctata is associated with three biochemical defects: a severe impairment of peroxisomal plasmalogen synthesis, impaired oxidation of phytanic acid, and failure to process peroxisomal 3-oxo-acyl thiolase (61). VLCFA, pipecolic, and bile acid metabolism are normal, and peroxisomes are present although their structure may not be normal. Clinical manifestations are shortening of proximal limbs, cataracts, mental retardation, ichthyosis, and chondrodysplasia punctata. Its nosology is uncertain. More than one peroxisomal function is impaired but the organelle is present; possibly it will be shown to involve a unique set of targeting or import mechanisms.

DIAGNOSIS OF PEROXISOMAL DISORDERS

Prompt and accurate diagnosis of the peroxisomal disorders is important since they are genetically determined. X-linked ALD is an X-linked disorder; all others are autosomal recessive, so that recurrence risk is 25%. All of the disorders can be identified prenatally and genetic counseling is possible and essential.

The diagnosis of peroxisomal disorders may be suspected in the following clinical settings:

1. Neonates with hypotonia, seizures, and failure to thrive or with liver disease
2. Infants with chondrodysplasia punctata
3. A boy with a dementing illness
4. Males with Addison disease
5. Men with progressive paraparesis, with or without adrenal insufficiency
6. Women with progressive paraparesis
7. Oxalic acid urinary stones and renal failure

Measurement of the levels of VLCFA in plasma (62) is the most widely used diagnostic assay for X-linked ALD, the disorders of peroxisome biogenesis, and the defects of peroxisomal β-oxidation. We have performed this assay in 19,000 persons and have identified more than 2,200 patients with peroxisomal disorders (Table 3).

Demonstration of diminished plasmalogen levels in red blood cells (63) or of impaired peroxisomal plasmalogen synthesis in cultured skin fibroblasts (64) is a valuable diagnostic technique for rhizomelic chondrodysplasia punctata and the disorders of peroxisome biogenesis. Other important diagnostic techniques are the measurement of the levels of pipecolic acid (65) and phytanic acid (66) and of bile acid intermediates (67). Table 4 lists the clinical indications for these various assays. Techniques for prenatal diagnosis are discussed in a recent review (14).

TREATMENT OF PEROXISOMAL DISORDERS

Therapy for the disorders of peroxisome biogenesis is limited because of the severe damage already present at time of birth. This limitation does not apply to X-linked

TABLE 3. *Experience with VLCFA assay at the Kennedy Institute, October 1990*

Total number of patients tested since 1980	19,000
X-linked ALD hemizygotes	874
X-linked ALD heterozygotes	1031
Other peroxisomal disorders	
Zellweger syndrome	180
Neonatal ALD	85
Infantile Refsum	19
Hyperpipecolic acidemia	5
RCDP	29
Single β-oxidation defects	18
Unusual phenotypes	9
Phenotype uncertain	37
Total peroxisome disease patients identified	2287

VLCFA, very long chain fatty acids; ALD, adrenoleucodystrophy; RCDP, rhizomelic chondrodysplasia punctata.

TABLE 4. *Peroxisomal disorders: biochemical diagnostic assays*

Disease	Assay	
Disorders of peroxisome biogenesis: Zellweger syndrome, neonatal ALD, infantile Refsum disease, hyperpipecolic acidemia	Plasma:	VLCFAs pipecolic acid phytanic acid bile acids
	RBCs:	Plasmalogens
	Fibroblasts:	Plasmalogen synthesis Catalase subcellular localization
X-linked ALD hemizygote	Plasma/RBCs:	VLCFAs
	Fibroblasts:	VLCFAs
X-linked ALD heterozygote	Plasma:	VLCFAs
	Fibroblasts:	VLCFAs
	DNA probe	
Rhizomelic chondrodysplasia punctata	Plasma:	Phytanic acid
	RBCs:	Plasmalogens
	Fibroblasts:	Plasmalogen synthesis Phytanic acid oxidation
Classic Refsum disease	Plasma:	Phytanic acid
	Fibroblasts:	Phytanic acid oxidation
Isolated defects of VLCFA degradation	Plasma:	VLCFAs
	Fibroblasts:	VLCFAs VLCFA oxidation Immunoblot of peroxisomal fatty acid oxidation enzymes
Hyperoxaluria, type I	Urine:	Organic acids
	Liver:	Alanine: Glyoxalate amino transferase in percutaneous liver biopsy
Acatalasemia	RBCs:	Catalase

ALD, adrenoleukodystrophy; VLCFA, very long chain fatty acids; RBC, red blood cells.

ALD since boys with this disorder are entirely normal until age 4 years or later. Diagnosis can be achieved prenatally or at birth. There thus is a 4-year or longer "window of opportunity" for preventive therapy.

Two approaches are under active investigation. There now exists a dietary regimen that can normalize the levels of saturated VLCFA in plasma within 4 weeks (68). The regimen combines dietary restriction of VLCFA with the administration of large amounts of oils that contain the monounsaturated fatty acids esterified with glycerol. The fatty acids are oleic acid (C18:1) and erucic acid (C22:1). The monounsaturated fatty acids have been shown to inhibit the synthesis of saturated VLCFA in ALD cultured skin fibroblasts (69). Figure 2 shows the effects of this regimen on the plasma level of C26:0 in 75 patients with X-linked ALD. The regimen has resulted in a statistically significant improvement of peripheral nerve function in patients with adrenomyeloneuropathy, and an international trial is now in progress to determine whether it can prevent the onset of neurological disability in persons with the biochemical defect of ALD who are neurologically intact. Dietary therapy does not alter

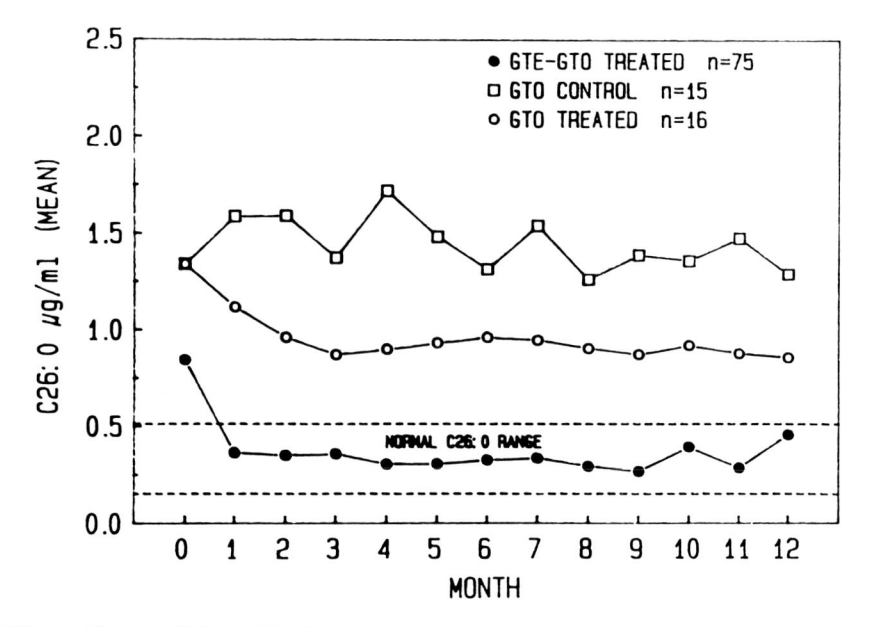

FIG. 2. Effect of GTO and GTE-GTO diets on plasma C26:0 levels. The abscissa shows duration of dietary therapy in months. Plasma C26:0 levels were measured as described previously (62). The figure compares the mean C26:0 levels in 15 male AMN patients (*open circles*) who continued their customary diet, 16 AMN patients who received GTO oil and a VLCFA-restricted diet (*squares*), and 75 male AMN or childhood ALD patients who received the GTE/GTO oils and the VLCFA-restricted diet (*solid circles*). The *horizontal dotted lines* indicate the zone of normal plasma C26:0 levels (0.33 ± 0.18 μg/ml). Note the rapid normalization of the C26:0 level in the GTE/GTO treated group. The mean baseline level in the control and GTO group happened to be identical. The baseline value in the GTE/GTO group was lower than in the other two groups because the last group included some individuals who had previously been on the GTO diet. GTE/GTO oil normalized plasma C26:0 levels irrespective of prior dietary history.

the course of the rapid neurological progression of boys with the severe cerebral childhood form of ALD.

Much interest has been evoked by a recent report that bone marrow transplantation brought about reversal of early neurological abnormalities in a 7½ year old boy with X-linked ALD (70). Bone-marrow-derived cells contain the enzyme that is deficient in ALD and do cross the blood-brain barrier at least to some extent. It was of particular interest that following the transplant plasma VLCFA levels were normalized without the need for a special diet. Bone marrow transplant was ineffective in more advanced cases and under those circumstances appeared to aggravate the pre-existing neurological deficit. Because of the need for matched donors and the risk of the procedure, bone marrow transplant is considered only under carefully selected circumstances. The highly favorable outcome of this approach in the one case, combined with the boys' normal status before symptoms begin and the serious prognosis of the disease, make X-linked ALD a strong potential candidate for gene therapy.

FUTURE DIRECTIONS

The combined incidence of the genetically determined peroxisomal disorders is estimated at 1:25,000. It is anticipated that general awareness of these disorders will increase, that their incidence will be reduced through genetic counseling, and that effective therapy will be developed for those forms in which pathological changes commence postnatally.

This chapter has focused on those reactions that take place mainly or exclusively in the peroxisome. For other reactions, such as the oxidation of long chain fatty acids, the peroxisomal pathway appears to represent a relatively minor duplication of the mitochondrial pathway. A recent and surprising finding is that the peroxisome also appears to be the site of a duplicate pathway for cholesterol biosynthesis (71). The physiological role and the mechanisms that regulate these duplicate pathways are not known. The observation that patients with disorders of peroxisome biogenesis have abnormally low plasma cholesterol and lipoprotein levels (41) suggests that the peroxisome is involved in cholesterol homeostasis. While the genetically determined peroxisome disorders discussed in this chapter are dramatic and at this time command all our personal research efforts, we believe that future research should focus to an increasing extent on the interaction between the peroxisome and other subcellular organelles in the control of normal metabolism.

ACKNOWLEDGMENT

This work was supported in part by grants HD24061, RR00035, RR00052, and RR00722 from the National Institutes of Health.

REFERENCES

1. Lazarow PB, De Duve C. A fatty acyl-CoA oxidizing system in rat liver peroxisomes: enhancement by clofibrate, a hypolipidemic drug. *Proc Natl Acad Sci USA* 1976; 73: 2043–6.

2. Lazarow PB. Rat liver peroxisomes catalyze the β-oxidation of fatty acids. *J Biol Chem* 1978; 253: 1522–8.
3. Osmundsen H, Neat CE, Norum KR. Peroxisomal oxidation of long chain fatty acids. *FEBS Lett* 1979; 99:292–6.
4. Hashimoto T. Individual peroxisomal beta-oxidation enzymes. *Ann NY Acad Sci* 1982; 386: 5–12.
5. Mannaerts GP, Debeer LJ, Thomas J, De Schepper PJ. Mitochondrial and peroxisomal fatty acid oxidation in liver homogenates and isolated hepatocytes from control and clofibrate-treated rats. *J Biol Chem* 1979; 254: 4585–95.
6. Kondrupf J, Lazarow PB. Peroxisomal β-oxidation in intact rat hepatocytes: quantitation of its flux. *Ann NY Acad Sci* 1982; 386: 404–5.
7. Igarashi M, Schaumburg HH, Powers J, Kishimoto Y, Kolodny E, Suzuki K. Fatty acid abnormality in adrenoleukodystrophy. *J Neurochem* 1976; 26: 851–60.
8. Ulrich J, Hershkowitz N, Heits P, Sigrist T, Baerlocher P. Adrenoleukodystrophy: preliminary report of a connatal case, light- and electron microscopical, immunohistochemical and biochemical findings. *Acta Neuropathol (Berl)* 1978; 43: 77–83.
9. Kelley RI. The cerebrohepatorenal syndrome of Zellweger: morphologic and metabolic aspects. *Am J Med Genet* 1983; 16: 503–17.
10. Moser AB, Singh I, Brown III FR, *et al.* The cerebro-hepato-renal (Zellweger) syndrome: increased levels and impaired degradation of very long chain fatty acids, and prenatal diagnosis. *N Engl J Med* 1984; 310: 1141–5.
11. Goldfischer S, Moore CL, Johnson AB, Peroxisomal and mitochondrial defects in the cerebro-hepato-renal syndrome. *Science* 1973; 182: 62–4.
12. Singh I, Moser AB, Goldfischer S, Moser HW. Lignoceric acid is oxidized in the peroxisomes: implications for the Zellweger cerebro-hepato-renal syndrome and adrenoleukodystrophy. *Proc Natl Acad Sci USA* 1984; 81: 4203–7.
13. Hruban Z, Vigil EL, Slesers A, Hopkins E. Microbodies: constituent organelles of animal cells. *Lab Invest* 1972; 27: 184–91.
14. Lazarow P, Moser HW. Disorders of peroxisomal biogenesis. In: Scriver CR, Beaudet AL, Sly WS, Valle D, eds. *The metabolic basis of inherited disease*. New York: McGraw Hill; 1989: 1479–509.
15. Zoeller RA, Allen LA, Santos NJ, *et al.* Chinese hamster ovary cell mutants defective in peroxisome biogenesis—comparison to Zellweger syndrome. *J Biol Chem* 1989; 264: 21872–8.
16. Tolbert NE. Metabolic pathways in peroxisomes and glyoxysomes. *Annu Rev Biochem* 1981; 50: 133–57.
17. Roels F, Goldfischer S. Cytochemistry of human catalase. *J Histochem Cytochem* 1979; 27: 1471–7.
18. Santos MJ, Imanaka T, Shio H, Small GM, Lazarow PB. Peroxisomal membrane ghosts in Zellweger syndrome—aberrant organelle assembly. *Science* 1988; 239: 1536–8.
19. Lazarow PB, Fujiki Y. Biogenesis of peroxisomes. *Annu Rev Cell Biol* 1985; 1: 489–530.
20. Small GM, Santos MJ, Imanaka T, *et al.* Peroxisomal integral membrane proteins in livers of patients with Zellweger syndrome, infantile Refsum's disease and X-linked adrenoleukodystrophy. *J Inherited Metab Dis* 1988; 11: 358–71.
21. Schram A, Strijland A, Hashimoto T, *et al.* Biosynthesis and maturation of peroxisomal β-oxidation enzymes in fibroblasts in relation to the Zellweger syndrome and infantile Refsum disease. *Proc Natl Acad Sci USA* 1986; 83: 6156–8.
22. Gould SJ, Keller G-A, Subramani S. Identification of peroxisomal targeting signals located at the carboxy terminus of four peroxisomal proteins. *J Cell Biol* 1988; 107: 897–905.
23. Gould SJ, Krisans S, Keller GA, Sibramani S. Antibodies directed against the peroxisomal targeting signal of firefly luciferase recognize multiple mammalian peroxisomal proteins. *J Cell Biol* 1990; 110: 27–34.
24. Osumi T, Fujiki Y. Topogenesis of peroxisomal proteins. *Bioessays* 1990; 12: 217–22.
25. Lazarow PB, Small GM, Santos M, *et al.* Zellweger syndrome amniocytes: morphological appearance and a simple sedimentation method for prenatal diagnosis. *Pediatr Res* 1988; 24: 63–7.
26. Tager JM, van der Beek WATH, Wanders RJA, *et al.* Peroxisomal beta oxidation enzyme proteins in the Zellweger syndrome. *Biochem Biophys Res Commun* 1985; 126: 1269–75.
27. Martinez M. Polyunsaturated fatty acid changes suggesting a new enzymatic defect in Zellweger syndrome. *Lipids* 1989; 24: 261–5.
28. Poulos A, Sharp P, Singh H, Johnson D, Fellenberg A, Pollard A. Detection of a homologous series of C26-C38 polyenoic fatty acids in the brain of patients without peroxisomes (Zellweger's syndrome). *Biochem J* 1986; 235: 607–10.
29. Heymans HSA, Schutgens RBH, Tan R, van den Bosch H, Borst P. Severe plasmalogen deficiency in tissues of infants without peroxisomes (Zellweger syndrome). *Nature* 1983; 306: 69–70.

30. Hajra AK, Bishop JE. Glycerolipid biosynthesis in peroxisomes via the acyl dihydroxyacetone phosphate pathway. *Ann NY Acad Sci* 1982; 386: 170–81.
31. Kase BF, Pedersen JI, Standvik B, Björkheim I. In vivo and in vitro studies on formation of bile acids in patients with Zellweger syndrome. *J Clin Invest* 1985; 76: 2393–402.
32. Pedersen JI, Gustafsson J. Conversion of 3α, 7α, 12α-trihydroxy-5β-cholestanoic acid into cholic acid by rat liver peroxisomes. *FEBS Lett* 1980; 121: 345–8.
33. Poulos A, Sharp P, Fellenberg AJ, Danks DM. Cerebro-hepato-renal (Zellweger) syndrome, adrenoleukodystrophy, and Refsum's disease: plasma changes and skin fibroblast phytanic acid oxidase. *Hum Genet* 1985; 70: 172–7.
34. Poulos A, Johnson D, Singh H. Defective oxidation of pristanic acid by fibroblasts from patients with disorders in propionic acid metabolism. *Clin Genet* 1990; 37: 106–10.
35. Wanders RJA, ten Brink HJ, van Roermund CWT, Schutgens RBH, Tager JM, Jakobs C. Identification of pristanoyl-CoA oxidase activity in human liver and its deficiency in the Zellweger syndrome. *Biochem Biophys Res Commun* 1990; 172: 490–5.
36. Steinberg D. Refsum disease. In: Scriver CR, Beaudet AL, Sly WS, Valle D, eds. *The metabolic basis of inherited disease*. New York: McGraw Hill; 1989: 1533–50.
37. Danks DM, Tippett P, Adams C, Campbell P. Cerebro-hepato-renal syndrome of Zellweger: a report of eight cases with comments upon the incidence, the liver lesion, and a fault in pipecolic acid metabolism. *J Pediatr* 1975; 86: 382–7.
38. Mihalik SJ, Moser HW, Watkins PA, Dans DM, Poulos A, Rhead WJ. Peroxisomal L-pipecolic acid oxidation is deficient in liver from Zellweger syndrome patients. *Pediatr Res* 1989; 25: 548–52.
39. Bowen P, Lee CSN, Zellweger H, Lindenberg R. A familial syndrome of multiple congenital defects. *Bull Johns Hopkins Hosp* 1964; 114: 402–14.
40. Kelley RI, Datta NS, Dobyns WB, *et al*. Neonatal adrenoleukodystrophy: new cases, biochemical studies, and differentiation from Zellweger and related peroxisomal polydystrophy syndromes. *Am J Med Genet* 1986; 23: 869–901.
41. Scotto JM, Hadchouel M, Odievre M, *et al*. Infantile phytanic acid storage disease, a possible variant of Refsum's disease: three cases, including ultrastructural studies of the liver. *J Inherited Metab Dis* 1982; 5: 83–90.
42. Gatfield PD, Taller E, Hinton GG, Wallace AC, Abdelnour GM, Haust MD. Hyperipipecolatemia: a new metabolic disorder associated with neuropathy and hepatomegaly. *Can Med Assoc J* 1968; 99: 1215–33.
43. Evrard P, Caviness VS, Prats-Vinas J, Lyon G. The mechanism of arrest of neuronal migration in the Zellweger malformation: an hypothesis based upon cytoarchitectonic analysis. *Acta Neuropathol (Berl)* 1978; 41: 109–17.
44. Brul S, Westerveld A, Strijland A, *et al*. Genetic heterogeneity in the cerebrohepatorenal (Zellweger) syndrome and other inherited disorders with a generalized impairment of peroxisomal functions— a study using complementation analysis. *J Clin Invest* 1988; 81: 1710–5.
45. Roscher AA, Hoefler A, Hoefler G, *et al*. Genetic and phenotypic heterogeneity in disorders of peroxisome biogenesis—a complementation study involving cell lines from 19 patients. *Pediatr Res* 1989; 26: 67–72.
46. Poll-The BT, Skjeldal OH, Stokke O, Poulos A, Demaugre F, Saudubray J-M. Phytanic acid alpha-oxidation and complementation analysis of classical refsum and peroxisomal disorders. *Hum Genet* 1989; 81: 175–81.
47. McGuinnes MC, Moser AB, Moser HW, Watkins PA. Peroxisomal disorders: complementation analysis using beta-oxidation of very long chain fatty acids. *Biochem Biophys Res Commun* 1990; 172: 364–9.
48. Tager JM, Brul S, Wiemer EAC, *et al*. Genetic relationship between the Zellweger syndrome and other peroxisomal disorders characterized by an impairment in the assembly of peroxisomes. In: Tanaka K, Coates PM, eds. *Fatty acid oxidation*. New York: Wiley-Liss 1990: 545–58. (*Progress in clinical and biological research*; vol 321).
49. Moser HW, Moser AB, Singh I, O'Neill BR. Adrenoleukodystrophy: survey of 303 cases: biochemistry, diagnosis and therapy. *Ann Neurol* 1984; 16: 628–41.
50. Lazo O, Contreras M, Hashmi M, Stanley W, Irazu C, Singh I. Peroxisomal lignoceroyl-CoA ligase deficiency in childhood adrenoleukodystrophy and adrenomyeloneuropathy. *Proc Natl Acad Sci USA* 1988; 85: 7647–51.
51. Wanders RJA, van Roermund CWT, van Wijland MJA, *et al*. Direct evidence that the deficient oxidation of very long chain fatty acids in X-linked adrenoleukodystrophy is due to an imparied ability of peroxisomes to activate very long chain fatty acids. *Biochem Biophys Res Commun* 1988; 153: 618–24.

52. Lazo O, Contreras M, Singh I. Topographical localization of peroxisomal acyl-CoA ligases—differential localization of palmitoyl-CoA and lignoceroyl-CoA ligases. *Biochemistry* 1990; 29: 3981–6.
53. Aubourg P, Sack GH, Meyers DA, Lease JJ, Moser HW. Linkage of adrenoleukodystrophy to a polymorphic DNA probe. *Ann Nuerol* 1987; 21: 240–9.
54. Miyazawa W, Hayashi H, Hijikata M, *et al*. Complete nucleotide sequence of cDNA and predicted amino acid sequence of rat acyl-CoA oxidase. *J Biol Chem* 1987; 262:8131–7.
55. Hijikata M, Ishii N, Kagamiyama H, Osumi T. Hashimoto T. Structural analysis of cDNA for rat peroxisomal 3-ketoacyl-CoA thiolase. *J Biol Chem* 1987; 262: 8151–8.
56. Palosaari PM, Hiltunen JK. Peroxisomal bifunctional protein from rat liver is a trifunctional enzyme possessing s-eonyl-CoA hydratase, 3-hydroxyacyl-CoA dehydrogenase, and delta-3, delta-2-enoyl-CoA isomerase activities. *J Biol Chem* 1990; 265: 2446–9.
57. Poll-The BT, Roels F, Ogier H, *et al*. A new peroxisomal disorder with enlarged peroxisomes and a specific deficiency of acyl-CoA oxidase (pseudo-neonatal adrenoleukodystrophy). *Am J Hum Genet* 1988; 42: 422–34.
58. Watkins PA, Chen WW, Harris CJ, *et al*. Peroxisomal bifunctional enzyme deficiency. *J Clin Invest* 1988; 83: 771–7.
59. Schram AW, Goldfischer S, van Roermund CT, *et al*. Human peroxisomal 3-oxoacyl-coenzyme A thiolase deficiency. *Proc Natl Acad Sci USA* 1987; 84: 2494–6.
60. Goldfischer S, Collins J, Rapin I, *et al*. Pseudo-Zellweger syndrome: deficiencies in several peroxisomal oxidative activities. *J Pediatr* 1986; 108: 25–32.
61. Hoefler G, Hoefler S, Watkins P, *et al*. Biochemical abnormalities in rhizomelic chondrodysplasia punctata. *J Pediatr* 1988; 112: 726–33.
62. Moser HW, Moser AB, Frayer KK, *et al*. Adrenoleukodystrophy: increased plasma content of saturated very long chain fatty acids. *Neurology* 1981; 31: 1241–9.
63. Bjorkhem I, Sisfontes L, Bostrom B, Kase BF, Blomstrand R. Simple diagnosis of the Zellweger syndrome by gas-liquid chromatography of dimethylacetals. *J Lipid Res* 1986; 27: 786–91.
64. Roscher A, Molzer B, Bernheimer H, Stockler S, Mutz I, Paltauf F. The cerebrohepatorenal (Zellweger) syndrome: an improved method for the biochemical diagnosis and its potential value for prenatal detection. *Pediatr Res* 1985; 19: 930–3.
65. van den Berg GA, Breukelman H, Elzinga H, Trijbels JMF, Monnens LAH, Muskiet FAJ. Determination of pipecolic acid in urine and plasma by isotope dilution mass fragmentography. *Clin Chim Acta* 1986; 159: 229–37.
66. Moser HW, Moser AB. Measurement of phytanic acid levels. In: Hommes F, ed. *Techniques in diagnostic human biochemical genetics, a laboratory manual.* New York: Wiley-Liss; 1991: 193–203.
67. Setchell KDR, Vestal CH. Thermospray ionization liquid chromatography-mass spectrometry—a new and highly specific technique for the analysis of bile acids. *J Lipid Res* 1989; 30: 1459–69.
68. Rizzo WB, Leshner RT, Odone A, *et al*. Dietary erucic acid therapy for X-linked adrenoleukodystrophy. *Neurology* 1989; 30: 1415–22.
69. Rizzo WB, Watkins PA, Phillips MW, Cranin D, Campbell B, Avigan J. Adrenoleukodystrophy: oleic acid lowers fibroblast saturated C22-C26 fatty acids. *Neurology* 1986; 36: 357–61.
70. Aubourg P, Blanche S, Jambaque I, *et al*. Reversal of early neurologic and neuroradiologic manifestations of X-linked adrenoleukodystrophy by bone marrow transplantation. *N Engl J Med* 1990; 322: 1860–6.
71. Thompson SL, Krisans SK. Rat liver peroxisomes catalyze the initial step in cholesterol synthesis: the condensation of acetyl-CoA units into acetoacetyl-CoA. *J Biol Chem* 1990; 265: 5731–5.

DISCUSSION

Dr. Galli: Can these enzymes be induced by compounds such as clofibrate? And do n-3 fatty acids have an effect similar to erucic acid in your patients?

Dr. H. W. Moser: We have treated patients with X-linked ALD with clofibrate and saw no lowering of VLCFA. Lazarow's group treated patients with Zellweger syndrome with clofibrate but without effect.

Oleic acid and erucic acid were chosen because in studies of cultured skin fibroblasts these were the most effective in lowering the rate of synthesis of the saturated VLCFA. We have not tested the effect of other unsaturated acids.

Dr. Bazan: Is there any information on the reason why neuronal migration is altered? We know that migration is highly dependent on the glial surface for the navigation events and for signal recognition and signal information. Although it might not help these patients, this might be a unique opportunity to address this fundamental question. Do we know if the glial cells are affected?

Dr. H. W. Moser: Glial cells are affected. Dr. J. M. Powers showed that the radial glia in the fetus has inclusions characteristic of VLCFA. We have also compared neuronal migration in the various types of peroxisomal diseases. In classical rhizomelic chondrodysplasia, where there is a profound defect in plasmalogen synthesis but where VLCFA are metabolized normally, Margaret Norman in Vancouver found that there was no migrational defect. Conversely, in a patient with bifunctional enzyme defect, where VLCFA are increased but plasmalogens are normal, there was a profound neuronal migration abnormality (1). At this time, the VLCFA and the bile acid intermediates are under the greatest suspicion.

Dr. Gualde: Do these patients have any immunologic dysfunction?

Dr. H. W. Moser: Patients with X-linked ALD have profound perivascular accumulation of lymphocytes in the nervous system. The pattern is compatible with an immunologic reaction to an antigen within the nervous system (2). We also found that the ganglioside fatty acid composition is highly abnormal, as is the fatty acid composition of phosphatidylcholine. It is our working hypothesis that the abnormal brain fatty acid composition leads to an autoimmune response with a "final common pathway" resembling that in multiple sclerosis.

Dr. Small: In your statement about the viscosity of the red cell membranes you imply that the VLCFA are esterified into the phospholipids of the red cell membranes and that this increases the viscosity. If this is true these phospholipids must be in many others cells, in other organelles. Perhaps that is part of the problem.

Dr. H. W. Moser: When adrenal cells are cultured in a medium containing docosahexanoic acid in a concentration equivalent to that in ALD plasma their capacity to release cortisone is diminished. The hypothesis is that the abnormality in the plasma membrane interferes with ACTH receptor function. The cholesterol ester abnormality in the brain appears to be a secondary phenomenon. We have examined tissues from ALD patients in whom there were parts of the brain that were not yet affected pathologically. In that part of the brain the cholesterol esters were normal and the main excess of hexacosanoic acid was found in the phosphatidylcholine fraction. The abnormal phosphatidylcholine fatty acid composition may play a role in the pathogenesis.

Dr. Heim: Long chain dicarboxylic acid urea is a typical phenomenon in peroxisomal disorders. Does it occur in every kind of disorder or is it more characteristic of ALD?

Dr. H. W. Moser: It is a relatively small abnormality compared to that seen in the mitochondrial disorders and it is not always present. The abnormality is present in neonatal ALD but not in X-linked ALD.

REFERENCES

1. Watkins PA, Chen WW, Harris CJ, *et al.* Peroxisomal bifunctional enzyme deficiency. *J Clin Invest* 1988; 83: 771–7.
2. Griffin DE, Moser HW, Mendoza Q, Moench T, O'Toole S, Moser AB. Identification of the inflammatory cells in the nervous system of patients with adrenoleukodystrophy. *Ann Neurol* 1985; 18: 660–3.

Long Chain Polyunsaturated Fatty Acid Metabolism and Cellular Utilization: Regulation and Interactions

Claudio Galli, Cristina Mosconi, and Franca Marangoni

Institute of Pharmacological Sciences, School of Pharmacy, University of Milano, 20133 Milano, Italy

The unique presence of the long chain highly unsaturated fatty acids (HUFA) of the linoleic (LA) and the α linolenic (LNA) acid series in the animal kingdom underlines the existence of specialized mechanisms for the incorporation and maintenance of these compounds, which are present in biological systems mainly as esters of glycerol in phospholipids, as structural components of biomembranes. The fact that the 18-carbon polyunsaturated fatty acids (PUFA), LA and α LNA, are present in large excess in modern food, when compared with the trace concentrations of the HUFA, has led to the concept that the major process responsible for the availability of HUFA in higher organisms is their metabolic formation from the 18-carbon PUFA of dietary origin. Biochemical studies have shown that enzymatic desaturation and elongation of LA and α LNA occur in tissues, the liver being the most relevant site of fatty acid metabolism. In addition, nutritional studies carried out mostly on laboratory animals have shown that modifications of the absolute amounts and relative proportions of LA and α LNA in the diet induce changes of HUFA profiles in lipids of various tissues that can be attributed to the fatty acid desaturation and elongation reactions disclosed in biochemical investigations.

On the other, studies carried out in various types of cells show that data on the desaturation and elongation of unsaturated fatty acids do not quantitatively account for the accumulation of selected PUFA in different tissues nor for the incorporation of specific HUFA in selected lipid pools. Hence, metabolic studies do not allow an accurate prediction of the effects of manipulations of dietary fatty acids on the fatty acid profiles of different cells (1). A number of integrated processes, in cells and in their membranes, responsible for the continuous remodeling of structural lipids, appear to be involved in the maintenance of selected fatty acid profiles, while allowing a turnover of the lipid components.

In addition, the intake of preformed HUFA in the diet plays important physiological and metabolic roles. For instance, tissue and organ development in physiological states, such as intrauterine growth of the embryo and fetus and the early postnatal growth of the suckling newborn, are highly dependent upon the availability of preformed HUFA obtained from the mother. Also, the presence of appreciable levels of HUFA of the n-3 and n-6 series in foods obtained from marine animals and from lean muscles of terrestrial animals, respectively, indicates that under various dietary conditions in the past and at present, the intake of preformed HUFA has contributed and is contributing to the availability of these structural components for organ development and function. The intake of appreciable amounts of long chain PUFA (LCPUFA) is typical of animal species that are predators, and this may have represented an important process for the development of specialized functions in organs requiring an adequate availability of HUFA, and, more generally, for the evolution of species endowed with more developed organs and functions (2).

It appears, thus, that the maintenance of the proper amounts and proportions of HUFA in biological systems is based on a number of processes, such as 1) metabolic conversion of the major polyunsaturated fatty acids of the diet, LA and α LNA, to HUFA; 2) intake of preformed HUFA with the diet; 3) phospholipid biosynthesis coupled with membrane formation; 4) uptake and incorporation of selected fatty acids in tissue lipids and in lipid classes; 5) and remodeling of glycerophospholipids in biomembranes through reactions (deacylation, reacylation) involving hydrolysis and re-esterification of these compounds within the membrane.

These combined processes will ultimately affect levels of HUFA in biomembranes and, as a result, their physicochemical properties, the availability of substrates for eicosanoid synthesis, and the activity of enzymes involved in lipid metabolism and in the generation of lipid-derived mediators.

This chapter is devoted to a brief discussion of some of the factors which appear to modulate HUFA profiles in tissues (dietary intake; differential tissue responses to fatty acid intakes with particular relevance to the relationships between liver and extrahepatic tissues; relations between the intake and incorporation of HUFA into plasma and cell lipids and the dietary energy intake; interactions between fatty acid series and between HUFA and antioxidants). We also discuss the influences of modified HUFA profiles in various cells on functional parameters, assessed in response to cell activation.

FACTORS AFFECTING HUFA PROFILES IN TISSUES

Fatty Acid Metabolism

The major site of the metabolism of PUFA is the liver, where, in the endoplasmic reticulum, dietary unsaturated fatty acids are modified through desaturation and elongation reactions. These types of reactions are discussed in detail in Dr. Sprecher's chapter. Although data on desaturation and elongation rates may be useful for appreciating the rates of fatty acid metabolism under various conditions, as has been pointed out by Sprecher (1), they do not allow us to predict the effects of supplementation with unsaturated fatty acids on the fatty acid profiles of cell membranes. Other parameters, such as specificity for acylation processes, may prevail in determining the preferential incorporation of certain fatty acids in phospholipids. Rates of acylation reactions are undoubtedly much higher than those for desaturation and elongation (see Dr. Sprecher's chapter) and thus acylation processes may play a more important role in modulating the incorporation of fatty acids in selected phospholipid pools.

Coupling of the metabolism of PUFA to membrane lipid biosynthesis appears also to be an important process in modifying tissue fatty acid composition, at least in the liver (1). Metabolic studies carried out in various laboratories by incubating liver microsomes with labeled substrates have shown different rates of conversion for fatty acids with different degrees of unsaturation and belonging to different series. Metabolic data coupled with data obtained in animal experiments carried out by feeding different fatty acids have also led to the concept of competition between substrates for the desaturation steps. More specifically, the well-known accumulation of 20:3 n-9 during essential fatty acid (EFA) deficiency (3) and that of 22:5 n-6 during a deficiency of n-3 fatty acids (4) are usually explained as a consequence of the released inhibition in the desaturation and elongation of oleic acid and 20:4 n-6, respectively. However, alternative explanations which have been proposed (1) are that competition between PUFA of the different series occurs in phospholipid acylation processes, or that different turnover rates of phospholipids with different types of PUFA may result in accumulation of certain fatty acids.

A generally accepted concept concerning fatty acid metabolism is that the liver is the major site of formation and that extrahepatic cells and tissues take up fatty acids from plasma for further modification by metabolic conversion and by additional processes.

The types of mechanisms which control the fatty acid profiles in cells (for an overview, see ref. 5) are listed in Table 1. Reactions taking place in the endoplasmic reticulum appear to predominate in the liver, whereas reactions in the plasma membranes and other organelles are relevant in extrahepatic tissues and especially in circulating cells.

TABLE 1. *Enzymes involved in maintenance of fatty acyl group composition*

Reactions occurring in endoplasmic reticulum
  Elongation and desaturation of precursor fatty acids
  Formation of phosphatidate and other phosphoglycerides
  Phospholipid exchange enzymes
Membrane synthesis
  Transport of lipids and proteins to plasma membrane
Reactions taking place in plasma membrane and other organelle membranes
  Phospholipase action
  Acylation
  Transacylation
  Headgroup exchange

HUFA in Liver and Extrahepatic Tissues

An understanding of the role of liver as key organ for fatty acid metabolism and as a store of PUFA for supply to other tissues comes from nutritional and metabolic studies. In rats born to mothers fed an EFA-deficient diet during pregnancy and lactation, and subsequently fed the EFA-deficient diet after weaning (6), levels of arachidonate in liver (mg/g tissue) decline within a few weeks, reaching at 40 days a value of about 10% of the values at birth (Fig. 1). This value was not subsequently reduced any further. Levels of 20:3 n-9 increased very slowly during the same period of time. In brain, in contrast to the situation in liver, arachidonate continued to accumulate after birth, though reaching, at 40 days, a value about 20% lower than in EFA-supplemented animals. After 40 days of age, when the concentration of arachidonate in liver reached its minimum value, 20:3 n-9 started to accumulate in brain. These results indicate that during EFA deficiency the liver supplies arachidonate to the brain, where it accumulates until liver stores are available. After the liver is depleted of n-6 PUFA, the brain starts accumulating n-9 PUFA. The central role of the liver in synthesizing and providing arachidonate to extrahepatic tissues for membrane synthesis has been confirmed in a more recent study (7), showing decline of arachidonate in liver lipids, but conservation in heart and kidney cortex phospholipids in EFA-deficient mice. In the same study it was shown that labeled arachidonate, which was rapidly taken up in the liver, was released over a period of time by this organ, being mobilized for acylation into heart and kidney phospholipids. In this and other studies on the effects of EFA deficiency on tissue fatty acids it was shown that the total level of unsaturation (unsaturation index) of individual phospholipids was not modified in extrahepatic tissues such as the brain, due to the replacement of HUFA of the n-6 series (mainly arachidonate) by 20:3 n-9, whereas reduction of total unsaturation occurred in liver as a consequence of the marked decrease of arachidonate compensated by only a modest accumulation of the n-9 PUFA.

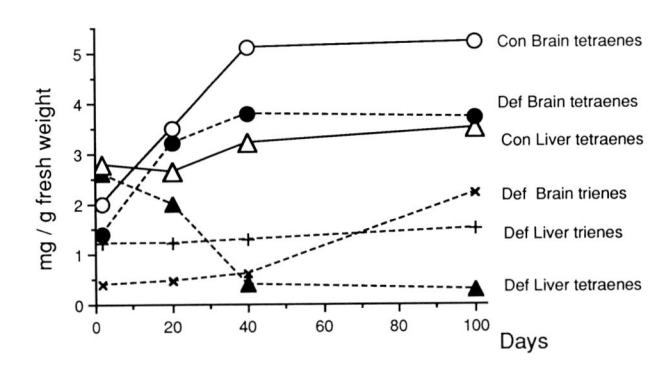

FIG. 1. Time course of the levels (mg/g fresh weight) of tetraenoic fatty acids (20:4 + 22:4 n-6) and of trienoic fatty acids (20:3 + 22:3 n-9) in brain and liver of control and EFA-deficient rats. Con, control; Def, deficient.

Although the uptake of fatty acids by various types of cells from plasma is a generally recognized process, limited information is available concerning the incorporation into tissues of fatty acids mobilized from the liver. In fact, the mechanisms responsible for the delivery from plasma to extrahepatic cells of linoleic acid, which is not synthesized by animal cells, and of arachidonic acid, which is not easily formed from its precursor, have not been fully elucidated. It has been recently shown, however, that low density lipoproteins (LDL) deliver arachidonate for prostaglandin synthesis to fibroblasts through high affinity receptor-mediated mechanisms (8). This is, possibly, a general mechanism for arachidonate delivery to cells expressing high numbers of LDL receptors and also a high activity of PGH synthetase.

The liver plays also a central role in supplying the long chain n-3 fatty acids— e.g., docosahexaenoic acid (DHA), which is primarily generated in this organ from dietary α linolenic acid (18:3 n-3) through desaturation and elongation reactions— to the brain and the retina (9). The highly unsaturated n-3 fatty acids are utilized for the synthesis of phospholipids which are released from the liver in the bloodstream in the form of lipoproteins. It has been proposed that the uptake of the n-3 HUFA in the retina operates through an apolipoprotein E LDL receptor, which has been found in developing photoreceptor cells (10).

Liver-Extrahepatic Tissue Relationships in Feeding Studies

The different balance between the reactions listed in Table 1 (mainly FA metabolism *vs.* phospholipid remodeling in membranes) in liver and extrahepatic tissues, explains why the patterns of tissue fatty acids are changed in different ways in the liver and in other tissues after feeding PUFA. For instance, after feeding diets (11) with high (10% of energy) (HL) or low (2.5%) (LL) LA content to rabbits, it was observed, when comparing the HL with the LL group, that both LA and arachidonate accumulated in livers of the HL group, as expected, but in platelets, in contrast, arachidonate was depleted, being replaced by LA. Somewhat similar findings were observed in human studies (12) in which elevation of the LA content in the diet resulted in a lower arachidonate/linoleate ratio in platelets. In addition it was found that the unsaturated index (UI) of platelet lipids was not affected in either study by the change in the LA content in the diet, whereas in the animal study it appeared that this index was affected by the diet in liver. These data indicate that the prevailing process concerning PUFA metabolism in liver is the conversion of LA to arachidonate; so after high LA, the more LA that enters the liver, the more is converted to arachidonate, with only slight effects on the arachidonate/linoleate ratio. The accumulation of both PUFAs in liver also results in elevation of the UI. In platelets, by contrast, the prevailing process appears to be replacement of arachidonate by LA, the total level of PUFA and the UI of lipids remaining constant.

A more detailed picture of the differences in fatty acid accumulation in liver *vs.* other tissues after feeding, e.g., increasing levels of LA, is presented in Fig. 2, which shows the relationships between relative LA and arachidonate levels in liver and in

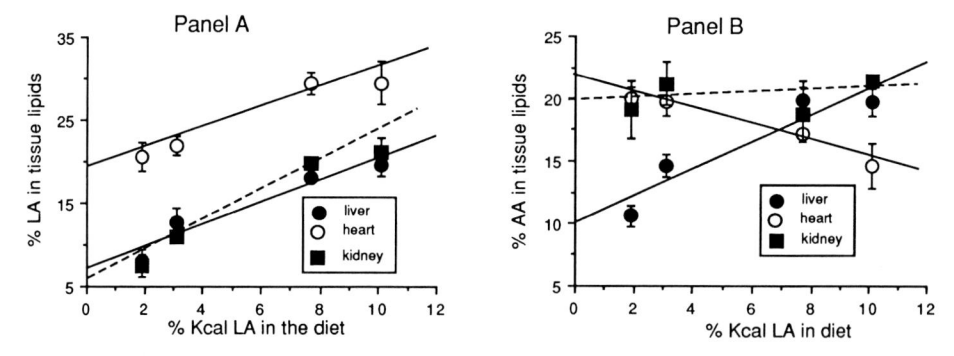

FIG. 2. Relationships between levels of linoleic acid (LA) in the diet as % of energy intake and levels, as % of tissue fatty acids, of LA (*Panel A*), and of arachidonic acid (AA) (*Panel B*) in liver, heart, and kidneys.

other organs of rats fed isoenergetic, semisynthetic diets containing from 2% to 10% of energy as LA (from 9% to 48% of dietary fatty acids). It is evident that, while LA increased as percentage of total fatty acids in liver, heart, and kidney with increasing intake of LA in the diet, changes of arachidonate levels followed very different trends in the various organs. Arachidonate was increased in the liver, whereas it was not modified in kidney and tended to decrease in heart. Similarly, with increasing dietary LA, the total level of saturation (now shown) increased in liver and, somewhat less, in kidneys, but it decreased in heart. We have already mentioned that in EFA deficiency the UI is not modified in brain phospholipids, whereas it is reduced in liver phospholipids. The different types of interactions between PUFA in liver and other tissues, e.g., the heart, are also apparent when, in the above study with increasing amount of LA in the diet, we considered the relationships between dietary LA and the levels of n-3 fatty acids in liver and heart (Fig. 3). The levels of EPA and DHA in liver were not affected by dietary LA, whereas DHA levels, similar to those of arachidonate, were reduced with increasing dietary LA. This again

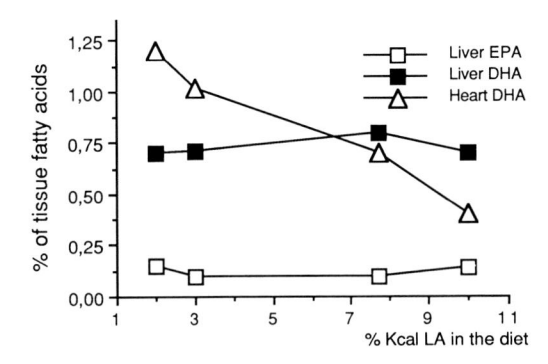

FIG. 3. Relationships between levels of linoleic acid (LA) in the diet as % of energy intake and levels of EPA and DHA, as percentage of tissue fatty acids, in liver and heart.

indicates that in heart, displacement of n-3 fatty acids by increasing dietary LA was the major process, whereas in liver, the enhanced LA pool did not interfere with n-3 fatty acid pools.

As shown by these examples, the different responses of PUFA profiles in liver and other tissues to changes of the intake of unsaturated fatty acids with the diet make it rather difficult to predict the impact of dietary manipulations on tissue fatty acids, and, indirectly, on functional parameters that are dependent upon or correlated with fatty acid pools. In addition, the metabolic relationships between liver and extrahepatic tissues may play a role in inducing alterations in the fatty acid profiles in tissues as a consequence of liver diseases. In liver cirrhosis (13), for instance, levels of arachidonate in platelet lipids are reduced, possibly as a result of impaired synthesis in the damaged organ.

ACCUMULATION OF HUFA IN PLASMA AND CELL LIPIDS IN HYPERCHOLESTEROLEMIA AND IN RELATION TO FAT INTAKE

Data on the favorable effects of dietary n-6 and/or n-3 fatty acids on plasma lipids and thrombotic parameters in animal and human studies have led to the generally accepted recommendation that the intake of these compounds should be increased in order to prevent a rise in serum cholesterol and its vascular complications. Limited information is, however, available on the status and metabolism of LCPUFA in hypercholesterolemic subjects. We have found that the levels of arachidonic acid in platelet phospholipids of type IIa hypercholesterolemic patients were higher than in normocholesterolemic subjects (14), suggesting that the processes responsible for uptake, incorporation, or utilization of this fatty acid are affected by altered lipoprotein metabolism.

In addition, we have treated both normocholesterolemic subjects (five healthy volunteers with serum cholesterol ranging from 165 to 220 mg/dl, and on a typical Western diet, with fat contributing about 36% of energy and about 2,400 kcal/day), and eight moderately hypercholesterolemic patients (type IIa with average serum cholesterol of 290 mg/dl, on a prudent diet with 1,700 kcal/day and 30% fat), for a period of 6 weeks, with highly enriched preparations of EPA + DHA ethyl esters (2.7 and 1.6 g/day, respectively). We found that, in the hypercholesterolemics, levels of EPA and DHA in plasma and circulating cells were considerably higher than in controls both before and after treatment (Fig. 4). This suggests that some aspect of n-3 fatty acid metabolism (e.g., plasma transport, incorporation into cells) is also modified by hypercholesterolemia. It should be borne in mind, however, that in the above treatment schedule, the patients were on a relatively low fat intake and this might have affected n-3 fatty acid incorporation in plasma and cell lipids, especially after supplementation.

PUFA AND ANTIOXIDANTS

Highly unsaturated fatty acids are susceptible to oxidative alterations, which are blocked by natural lipid-soluble compounds with antioxidant properties such as the

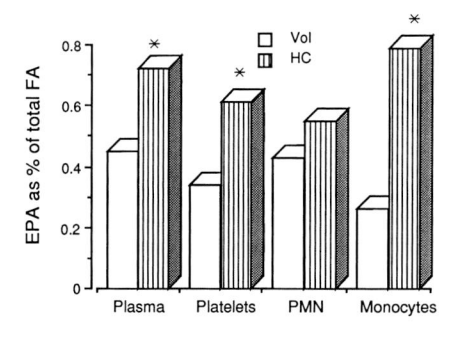

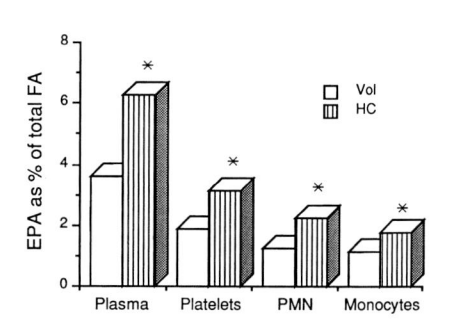

FIG. 4. Levels of EPA in plasma, monocyte, and polymorphonuclear leukocyte lipids in hypercholesterolemic (HC) subjects on a low fat diet or in normocholesterolemics (Vol) on a regular diet treated with 2.7 g/day of EPA and 1.6 g/day DHA for 6 weeks.

tocopherols, and, in biological systems, by enzymatic processes cooperating with lipid antioxidants in the prevention of and protection from oxygen-generated radicals.

In nature, fats rich in PUFA also contain high levels of lipid antioxidants, such as the tocopherols and other compounds, but in the preparation of oils and fats and in their use for cooking, some loss may occur. Adequate levels of vitamin E in the diet are recommended in order to control lipid peroxidation processes and to prevent cell damage resulting from generation of lipid peroxides. Dietary requirements for vitamin E are obviously dependent upon the intake of PUFA, and thus the use of preparations enriched with HUFA of the n-3 series, with five and six double bonds, may result in shortage of vitamin E in tissues.

The administration of fish oil concentrates has, indeed, been shown to induce a depletion of circulating levels of α-tocopherol (15). Furthermore we have observed (16) that the administration of n-3 fatty acids (MaxEPA) supplemented with additional α-tocopherol, up to 10 mg/ml *vs.* the original 1 mg/ml of the preparation, to rats fed a standard laboratory chow, induced a significant change in the proportion of n-6 PUFA in plasma and circulating cells, when compared to the n-6 fatty acid profiles obtained with the administration of MaxEPA without the vitamin supplement. In fact, levels (Table 2) of LA were significantly higher in plasma and those of arachidonate significantly higher in platelets, red blood cells, and especially in polymorphonuclear leukocyte lipids, after 8 weeks of administration with 3.2 ml/kg/day MaxEPA containing the α-tocopherol supplement. In contrast, vitamin E supplementation did not affect the levels of 20:5 and 22:6 in the same samples. It appears, thus, that the effects of n-3 fatty acids on the profile of n-6 in plasma and cells are modulated by the availability of lipid antioxidants, and this represents an additional type of interaction between dietary fatty acids, on the one hand, and the metabolism and accumulation of PUFA in cells and tissues on the other.

TABLE 2. Levels of n-6 and n-3 PUFA in plasma and cell lipids[a]

Fatty acids	Plasma		Platelets		Red blood cells		PMN	
	−Vit E	+Vit E	−Vit E	+Vit E	−Vit E	+Vit E	−Vit E	+Vit E
18:2	25.6	**28.7**	11.3	10.5	11.9	11.8	10.0	10.1
20:4	9.4	**10.7**	19.8	**20.9**	18.4	**19.6**	11.2	**17.4**
20:5	1.2	1.0	4.4	3.9	1.9	1.8	2.0	1.7
22:6	3.0	3.0	2.6	2.6	4.1	4.0	6.2	6.4

[a] Values in bold differ from the corresponding values in regular typeface.
PUFA, polyunsaturated fatty acids; PMN, polymorphonuclear leukocytes.

PUFA AND CELL FUNCTION

This aspect is discussed by other authors in this volume. However, some consideration should be given in this chapter to the type of relationship between HUFA in cell lipids and functional parameters, which can be studied, for instance, during cell activation.

The impact of diet-induced modifications of the fatty acid profiles in cells on cell functions is generally attributed to alterations of the eicosanoid pathway, as a consequence of variations of the fatty acid precursor levels. Modified formation of metabolites derived from arachidonate and/or formation of compounds derived from EPA, when this fatty acid accumulates in cell lipids, have been shown as a consequence of manipulation of dietary fatty acids. It becomes, however, evident from various studies that other processes, in addition to those mediated by the eicosanoid system, are affected by diet-induced changes in cell fatty acids. Furthermore, different types of cells are differently affected by modifications of dietary fatty acids.

Among the processes involved in cell activation which have been reported to be modified by changes of the fatty acid composition of the diet, we wish to highlight in particular those concerning the formation of inositol phosphates by stimulated cells. The administration of isoenergetic diets enriched in either n-9 (olive oil), or n-6 (corn oil), or n-3 (MaxEPA) fatty acids to rabbits for a period of 5 weeks resulted in corresponding changes of the fatty acid profiles in plasma and platelet lipids (17). The formation of total inositol phosphates (IP) and the proportions among the various components (IP_3, IP_2, and IP) by platelets stimulated with thrombin were also significantly modified by the types of fatty acid in the diet. The lowest accumulation of IP_3, the product which is involved in the activation of calcium mobilization in the stimulated cell, was observed in platelets enriched in the n-3 fatty acids. This modification, which in the particular dietary conditions of the study was independent of changes in thromboxane formation by stimulated platelets, indicates that the phospholipase C pathway was affected by dietary fatty acids in a way which was not directly related to the eicosanoid system. We have also observed a reduction in total inositol phosphate production by thrombin-stimulated platelets and a change in the balance among the various products, in male volunteers treated for 6 weeks, while remaining on a conventional diet, with EPA plus DHA ethyl ester preparations (6 capsules/day containing a total of 2.7 g EPA and 1.6 g DHA) (18).

In another recent study, the incorporation of EPA or arachidonate in cultured myocardial cells resulted in gross differences in the fluctuations of cytosolic free calcium concentrations and of the changes in amplitude and frequency of contraction following exposure to ouabain (19). These, and other examples indicate that the proportions of HUFA in cell lipids, which can be modified by diet, influence a number of incompletely explored functional parameters. An additional point concerning the influence of diet-induced modifications of cell fatty acids on cell function is that different cells may be differently affected. In the above study carried out by administering EPA and DHA ethyl esters to volunteers, we have observed, for instance, that after treatment the production of superoxide anion by stimulated monocytes, but not from polymorphonuclear leukocytes, was significantly reduced.

CONCLUSION

In conclusion, the relationships between dietary PUFA and the fatty acid profiles of different cells and tissues are complex and appear to be dependent upon various factors and processes. Among them, the following appear to be relevant: 1) in the diet, the absolute amounts, the relative proportions among different PUFA, and their relationships with the energy intake and with dietary antioxidants; 2) in the body, the combined effects of desaturation and elongation reactions (mainly occurring in the liver) with processes at the membrane level, predominant in extrahepatic tissue, responsible for phospholipid remodeling and based upon deacylation-reacylation reactions, and coupled with membrane lipid synthesis. The relationships between the supply of PUFA by the liver to extrahepatic tissues, through poorly studied mechanisms, and the processes at membrane level, dictate the fatty acid profile in lipids of different cell types.

Alterations in lipid and lipoprotein transport, such as the hyperlipemias, appear to affect the metabolism and turnover of n-6 and n-3 PUFA. This aspect deserves investigation since supplementation of the diet with high levels of these fatty acids is recommended as an important step for the prevention of atherosclerosis and cardiovascular diseases.

Finally, modified HUFA levels in cell membranes affect functional parameters through mechanisms which indicate that fatty acids in membranes modulate processes in the transduction of stimuli and in the early activation phase in response to various agents.

REFERENCES

1. Sprecher H, Voss AC, Careaga M, Hadjiagapiou. Interrelationships between polyunsaturated fatty acid and membrane lipid synthesis. In: Lands WEM, ed. *Polyunsaturated fatty acids and eicosanoids*. Champaign, IL: AOCS; 1987: 154–68.
2. Crawford M, Marsh D. *The driving force. Food, evolution and the future*. London: Heinemann; 1989.

3. Mead JF. The metabolism of the polyunsaturated fatty acids. *Prog Chem Fats Other Lipids* 1971; 9: 159–92.
4. Galli C, Agradi E, Paoletti R. The (n-6) pentaene: (n-3) hexaene-fatty acid ratio as an index of linolenic acid deficiency. *Biochim Biophys Acta* 1974; 369: 142–5.
5. Stubbs CD, Smith AD. The modification of mammalian membrane polyunsaturated fatty acid composition in relation to membrane fluidity and function. *Biochim Biophys Acta* 1984; 779: 89–137.
6. Galli C, Agradi E, Paoletti R. Accumulation of trienoic fatty acids in rat brain after depletion of liver (n-6) polyunsaturated fatty acids. *J Neurochem* 1975; 24: 1187–90.
7. Lefkowith JB, Flippo V, Sprecher H, Needleman P. Paradoxical conservation of cardiac and renal arachidonate content in essential fatty acid deficiency. *J Biol Chem* 1985; 260: 15736–44.
8. Habenicht AJR, Salbach P, Goerig M, et al. The LDL receptor pathway delivers arachidonic acid for eicosanoid formation in cells stimulated by platelet-derived growth factor. *Nature* 1990; 345: 634–6.
9. Scott BL, Bazan NG. Membrane docosahexaeonate is supplied to the developing brain and retina by the liver. *Proc Natl Acad Sci USA* 1989; 86: 2903–7.
10. Bazan NG, Cai F. Internalization of apolipoprotein E (APO E) in rod photoreceptor cells by a low-density lipoprotein receptor. *Invest Ophthalmol Vis Sci [Suppl]* 1990; 31: 471.
11. Galli C, Agradi E, Petroni A, Tremoli E. Differential effects of dietary fatty acids on the accumulation of arachidonic acid and its metabolic conversion through the cyclooxygenase and lipoxygenase in vascular tissues. *Lipids* 1981; 16: 165–72.
12. Tremoli E, Petroni A, Socini A, et al. Dietary interventions in North Karelia, Finland and South Italy: modification of thromboxane B_2 formation in platelets of male subjects only. *Atherosclerosis* 1986; 59: 101–11.
13. Owen JS, Hutton RA, Day RC, Bruckdorfer KR, McIntyre N. Platelet lipid composition and platelet aggregation in human liver disease. *J Lipid Res* 1981; 22: 423–30.
14. Mosconi C, Colli S, Tremoli E, Galli C. Phosphatidylinositol (PI) and PI-associated arachidonate are elevated in platelet total membranes of type II hypercholesterolemic subjects. *Atherosclerosis* 1988; 72: 129–34.
15. Meydani SN, Shapiro AC, Meydani M, Macauley JB, Blumberg JB. Effect of age and dietary fat (fish oil, corn oil, and coconut oil) on tocopherol status of c57/BL6 Nia mice. *Lipids* 1987; 22: 345–50.
16. Mosconi C, Colli S, Medini L, et al. Vitamin E influences the effects of fish oil on fatty acids and eicosanoid production in plasma and circulating cells in the rat. *Biochem Pharmacol* 1988; 37: 3415–21.
17. Medini L, Colli S, Mosconi C, Tremoli E, Galli C. Diets rich in n-9, n-6 and n-3 fatty acids differentially affect the generation of inositol phosphates and of thromboxane by stimulated platelets, in the rabbit. *Biochem Pharmacol* 1990; 39: 129–33.
18. Galli C, Colli S, Mosconi C, et al. Effects of EPA and DHA ethyl esters on plasma fatty acids, and on fatty acids, eicosanoid, inositol phosphate formation, and functional parameters in platelets, PMN and monocytes in healthy volunteers. Abstract 18, Post. Sect. I. *II International Conference on the Health Effects of Omega-3 Polyunsaturated Fatty Acids in Seafoods.* Washington, D.C. March 1990: 20–23.
19. Hallaq H, Leaf A. Effects of n-3 and n-6 polyunsaturated fatty acids on the action of cardiac glycosides on cultured rat myocardial cells. Abstract 14, Progr. Abst. *II International Conference on the Health Effects of Omega-3 Polyunsaturated Fatty Acids in Seafoods.* Washington, D.C. March 1990: 20–23.

DISCUSSION

Dr. Strandvik: When you presented the data about the different fatty acids in different organs in relation to the linoleic acid contained in the diet, did you look at lipids of different polarity, and have you looked at different phospholipid classes? There could be tremendous changes in these in the absence of major changes in the lipid contents of different fatty acids.

Dr. Galli: An important point. We have found very different relationships between the accumulation of linoleic acid and arachidonic acid in plasma and liver following increased dietary intake of linoleic acid. In plasma, linoleic acid accumulates mainly in triglycerides and arachidonic acid mainly in cholesterol esters, whereas in liver, arachidonic acid mainly enters in phospholipids. The accumulation of arachidonic acid in the cholesterol ester pool may be mediated by the plasma LCAT activity, which transfers arachidonic acid from phospholipids to cholesterol esters. There are also differences when the incorporation of exogenous fatty acids in lipid pools is studied in cell culture.

Dr. Jeremy: You showed that there was a change in lipid profiles in the heart and you mentioned that this may relate to functional changes. What functional changes?

Dr. Galli: I am referring to data showing that n-3 fatty acids in heart muscle have antiarrhythmic properties. It appears that the higher the 22:6 content in the heart the less sensitive is the organ to arrhythmogenic agents (1,2). When 22:6 is decreased in the heart, as occurs during high dietary linoleic acid intake, the heart muscle may become more sensitive to arrhythmogenic conditions. The effects of n-3 fatty acids appear to be mediated by changes in Ca^{2+} mobilization within the cell.

Dr. Jeremy: PUFA have also been shown to inhibit calcium-linked potassium channels.

Dr. Crawford: We have been studying the effects of GLA-rich oils on heart and liver tissue over time. In the first 1–8 days the concentrations of arachidonic acid increase in the choline phosphoglycerides and later in the ethanolamine phosphoglycerides, though not as much as in the choline. What is interesting is that in the first 8 days you don't see any change in heart tissue phosphoglycerides, although the liver has already responded during this time. So there is a distinct delay in the way in which the heart takes up these fatty acids, which is quite consistent with your data.

Dr. Strandvik: In rats with essential fatty acid deficiency we have found tremendous differences in uptake of labeled arachidonic acid and linoleic acid in the heart compared with control rats. The uptake was very different in the different fractions, the most significant increase being in phosphatidylethanolamine. There are profound changes in cardiolipin in the heart. We followed the incorporation for 4 hours after giving labeled essential fatty acids orally or in chylomicrons. The increase occurs within 4 hours and the proportion of linoleic is 22% compared with 2% in controls.

Dr. Crawford: You are looking at a situation where there is severe arachidonic acid deficit in the cell membranes. We are looking at something quite different—that is, the effect of increasing the levels of arachidonic acid in different membrane fractions in animals receiving a normal diet. This is a different situation from essential fatty acid deficiency.

REFERENCES

1. Gudbjarnason S. Dynamics of n-3 and n-6 fatty acids in phospholipids of heart muscle. *J Int Med* 1989; 225[Suppl 1]: 117–28.
2. McLennan PL, Abeywardena MY, Charnock JS. Reversal of the arrhythmogenic effects of long-term saturated fatty acid intake by dietary n-3 and n-6 polyunsaturated fatty acids. *Am J Clin Nutr* 1990; 51: 53–8.

Polyunsaturated Fatty Acids in Human Nutrition,
edited by U. Bracco and R. J. Deckelbaum,
Nestlé Nutrition Workshop Series, Vol. 28,
Nestec Ltd., Vevey/Raven Press, Ltd., New York © 1992.

Essential Fatty Acids in Early Development

Michael A. Crawford, *K. Costeloe, W. Doyle, A. Leaf,
M. J. Leighfield, *N. Meadows, and A. Phylactos

*Institute of Brain Chemistry and Human Nutrition, Hackney Hospital,
London E9 6BE, England; and *The Department of Paediatrics, Medical College,
St. Bartholomew's Hospital, London EC1A 7BE, England*

From Swedish and British data, the incidence of cerebral palsy in low birthweight and premature infants has risen nearly threefold since the mid 1960s. It is important to know if the prenatal provision of nutrients, including arachidonic (AA) and docosahexaenoic acids (DHA), during fetal development and in the postnatal period is related to low birthweight and offers a route for the prevention of neurodevelopmental damage.

The study of maternal diets during pregnancy revealed significant nutrient deficits in mothers whose babies were born of low birthweight (<2,500 g) compared to mothers whose babies were in the range of 3,500–4,500 g where morbidity and mortality is at its lowest (48). From the study of the umbilical artery used as a sample of fetal tissue, it appears that individual low birthweight and premature babies may have had different intrauterine nutritional histories (50). This finding is particularly relevant to the interpretation of postnatal nutrition and prognosis.

Arachidonic acid concentrations in cord blood and umbilical artery blood were strikingly correlated with birthweight and head circumference, while negative correlations were found between these growth variables and the triene/tetraene ratio and the pentaene/tetraene ratio in umbilical artery endothelium. The possibility of using the umbilical artery as a diagnostic tool is discussed.

THE STRUCTURAL FUNCTION OF LIPIDS

Comparative Evidence

There are wide species differences in the metabolic efficiency in the conversion of parent essential fatty acids linoleic (LA) and α linolenic (α LNA) acids to the long chain more unsaturated derivatives. This, together with differences in food selection patterns, leads to differences in membrane composition. However, the composition of the brain does not vary in this way. In the 42 species we have so far studied the ethanolamine phosphoglycerides are consistently dominated by arachidonic and docosatetraenoic acids in the n-6 family and docosahexaenoic acid in the n-3 family with a balance of n-6 to n-3 between 1 and 2 to 1 (1).

Again, the composition of the liver, adrenal, heart muscle, or kidney phosphoglycerides are different in the same species. Even subcellular particles have characteristic compositions (e.g., endoplasmic reticulum, mitochondria, and synaptic junctions). Hence, there is both species and tissue specificity. The unique feature of the differences in the brain between species is that it is not the composition that varies but the extent to which it is developed, which implies that the composition is conserved and is a determinant of brain development (2), a concept which now finds much support from the experimental data and that may well have evolutionary implications (3). As it is the brain which is developed to the most outstanding degree in the human species, the implications of this concept could be particularly relevant to considerations of human brain development.

Compositional Conservation

There are at least two reasons that can be suggested for the "conservation" of fatty acid profiles. 1) Protein synthesis is specifically dictated by the genetic code. Hence the lipid/protein interface will seek a preferred lipid configuration. 2) Lipids are stored, unlike the water-soluble nutrients. Experience gained from deficiency experiments with vitamin B-1 or C led to an expectation of the response to deficiency which is inappropriate to lipid deficiency. The use of stores during dietary deficiency explains conservation on the one hand and the need for a different perspective of lipid or essential fatty acid (EFA) deficiency on the other.

An additional distinction needs to be made between lipid deficiency and the more widely understood deficiencies of proteins, water-soluble vitamins, and minerals. Desaturation and chain elongation are involved in the transformation of linoleic and αLNA to their long chain derivatives arachidonic acid and DHA (4,5). Mead and Slaton (6) showed that in EFA deficiency, oleic acid was desaturated and chain-elongated to an eicosatrienoic acid. In the absence of EFA, this "Mead acid" (20:3, n-9) provides some degree of polyunsaturation for cell membranes and a buffer against fat deficiency. There is no such parallel in the water-soluble nutrients.

The concept of conservation has important implications in that deficits which are nutritionally significant but not severe enough to disrupt cellular architecture might be expected to modify cell regulatory activity before conformational change becomes apparent. This was tested by Hassam et al. (7) who found that deficiency in rabbits led initially to striking reduction in eicosanoid synthesis before there were significant changes in membrane lipid composition.

METABOLIC STUDIES

Differences Between 18-Carbon and Long Chain Unsaturated Fatty Acids

The key issue regarding brain development is that the brain does not use the parent 18-carbon chain length fatty acids and only uses 20:4, n-6, 22:4, n-6, and 22:6, n-3. Consequently the mechanism and efficiency of conversion becomes a crucial issue.

Enzyme studies showed that the rate of conversion of linoleic to arachidonic acid was limited *in vitro* by the first desaturation (6-desaturase) (4,8). However, the *in vivo* studies (9) gave a different view. The desaturation *in vitro* operated four times slower than the chain elongation (5). On the other hand, the conversion to arachidonic acid *in vivo* operated to produce an order of magnitude in the difference between simultaneous incorporation of arachidonic acid compared to arachidonic acid synthesized from linoleic acid in the liver and a 30-fold difference for the developing brain (9,10).

Desaturation and Compartmentalization

The distribution of radioactively labeled linoleic acid or arachidonic acid in the metabolic pools happens quickly. 1) Some 50–60% of linoleic acid can be recovered from the triglyceride pool and 40–50% from the phosphoglyceride pool. By contrast some 90% of arachidonic acid is recovered from the membrane phosphoglycerides. 2) The triglyceride and free fatty acid pools supply substrate for oxidation. In rat studies, some 50–60% of radioactive ^{14}C from αlinolenic acid and linoleic acid was found in expired air as CO_2, but only 12–15% of arachidonic acid and DHA after a 24 h period (10,11). 3) The fraction incorporated into phosphoglycerides will become a part of cell membrane structures. Less will thus be available for oxidation or desaturation and so it will be conserved. 4) This leaves the free fatty acid fraction from the triglyceride pool as that which is available for conversion to arachidonic acid. However, the proportion of ^{14}C in this pool drops to less than 1% in a matter of 10–20 minutes so there is relatively little available for desaturation. It is this process of compartmentalization which seems to cause the striking difference between the *in vitro* and *in vivo* rates of linoleic conversion to arachidonic acid. Compartmentalization involves several selective but rapid steps, including preferential activation and esterification. The rate of conversion is limited by the desaturations.

The species differences play a part in the conversion of linoleic acid to arachidonic acid. The cat family apparently expresses little or no 6-desaturation activity (12). There are also differences in the proportion compartmentalized into the free fatty acid fraction (13). Hence, *in vivo*, it would seem that the influence of the desaturation has been overemphasized. The key issue is compartmentalization.

Compartmentalization and Placental Delivery

The important period for brain development is during early cell division when the fetus is nourished by the placenta. It is known from studies at term (14) and at midterm (15), that the human placenta concentrates arachidonic acid and DHA and lowers the amount of linoleic acid in the blood supply to the fetus. It does not, however, appear to do this by improved desaturation but rather by recompartmentalization of the fatty acids, which means a preferential selection of the long chain polyunsaturated fatty acids for transfer to the fetus (16, and unpublished data of D. Fornel).

INTEGRITY OF THE BRAIN: ANIMAL STUDIES

Summary of General Evidence

The integrity and function of the brain depends on a specific profile of membrane lipids and their fatty acids (1). Depletion of the EFA used in brain or neural lipids results in loss of integrity (17), cell DNA (2), and cell function (18–22) in rats, dogs, chickens, and primates, and suggestions of similar effects in a human infant (23). The functional effects documented include neurodevelopmental deficits in visual and cognitive development as well as an effect on life span (24).

Nutritional Encephalomalacia and Peroxidation

Crazy chick disease or nutritional encephalomalacia (NE) was originally thought to be caused by vitamin E deficiency. However, in the experimental model vegetable oils containing a high proportion ($>50\%$) of linoleic acid but very little linolenic acid ($< 0.5\%$) were used. Budowski et al. (17,25) found that linolenic acid dramatically protected against encephalomalacia. In the chicken, the cerebrum is formed before hatching whereas the cerebellum undergoes a growth spurt between 12 and 28 days after hatching, which is the time it acquires its polyunsaturated fatty acids and is the same time at which NE occurs (25). This disease is therefore an example of Dobbing's notion that the brain is most vulnerable to distortion during the growth phase (27), but is applied to a specific part of the brain and to a specific n-3 deficiency.

Encephalomyelitis

A form of inflammatory brain damage, experimental allergic encephalomyelitis (EAE), occurs in guinea pigs in response to the injection of brain tissue. It was not possible to induce the same disease in rats until Clausen & Moller (16) hit on the idea that depletion of EFA in the diet might weaken the brain cell membranes and render them susceptible. This proved to be the case and has been repeated by Selivonchick and Johnston in 1975 (28). The original experiment of Clausen and Moller was perhaps the first example of the requirement for EFAs for maintenance of neural integrity, showing that depletion of EFA can make the brain vulnerable to neurally offensive agents and a T-cell-mediated reaction (29).

HUMAN DEVELOPMENT-FETAL GROWTH

Preparation in Advance of Reproduction

The evidence for an essential fatty requirement during pregnancy has been reviewed previously (30–32). It is a general principle in animal reproduction that preparation takes place in advance of the event and the same appears to apply to the human (33). A test of this concept has been done with rats where it was found that a certain proportion of the body as fat needs to be present before conception will occur (34). There is experimental support that nutritional deficiencies are most likely to affect fetal growth and development very early in pregnancy in many if not all mammals (35–37).

Retrospective studies on food shortages resulting from World War II show that mothers entering the shortage pregnant experienced substantially less neurological damage to their babies than those who became pregnant during the shortage. In the latter, there was an increase in low birthweight babies, perinatal mortality, and neonatal mortality, as well as an increase in congenital abnormalities of several kinds, especially neurodevelopmental defects (38). Such data suggest that fetal growth retardation is a function of maternal nutrition at or prior to conception.

Neurodevelopmental Distortions

The major focus during human embryonic and fetal growth is on brain development; 70% of its cells divide during fetal growth. Retardation of fetal growth is associated with deficits and distortions of brain cell growth and functional development; in general, these deficits cannot be made good later (27). Low head circumference at birth has been found to be associated with poor cognitive development (39). With falling birthweight, the risk of serious neurological and other developmental handicaps increases dramatically. In a study of 811,613 births in the former East Germany, the incidence was 1.6/1,000 births in the 3,500–4,500 g range rising to more than 200/1,000 of those born below 1,000 g (38).

A baby born to a mother whose previous child was born at low birthweight has three times the risk of still birth, neonatal death, and neurological abnormality (40). In spite of improvements in perinatal care, the prevelance of neurodevelopmental handicap and cerebral palsy has remained static or increased in low birthweight infants (41–44). On current data from eight studies published in the 1980s, some 20–30% of surviving extremely low birthweight infants (<1,000 g) have a major neurodevelopmental handicap (40). The impact of the grey area of functional and cognitive disability is in a larger dimension. In England and Wales some 47,500 low birthweight babies were born in 1988 (41) and 10% of these are expected to have a severe neurodevelopmental handicap (42). A high proportion of the remainder will have some form of deficit or disturbance.

Multiple Handicaps

The principle that deficits and distortions in early development have lasting effects on organ efficiency and function is not restricted to the brain but may include congenital heart defects and impairment of the immune system (45), with more than one deficit frequently occurring in the same individual (40).

Social Class, Nutrition, and Low Birthweight

The risks both of perinatal or neonatal mortality and of low birthweight and handicap are increased severalfold in the lower socioeconomic groups (46), a contrast which cannot be explained by a genetic difference. Our prospective studies show that there are significant differences across the social classes in nutrient intakes of pregnant mothers in relation to vitamins, energy, and EFA (47).

Evidence Relative to Preconceptional Nutrition

Our more recent studies showed that poor nutrition around the time of conception was associated with low birthweight and head circumference (48) (Tables 1–3). There was a wide range of nutrient intake deficits in the habitual diet of the mother in which dietary energy, B vitamins, magnesium (48,49), and the EFAs (50) all correlated strongly with low birthweight and head circumference. Analysis of the data on the basis of the prevention of low birthweight was done (51) and showed that significantly fewer low birthweight babies were born in the test group who had received prenatal nutrition counseling compared to the controls.

The statistics on nutrients and birthweight in our studies correlated better with maternal diet close to the time of conception than in the latter part of pregnancy,

TABLE 1. *General data: nutrient intakes and birthweight**

	Birthweight range			
Birthweight range	<2,500 g, n = 28	<3,000 g, n = 161	3,000–3,449 g, n = 168	3,500–4,500 g, n = 165
Height (cm)	158 (3.0)	161 (0.7)	163 (0.5)	163 (0.5)
Prepregnancy Wt (kg)	57.2 (2.4)	56.8 (0.85)	57.9 (0.71)	62.5 (0.88)
Nonsmokers (%)	79	70	72	76

	Birthweight range		
	Low birthweight mothers: <2,500 g, n = 28	Reference mothers: 3,500–4,500 g, n = 165	p = 2-tailed
Nutrients			
Kcalories	1,642 (89)	1,974 (34)	0.001
Protein (g)	62.8 (4.0)	74.4 (1.3)	0.006
Fat (g)	72.4 (4.4)	88.9 (1.7)	0.002
Carbohydrate (g)	195 (11)	231 (4.6)	0.004

* Mean (SEM) heights, prepregnancy weights, and nutrient intakes of mothers with infants of birthweights at or below 2,500 g, and 3,500 to 4,500 g (reference mothers). The "reference mothers" were those in the study who produced babies in the range where mortality and morbidity is reported to be at its lowest.

TABLE 2. *Mean (SEM) and median daily intakes of fatty acids of mothers of low birthweight babies (<2,500 g) and mothers with optimum birthweight babies (3,500–4,500 g)**

	<2,500 g, n = 28			3,500–4,500 g, n = 165			
	Mean	SEM	Median	Mean	SEM	Median	p = 2-tailed
n-6 family							
18:2,n-6 (g)	8.45	(851)	8.15	11.6	(408)	11.0	0.005
20:3,n-6 (mg)	24	(4)	20	36	(2)	30	0.003
20:4,n-6 (mg)	140	(17)	140	178	(7)	170	0.030
22:4,n-6 (mg)	11	(2)	10	12	(1)	10	0.323
22:5,n-6 (mg)	11	(5)	10	7	(1)	10	0.855
n-3 family							
18:3,n-3 (mg)	754	(82)	720	1,029	(33)	930	0.001
20:5,n-3 (mg)	79	(15)	50	124	(11)	70	0.046
22:5,n-3 (mg)	93	(36)	60	70	(3)	70	0.287
22:6,n-3 (mg)	140	(22)	115	160	(10)	130	0.453
Positional and trans isomers							
18:1t (mg)	1,620	(122)	1,600	1,911	(63)	1,780	0.128
18:2tt (mg)	68	(6)	65	76	(3)	70	0.524
18:2tc+ct (mg)	147	(12)	145	171	(5)	170	0.093
Totals							
PUFA (mg)	9,960	(850)	9,570	13,300	(430)	12,750	0.004
n-6 fats (mg)	8,880	(810)	8,360	11,900	(410)	11,280	0.006
n-3 fats (mg)	1,090	(100)	930	1,400	(40)	1,280	0.003
Trans (mg)	2,835	(213)	2,630	3,384	(115)	3,090	0.101
P/S ratio	0.33	(0.03)	0.32	0.39	(0.01)	0.36	0.119
% energy from EFA, %	5.28	(0.35)	4.97	6.04	(0.16)	5.80	0.073

* Minor components are included in totals but not listed individually. Significance test = Mann-Whitney U test. The fatty acid data are calculated from a computerized database on fat and fatty acid composition of foods, constructed in our laboratory from direct analysis by capillary gas-liquid chromatography of the foods eaten in London.
t, trans; tt, trans trans; ct, cis trans.

implying that maternal nutrition at or before the time of conception is important. This conclusion is consistent with the fact that cell number will be determined very early during embryonic development and in the first phases of fetal growth. While dietary intervention during pregnancy may yield modest gains, it is likely that preconceptional intervention would be more rewarding; this has the logical advantage of preparing for the period of brain cell division and organogenesis.

A DIAGNOSTIC TECHNIQUE FOR FETAL GROWTH RETARDATION

Placental Growth

To assess the tissue EFA status of low birthweight babies, several studies were done on placental tissue, maternal blood, and cord blood which suggested that arachidonic acid levels were less in the maternal and cord blood from babies of low birthweight, low placental weight, and small head circumference (50). To further test

TABLE 3. *Pearson's correlation coefficients between birthweights and nutrient intakes of mothers with babies above and below the median birthweight (3,270 g); 513 London mothers**

	Correlation coefficients for			
	255 mothers with babies <3,270 g		258 mothers with babies >3,270 g	
	r	p	r	p
Minerals				
Magnesium	0.253	<0.001	0.057	NS
Iron	0.247	<0.001	0.079	NS
Phosphorus	0.243	<0.001	0.005	NS
Zinc	0.238	<0.001	0.007	NS
Sodium	0.237	<0.001	0.052	NS
Potassium	0.208	<0.001	0.068	NS
Calcium	0.184	0.002	0.024	NS
Vitamins				
Thiamin (B-1)	0.200	<0.001	0.025	NS
Niacin	0.198	<0.001	0.011	NS
Pantothenic acid	0.186	0.002	0.050	NS
Riboflavin (B-2)	0.183	0.002	0.036	NS
Folic acid	0.173	0.003	0.081	NS
Pyridoxine (B-6)	0.168	0.004	0.048	NS
Protein	0.238	<0.001	0.024	NS
Energy	0.225	<0.001	0.015	NS
Fiber	0.212	<0.001	0.028	NS

* Nutrient intakes above 3,270 g were unrelated to birthweight. Many previous studies on nutrition and pregnancy outcome have used "mean birthweight" to test for specific effects. If, however, there is no nutrient relationship in the large part of the population then the effect of nutrition will be substantially diluted. In terms of preventing neurodevelopmental handicap, what matters is a reduction in the incidence of low birthweight and prematurity, not an increase in the mean birthweight of a population.

the evidence on maternal nutritional status in relation to birthweight, we then examined the endothelium from umbilical arteries, as a representative piece of fetal tissue, from babies of different birthweights. It was surprising to find significant amounts of Mead acid in the arteries of normal birthweight babies. However, more impressive was the extent to which the Mead acid and its elongation product (23:3, n-9) were increased in low birthweight babies. Associated with the raised long chain n-9 fatty acids was a reduced proportion of arachidonic acid.

As mentioned previously, the Mead acid (20:3, n-9) is synthesized from oleic (18:1, n-9) acid during EFA deficiency to compensate for the loss of polyunsaturation, and particularly of arachidonic acid, in cell membrane (52). Additionally, in a deficiency of DHA or n-3 fatty acids, the n-6 docosatetraenoate (22:4, n-6) is desaturated to its corresponding docosapentaenoate (22:5, n-6) which in the absence of n-3 fatty acids is thought to substitute for docosahexaenoic acid (22:6, n-3). Hence the ratio of the Mead acid to arachidonic acid is used as a marker of EFA deficiency (20:3,

TABLE 4. *Ranges of individual fatty acid, composition of umbilical artery choline phosphoglycerides (CPG), and ethanolamine phosphoglycerides (EPG), birthweights, and head circumferences**

Ranges of values for

Birthweights (g)   Head circumferences (cm)
Lowest 820   25.5
Highest 4,310   36.5

	Fatty acid									
	n-6					n-3				n-9	
	18:2	20:3	20:4	22:4	22:5	18:3	20:5	22:5	22:6	20:3	22:3
% of total EPG											
Lowest	0.45	0.37	10.8	2.29	2.91	tr	tr	tr	7.36	1.85	1.0
Highest	3.1	3.60	26.1	7.24	7.62	0.25	1.1	0.97	18.0	6.40	3.6
CPG											
Lowest	tr	1.26	5.63	1.17	1.66	tr	tr	tr	0.10	1.74	0.6
Highest	3.1	2.90	10.1	3.03	3.80	0.36	0.23	tr	5.20	4.46	2.1

* The fatty acids are expressed as a percentage of the total in the ethanolamine phosphoglycerides (EPG) and in the choline phosphoglycerides (CPG) from umbilical arteries. They represent the highest and lowest values for each fatty acid separately found in the data.
tr, trace.

n-9/20:4, n-6 or the triene/tetraene [T/T] ratio) and the ratio of docosapenta- to -tetraenoate (22:5, n-6/22:4, n-6 or P/T ratio) is used as a test for a DHA or n-3 deficit.

Both the P/T and the T/T ratios were raised in the tissues from low birthweight and low head circumference babies compared to babies in the normal birthweight range. Furthermore, there were strong correlations between these two markers and both birthweight and head circumference (Tables 4–6). If the fetus was failing to grow for genetic reasons, its demand for nutrients would be minimal. On the other hand, the presence of substantial amounts of Mead acid is consistent with an attempt to make good an inadequate supply. These data suggest that it is the failure of placental delivery which is responsible rather than a failure of the fetus to grow. Babies with fetal growth retardation are most frequently born with small placentas containing multiple infarctions (53). On the basis of this pathology, it can be argued that poor placental development is responsible for fetal growth retardation. A large part of placental growth occurs before the fetal growth spurt and since the placenta is mainly a rapidly developing vascular system it would not be surprising if the principles which relate to vascular disease also operate on the placenta, thereby explaining the concordance of the high incidence of vascular disease in men and low birthweight in women from the same socioeconomic group (54). Reduced prostacyclin synthesis has been reported in the umbilical arteries from low birthweight babies (55). It may be that inadequate supply of nutrients causes poor placental growth and function, and that EFA inadequacy specifically compromises the development of the placental endothelial tissue.

TABLE 5. *Regression of birthweight and head circumference with individual fatty acids**

	Pearson's coefficient	t	n	p
Ethanolamine phosphoglycerides				
Birth wt. vs. 20:4n-6	+0.53	2.98	14	<0.02
Head circ. vs. 20:4n-6	+0.44	2.34	12	<0.05
Birth wt. vs. 22n:6n-3	+0.54	2.19	14	<0.05
Head circ. vs. 22:6n-3	+0.49	1.78	12	—
Birth wt. vs. 16:0	−0.52	1.93	13	—
Head circ. vs. 16:0	−0.45	1.49	11	—
Birth wt. vs. 18:0	−0.52	2.11	14	—
Head circ. vs. 18:0	−0.48	1.68	12	—
Mead acid				
Birth wt. vs. 20:3n-9	−0.61	3.43	14	<0.01
Head circ. vs. 20:3n-9	−0.75	4.00	12	<0.01
Choline phosphoglycerides				
Birth wt. vs. 20:4n-6	+0.35	1.28	14	—
Head circ. vs. 20:4n-6	+0.37	2.08	12	—
Mead acid				
Birth wt. vs. 20:3n-9	−0.50	2.84	14	<0.02
Head circ. vs. 20:3n-9	−0.42	2.27	12	<0.05

* The data are presented only on fatty acids that correlated significantly with one of the birth dimensions. The strongest correlations were obtained in the ethanolamine phosphoglycerides.

TABLE 6. *Regression of birthweight and head circumference with indices of EFA status in cord arteries**

	Pearson's coefficient	t	n	p
Ethanolamine phosphoglycerides				
Triene/tetraene ratio (EFA deficiency)				
Birth wt. vs. 20:3n-9/20:4n-6	−0.87	6.46	14	<0.001
Head circ. vs. 20:3n-9/20:4n-6	−0.83	5.14	12	<0.001
Pentaene/tetraene ratio (n-3 deficiency)				
Birth wt. vs. 22:5n-6/22:4n-6	−0.79	5.07	14	<0.001
Head circ. vs. 22:5n-6/22:4n-6	−0.89	5.09	12	<0.001
Choline phosphoglycerides				
Triene/tetraene ratio (EFA deficiency)				
Birth wt. vs. 20:3n-9/20:4n-6	−0.68	3.86	14	<0.01
Head circ. vs. 20:3n-9/20:4n-6	−0.63	3.20	12	<0.01
Pentaene/tetraene ratio (n-3 deficiency)				
Birth wt. vs. 22:5n-6/22:4n-6	−0.66	3.74	14	<0.01
Head circ. vs. 22:5n-/22:4n-6	−0.46	2.42	12	<0.05

* The indices of EFA deficiency were negatively correlated with birthweights and head circumference. The relationship with the long chain EFA were positive and saturated fatty acids were negative. Levels of significance reported are for the two-tailed *t* test. Again the strongest correlations were found for the EPG fraction.

POSTNATAL DEVELOPMENT

The dietary distinction between the 18-carbon and longer chain length EFA is noticed in babies fed milk with and without the long chain EFA. We reported that infants fed cow's milk formulas with only linoleic acid and no long chain derivatives show a fall in the concentration of the long chain derivatives in the plasma, especially the triglycerides, in comparison with infants fed breast milk, which contains about 1% of the dietary energy as the long chain derivatives (56). Friedman et al. (57) found that infants fed intravenously with Intralipid, which contains little or no long chain derivatives, showed a reduction in the long chain derivatives and in prostaglandin synthesis both in the circulation and in liver in those who came to postmortem. Putnam et al. (58) compared infants fed two different infant formulas and breast milk. They showed that the levels of the long chain derivatives were not being maintained in the infants fed on the artifical formulas.

At birth, the blood levels of arachidonic acid and DHA are remarkably high as a result of the biomagnification process achieved by the normal placenta (15). In normal babies, there is a decline of red cell DHA and plasma arachidonic acid and DHA postnatally which is faster in the formula-fed baby compared to the breast-fed baby. A similar situation in premature babies has been described by Carlson et al. (59), Shires et al. (60), and Uauy et al. (61).

In premature infants fed conventional formula, the plasma choline phosphoglyceride arachidonate falls and the linoleate rises. In Figs. 1–3 we present data on plasma choline phosphoglyceride obtained from 10 premature babies illustrating the level at birth compared to the level at the expected date of delivery. The data illustrate the wide degree of variability from baby to baby in the extent of the fall in DHA and arachidonic acid and the rise in linoleic acid. Figure 4 shows how rapid is the replacement of arachidonic acid by linoleic acid.

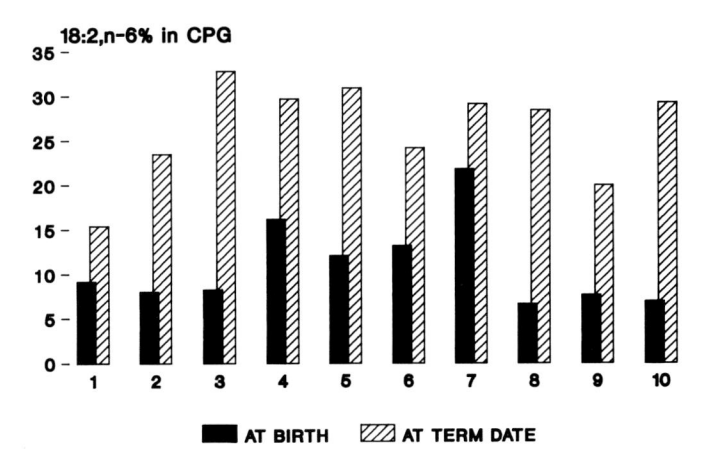

FIG. 1. The proportion of linoleic acid in the plasma choline phosphoglycerides (CPG) is low at birth but rises toward the expected day of delivery.

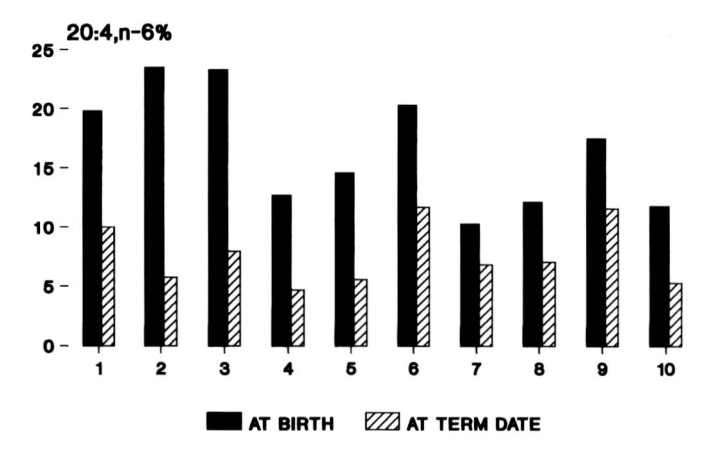

FIG. 2. The arachidonic acid porportions change in the opposite direction to linoleic acid as seen in Fig. 1.

In a previous study we tested the association between depressed EFA intakes and low birthweight by studying the circulating arachidonic acid in levels at term. We found these to be depressed both in cord and maternal plasma and in red cells in low birthweight babies (50). Among these infants, our data indicated that arachidonic acid levels correlated with birthweight although the T/T and P/T ratios had a greater significance when measured in the umbilical artery (Table 6). Maternal and cord plasma arachidonic acid (50) and endothelial arachidonic acid, together with the T/T ratio, were stronger predictors of birthweight than DHA, which might well be related to degree of prematurity (62,63).

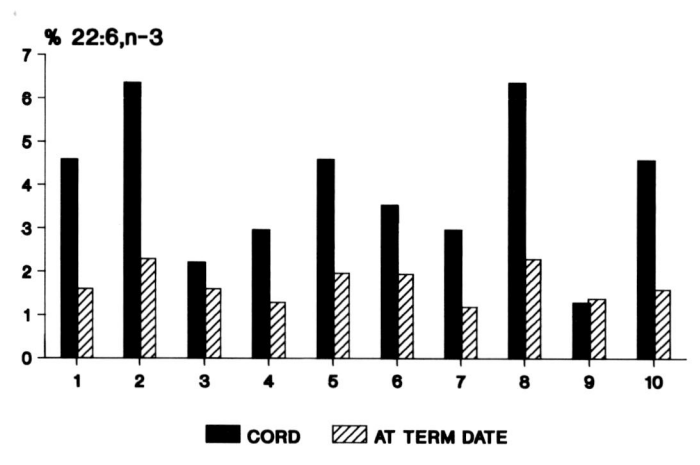

FIG. 3. The change in docosahexaenoic acid is similar to the arachidonic acid situation (Fig. 2). In these ten babies, which were from 8 to 13 weeks premature, there were wide variations in the levels at birth and in the proportionate change in levels of the fatty acids.

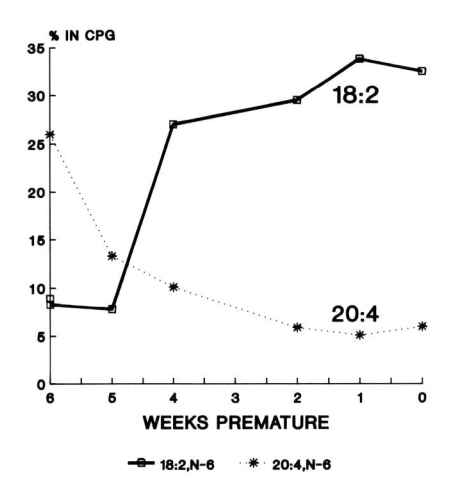

FIG. 4. The diagram illustrates the scale speed of the loss of arachidonic acid due to premature birth using data from a baby born 6 weeks prematurely. Had the baby remained as a fetus it would have continued with a high circulating level of CPG arachidonic acid. Although the infant was fed ample linoleic acid, the linoleic acid effectively and quickly replaced the arachidonic acid.

The data make two points: 1) The premature infant is denied a focused intake of neural fatty acids for a period during which it otherwise would have received such an intake had it remained as a fetus; 2) The provision postnatally during this period of even substantial amounts of linoleic acid does not guarantee its conversion to arachidonic acid and is not the same as providing arachidonic acid preformed.

NEURAL DAMAGE IN THE PREMATURE INFANT

The incidence of neurodevelopmental handicap begins to increase below 3,000 g birthweight but increases especially below 1,500 g birthweight. Three points suggest a link between nutrition and risk of neural damage. 1) The fat store in the premature infant is small. A baby born of normal birthweight will have a fat store of some 300 g which will contain the neural fatty acids and other nutrients provided by the placenta, which will contribute to and help to protect postnatal development. 2) Premature and low birthweight babies are born with widely different circulating levels of the neural fatty acids and also undergo a different postnatal experience. 3) Many of low birthweight and premature babies will have been exposed during fetal growth to deficits of neural fatty acids. Regardless of whether an EFA deprivation is caused by maternal or placental conditions or both, the signal of an EFA deficit also implies a historical shortage of other nutrients.

Because this evidence specifically relates to the neural fatty acids we suggest the hypothesis that it offers a mechanism for the neural disturbances which are so frequent in these low birthweight and premature infants, though in view of the intimate relationship between macronutrients and micronutrients, we would argue that several micronutrients would participate.

There is already some evidence that the method of feeding these premature babies postnatally may have an influence on their motor development (64). However, it is common pediatric experience that even those premature and low birthweight babies who escape severe handicap may have delayed development or minor disturbances such as concentration or behavioral difficulties. There may be areas where this new knowledge on neural composition could contribute to significant improvements by early nutrition intervention following identification of those likely to be at risk.

CONCLUSION

In the period up to the 1960s, many premature infants died and concepts of feeding them were primitive and associated with much morbidity (65). As an understanding of the need for the premature infant to gain weight developed, methods of feeding were improved and management technology advanced, so mortality and handicap declined. Since then, advanced technology has improved survival rate but at the same time the incidence of cerebral palsy in low birthweight babies has risen nearly threefold (43,44). It is difficult to argue that the technology is the cause of the increase in cerebral palsy, but from the data it is plausible that mothers who are ill prepared physiologically and nutritionally for pregnancy produce babies who themselves are ill prepared. As the focus in human fetal and neonatal development is the brain, it would not be surprising if the brain was effected by this ill-preparedness. This suggestion has four important implications:

1. The health care workers who are responsible for feeding the premature infant need to recognize that it is not simply a question of trying to improve weight gain when brain development is at stake.

2. Premature infants are born with widely different nutritional histories and nutrient stores. Therefore, in addition to the principle of providing nourishment designed for the premature infant, the individual needs should be identified to make good any nutritional backlog.

3. Where neural damage is suspected to be associated with nutrition, early dietary intervention, along with other forms of therapy, may allow the plasticity of the developing brain to be exploited, thus minimizing the final damage.

4. The strategy for the prevention of prematurity, low birthweight, and neurodevelopmental disturbances needs to start with the period before conception.

REFERENCES

1. Crawford MA, Casperd NM, Sinclair AJ. The long chain metabolites of linoleic and linolenic acids in liver and brain in herbivores and carnivores. *Comp Biochem Physiol* 1976; 54B: 395–401.
2. Crawford MA, Sinclair AJ. Nutritional influences on the evolution of the mammalian brain. In: Elliott K, Knights J, eds. *Lipids, malnutrition and the developing brain* (Ciba Foundation Symposium). Amsterdam: Elsevier; 1972: 267–87.
3. Crawford MA, Marsh DE. *The driving force: food, evolution and the future*. London: Heinemann; 1990.
4. Brenert JT, Sprecher H. Studies to determine the role, rates of chain elongation and desaturation play in regulating the unsaturated fatty acid composition of rat liver lipids. *Biochem Biophys Acta* 1975; 398: 354–63.
5. Sprecher H. Biochemistry of essential fatty acids. *Prog Lipid Res* 1981; 20: 13–22.
6. Mead JF, Slaton WH. Metabolism of essential fatty acids: III. Isolation of 5,8,11-eicosatrienoic acid from fat-deficient rats. *J Biol Chem* 1956; 219: 705–9.

7. Hassam AG, Willis AL, Denton JP, Stevens P, Crawford MA. The effect of essential fatty acid deficient diet on the levels of prostaglandins and their fatty acid precursors in the rabbit brain. *Lipids* 1979; 14: 78–80.
8. Brenner RR, Peluffo RO. Effect of saturated and unsaturated fatty acids on the desaturation in vitro of palmitic, stearic, oleic, linoleic and linolenic acids. *J Biol Chem* 1966; 241: 5213–9.
9. Hassam AG, Crawford MA. The differential incorporation of labelled linoleic, gamma-linolenic, dihomogamma-linolenic and arachidonic acids into the developing rat brain. *J Neurochem* 1976; 27: 967–8.
10. Sinclair AJ. The incorporation of radioactive polyunsaturated fatty acids into the liver and brain of the developing rat. *Lipids* 1975; 10: 175–84.
11. Leyton J, Drury PJ, Crawford MA. Differential oxidation of saturated and unsaturated fatty acids in vivo in the rat. *Br J Nutr* 1987; 57: 383–93.
12. Rivers JPW, Sinclair AJ, Crawford MA. Inability of the cat to desaturate essential fatty acids. *Nature* 1975; 285: 171–3.
13. Cunnane SC, Napoleon Keeling PW, Thompson RPH, Crawford MA. Linoleic acid and arachidonic acid metabolism in human peripheral blood leucocytes: comparison with the rat. *Br J Nutr* 1984; 51: 209–17.
14. Olegard R, Svennerholm L. Fatty acid composition of plasma and red cell phosphoglycerides in full term infants and their mothers. *Acta Paediatr Scand* 1970; 59: 637–47.
15. Crawford MA, Hassam AG, Williams G, Whitehouse WL. Essential fatty acids and fetal brain growth. *Lancet* 1976; i: 452–3.
16. Clausen J, Moller J. *Acta Neurol Scand* 1967; 43: 375–88.
17. Budowski P, Hawkey CM, Crawford MA. L'effet protecteur de l'acide alpha-linolenique sur l'enceohalomalaciie chez le poulet. *Ann Nutr Anim* 1980; 34: 389–400.
18. Lamptey MS, Walker BL. A possible essential role for dietary linolenic acid in the development of the young rat. *J Nutr* 1976; 106: 86.
19. Galli C, Galli G, Spagnuolo C, et al. In: Bazan NG, Brenner RR, Giusto NM, eds. *Function and biosynthesis of lipids*. New York: Plenum Press; 1977: 561–73.
20. Sun GY, Sun AY. Synaptosomal plasma membranes: acyl group composition of phosphoglycerides and (Na^-09+^- plus K^-09+^-)-ATP-ase activity during fatty acid deficiency. *J Neurochem* 1974; 22: 15–18.
21. Yamamoto N, Saitoh M, Moriuchi A, Nomura M, et al. Effect of dietary alpha-linolenate/linolleate balance on brain lipid composition and learning ability in rats. *J Lipid Res* 1987; 28: 144–51.
22. Neuringer M, Anderson GJ, Connor WE. The essentiality of n-3 fatty acids for the development and function of the retina and brain. *Annu Rev Nutr* 1988; 8: 517–41.
23. Holman RT, Johnstone SB, Hatch TE. A case of human linolenic acid deficiency involving neurological abnormalities. *Am J Clin Nutr* 1982; 35: 617–23.
24. Bazan NG. Supply of n-3 polyunsaturated fatty acids and their significance in the central nervous system. In: Wurtman RJ, Wurtman JJ, eds. *Nutrition and the Brain*. New York: Raven Press; 1990: 1–24.
25. Budowski P, Hawkey CM, Crawford MA. L'effet protecteur de l'acide apha-linolenique sur l'enceohalomalaciie chez le poulet. *Ann Nutr Anim* 1980; 34: 389–400.
26. Budowski P, Leighfield MJ, Crawford MA. Nutritional encephalomalacia in the chick: an exposure of the vulnerable period for cerebellar development and the possible need for both w6 and w3 fatty acids. *Br J Nutr* 1987; 58: 511–20.
27. Dobbing J. Vulnerable periods of brain development. In: Elliott K, Knights J, eds. *Lipids, malnutrition and the developing brain* (Ciba Foundation Symposium). Amsterdam: Elsevier; 1972: 1–7.
28. Selivonchick DP, Johnson PV. Fat deficiency in rats during development of the central nervous system and susceptibility to experimental allergic encephalomyelitis. *J Nutr* 1975; 105: 288–92.
29. Stackpoole A, Mertin J. The effect of prostaglandin precursors *in vivo* models of cell-mediated immunity. *Prog Lipid Res* 1981; 21: 649–54.
30. FAO/WHO. *The role of dietary fats and oils in human nutrition* (Report of an Expert Consultation). Rome: FAO; 1978.
31. Crawford MA, Hassam AG, Stevens PA. Essential fatty acid requirements in pregnancy and lactation with special reference to brain development. *Prog Lipid Res* 1981; 20: 30–40.
32. Galli C, Socini A. Dietary lipids in pre- and post-natal development. In: Perkins EG, Visek WJ, eds. *Dietary fats and health*. Chicago: 1983: 278–301. *Proceedings of American Oil Chemists Society Conference*; vol 16).

33. Crawford MA, Doyle W, Drury P. Relationship between maternal and infant nutrition, the special role of fat in energy transfer. *Trop Geogr Med* 1985; 37: S5, 1–16.
34. Frisch RE. In: Vigersky R, ed. *Anorexia Nervosa*. New York: Raven Press; 1977.
35. Hurley LS. Nutritional deficiencies and excesses. In: *Handbook of teratology*. New York: Plenum Press; 1979: 261–308.
36. Giroud A. *Nutrition of the embryo*. Springfield: Thomas; 1970.
37. Smithells RW. Multivitamins for the prevention of neural tube defects. *Drugs* 1989; 38: 849–54.
38. Wynn M, Wynn A. *The prevention of handicap of early pregnancy origin*. London: The Foundation for Education and Research in Child Bearing; 1981.
39. Dunn HG, ed. *Sequelae of low birth weight: The Vancouver Study*. Oxford: Blackwell Scientific Publications; 1986.
40. Marlow N, Chiswick ML. Neurodevelopmental outcome in extremely low birthweight survivors. *Recent Adv Perinat Med* 1985; 2: 181–205.
41. OPCS. *Congenital malformation statistics 1981–85: notifications. England and Wales*. London: Office of Population Censuses and Surveys; 1988, Series MB3, no 2.
42. NSO. The National Audit Office report on maternity services. London: HMSO; 1990.
43. Hagberg B, Hagberg G, Zetterstrom R. Decreasing perinatal mortality—increase in cerebral palsy morbidity. *Acta Pediatr Scand* 1989; 78: 664–70.
44. Pharoah POD, Cooke T, Cooke RWI, Rosenbloom L. Birthweight specific trends in cerebral palsy. *Arch Dis Child* 1990; 65: 602–6.
45. Chandra RK. Nutrition as a critical determinant in susceptibility to infection. *World Rev Nutr Diet* 1976; 25: 166–88.
46. Davie R, Butler N, Goldstein H. *From birth to seven—2nd report of the National Child Development Study (1958 Cohort)*. London: Longman; 1972.
47. Crawford MA, Doyle W, Craft IL, Laurance BM. A comparison of food intakes during pregnancy and birthweight in high and low socio-economic groups. *Prog Lipid Res* 1986; 25: 249–54.
48. Doyle W, Crawford MA, Wynn AH, Wynn SW. The association between maternal diet and birth dimensions. *J Nutr Med* 1990; 61: 9–17.
49. Doyle W, Crawford MA, Wynn AH, Wynn SW. Maternal nutrient intake and birthweight. *J Hum Nutr Diet* 1989; 62: 407–14.
50. Crawford MA, Doyle W, Drury P, Lennon A, Costeloe K, Leighfield M. n-6 and n-3 fatty acids during early human development. *J Int Med* 1989; 225[Suppl 1]: 159–69.
51. Orstead C, Arrington A, Kamath SK, Olsen R, Kohrs MB. Efficacy of prenatal nutrition counselling: weight gain, infant birthweight and cost effectiveness. *J Am Diet Assoc* 1985; 85: 40–5.
52. Holman RT. The deficiency of essential fatty acids. In: Kunau W, Homlan RT, eds. *Polyunsaturated fatty acids*. Cincinnatti: (*Proceedings of the Am Oil Chem Soc.*). 1977: 163–82.
53. Althabe O, Laberre C, Telenta M. Maternal vascular lesions in placentae of small for gestational age infants. *Placenta* 1985; 6: 265–76.
54. Marmot MG, McDowell ME. Mortality decline and widening social inequalities. *Lancet* 1986; ii: 274–6.
55. Ongari MA, Ritter JM, Orchard MA, Waddell KA, Blair IA, Lewis PJ. Correlation of prostacyclin synthesis by human umbilical artery with status of essential fatty acid. *Am J Obstet Gynecol* 1984; 149: 455–60.
56. Crawford MA, Hall B, Laurance BM, Munhambo A. Milk lipids and their variability. *Curr Med Res Opin* 1976; 4[Suppl 1]: 33–43.
57. Friedman Z, Frolich JC. Essential fatty acids and the major urinary metabolites of the E prostaglandins in thriving infants and infants receiving parenteral fat emulsions. *Pediatr Res* 1979; 13: 932–6.
58. Putnam JC, Carlson SE, Phillip WD, Barness linoleic acid. The effect of various dietary fatty acids on the fatty acid composition of erythrocyte phosphatidylcholine and phosphatidylethanolamine in human infants. *Am J Clin Nutr* 1982; 36: 106–14.
59. Carlson SE, Rhodes PG, Ferguson MG. Docosahexaenoic acid status of preterm infants at birth and following feeding with human milk formula. *Am J Clin Nutr* 1986; 44: 798–804.
60. Shires SE, Conway SP, Rawson I, Dear PRF, Keller J. Fatty acid composition of plasma and erythrocyte phospholipids in preterm infants. *Early Hum Dev* 1986; 1: 353–63.
61. Uauy R, Treen M, Hoffman D. Essential fatty acid metabolism and requirements during development. *Semin Perinatol* 1989; 13: 118–30.
62. Olsen SF, Hansen HS, Sorensen TIA, *et al.* Intake of marine fat, rich in (n-3)-polyunsaturated fatty acids, may increase birth weight by prolonging gestation. *Lancet* 1986; ii: 367–9.

63. Olsen FS, Secher NJ. A possible preventive effect of low-dose fish oil on early delivery and pre-eclampsia: indications from a 50 year old controlled trial. *Br J Nutr* 1990; 64: 599–609.
64. Lucas A, Morley R, Cole TJ, et al. Early diet in preterm babies and developmental status at 18 months. *Lancet* 1990; i: 1477–81.
65. Laurance BM, Smith HB. The premature babies' diet. *Lancet* 1962; i: 589–90.

DISCUSSION

Dr. Clandinin: In your reference to low birthweight infants in the group that correlates with maternal intake, are you referring to infants who are low birthweight and premature or who are just low birthweight?

Dr. Crawford: They are both. The evidence is that the highest risk groups are those which are fetal growth retarded and premature, and that comes out with the biochemical data as well.

Dr. Cunnane: Why can't the mother mobilize some of her linoleic acid to prevent or reverse fetal growth retardation?

Dr. Crawford: The fat the mother transfers from herself to the fetus is not rich in linoleic acid; but it is a fat which contains arachidonate and docosahexaenoate. A normal term baby is born with 300–400 g of fat which is a rich source of these fatty acids. In developing countries, where the mother may be surviving on minimal energy supply, fat deposition is reduced and so the ability of the baby to buffer an emergency situation in the neonatal period through the use of his own fat stores may be impaired, as it is when it is transferred from energy-dense human milk to energy-poor weaning foods.

Dr. Spector: In what form are these highly unsaturated fatty acids transferred to the fetus? I do not understand the mechanism of transport.

Dr. Crawford: This is a very difficult question. It appears from Douglas Kuhn's studies that the phosphoglycerides are attacked by phospholipase A2, are transferred as free fatty acids, and are resynthesized in a way which selectively incorporates the 20,22 polyenes, so that the emerging phosphoglycerides are rich in arachidonic and docosahexaenoic acids.

Dr. Guesry: Do you feel that your correlations between arachidonic acid and birthweight and between docosahexaenoic acid and prematurity suggest that EFA deficiency could be a cause of low birthweight and prematurity?

Dr. Crawford: I did not present the data as evidence of this, but as a signal of some nutritional problem that has occurred during fetal growth. We have a wide range of data showing that some 15 different nutrients track with low birthweight.

Dr. Guesry: Since δ-6-desaturase is immature in the low birthweight infant and will mature with gestational age it is not surprising that you find this type of correlation.

Dr. Crawford: We do not think so. The data on umbilical artery and cord blood were used as a test of the impact on the fetus of the differences we and others have found in maternal nutrient intakes in relation to low birthweight. The surprising feature is the amount of Mead acid. These are the only recorded cases where we have seen such amounts of Mead acid, which with its 22 carbon derivative (22:3, n-9) amounts to as much as 10% of the total fatty acids in the endothelial ethanolamine phosphoglycerides from our lowest birthweight baby. Secondly it seems as though the triene/tetraene ratio correlated more with birthweight than the docosahexaenoic acid content, which appeared to follow the degree of maturity. Hence arachidonic and docosahexaenoic acids, both key components of the most active membranes in the CNS and the peripheral nervous system, appear to be pointing in different directions.

These signals tell us about the intrauterine nutritional history of the neonate. Such information, especially in very low birthweight babies, may help to identify those most likely to be at risk of neurodevelopmental deficits or damage.

Dr. Koletzko: Your data on the correlations between maternal nutrition and infant birthweight look impressive but I really wonder what their meaning is. A significant correlation clearly does not always represent a causal relationship. For example, I cannot imagine how increasing the maternal dietary fiber intake could raise the birthweight of the infant. It is known that maternal body weight correlates closely with neonatal body weight. Could not this relationship explain part of the correlation between the maternal intake of most nutrients and birthweight? Mothers with higher body weights simply consume more food.

Dr. Crawford: It is the ponderal index that is related to the outcome of pregnancy rather than maternal weight *per se*. This suggests that conditions prior to pregnancy are more important than they have been given credit for. The reason why we started to investigate these issues was that we accepted that correlates between maternal nutrition and the outcome of pregnancy are simply correlates and nothing more. We now have fairly powerful tools for studying maternal nutrient intakes that were not available before, so these issues can be studied more fully. It is worth remembering the studies that were done in relation to human famines, particularly the Dutch famine during and after World War II. Mothers who were pregnant at the time food shortages began tended to produce healthy babies, while in mothers who conceived during the famine there was an increased incidence of congenital abnormality, low birthweight, and perinatal mortality. Other studies have supported these findings and our own correlates with maternal nutrition are strongest in relation to the situation around the time of conception. The data on the fetal umbilical tissue and the bloods at birth provide objective confirmation of the nutritional deficits.

Developmental Aspects of Long Chain Polyunsaturated Fatty Acid Metabolism: CNS Development

Michael Thomas Clandinin and Johny E. E. Van Aerde

Nutrition and Metabolism Research Group, Departments of Foods and Nutrition and Medicine, University of Alberta, Edmonton, Alberta, Canada T6G 2C2

Brain development is a sequential process characterized by stages of growth and maturation (1). Biochemical transitions in brain development are also sequential, paralleling anatomical changes (2). Alterations in the course of brain development can thus easily result in gross abnormalities of brain function, often associated with irreparable damage to the normal regulation of body activities or expression of behavior (3). Development in many tissues occurs uniformly and gradually, but in the brain development of neurons is characterized by several periods of "growth spurt" occurring in fetal and neonatal life (4). In human brain two separate periods of intense cell proliferation exist (5). During the first phase all macroneurons, most microneurons, and some glial elements are formed. The second phase principally involves development of glial cells. Rate of development in brain regions also differs. For example, the brainstem develops through fast prenatal and slow postnatal increases in cell numbers (6). Cell proliferation takes place in the forebrain area during the postnatal period, while cerebellar cell proliferation takes place at a later time.

Lipids, and as the focus for this discussion, fatty acids are major constituents of neural tissues comprising neuronal and glial membranes (reviewed in ref. 7). Thus in the developing brain the lipid composition also undergoes qualitative and quantitative changes with maturation. In general, during early stages of brain development brain lipid content increases as lipids are part of the general structure of brain cell membranes. With the onset of myelination other lipids accumulate in brain tissue (7). In humans myelination occurs during the perinatal period, continuing into the second decade of life (3). The motor and sensory roots are myelinated early whereas the reticular formation, nonspecific thalamic projections, and neocortex are myelinated later. Thus during brain development the quantitative content of phospholipid declines whereas the brain content of cholesterol, cerebrosides, and sulfatides increases (8).

TABLE 1. *Estimated tissue accretion of long chain polyenoic essential fatty acids during the last trimester of development*

	Long chain polyenoic essential fatty acids (mg/week)	
	ω-6	ω-3
Brain	30.8	14.4
Cerebellum	1.5	0.1
Liver	7.6	3.5
Brown adipose	145	15.8
White adipose	1,850	316
Total LCPE/week[a]	3,660	469

[a] Includes C18 fatty acids and amounts estimated to accrue in other tissues.

FATTY ACID ACCRETION IN HUMAN BRAIN

During the last trimester of human development, ω-3 and ω-6 fatty acids accrue in fetal tissues as an essential component of structural lipids (Table 1). Among the major fatty acid constituents to accrue are the chain elongation-desaturation products of 18:2ω6 and 18:3ω3 (Fig. 1) (9). For term infants during early postnatal brain

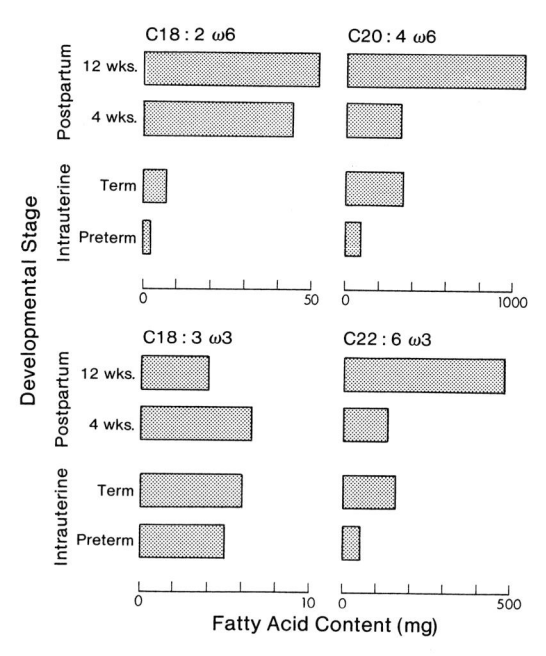

FIG. 1. Pattern of change in brain content of long chain polyenoic essential fatty acids.

TABLE 2. *Fatty acid content ($\mu g/ml$ plasma) of preterm infant plasma phospholipid fraction*[a]

	Mother's milk	Formula	Supplemented formula
$C18:2\omega 6$	270 ± 3.0	285 ± 26.4	435 ± 34.8***
$C20:4\omega 6$	140 ± 40.4	102 ± 10.7	82.2 ± 9.0***
$C20:5\omega 3$	8.2 ± 3.8	13.2 ± 1.2	3.6 ± 0.6***
$C22:6\omega 3$	40.8 ± 3.2	38.0 ± 2.5	13.2 ± 2.3***
C20 & $C22\omega 6$	197 ± 9.6	163 ± 13.7	119 ± 14.1***
C20 & $C22\omega 3$	56.9 ± 4.6	57.6 ± 4.0	19.5 ± 3.2***

*** $p < 0.001$.
[a] Values illustrated represent the mean ± SEM. While all fatty acid constituents were analyzed, only major essential fatty acid constituents are summarized above. "Supplemented" formula contained C20 and C22 $\omega 6$ and $\omega 3$ fatty acids. Overall = grand means; all samples all time periods.

development, the shorter chain precursors increase in brain tissue with little increase in levels of chain elongated products for several weeks postpartum (10,11). Intrauterine accretion of chain elongated-desaturated essential fatty acids occurs and as postnatal accretion of these components does not take place in tissues immediately after birth (12,13; Fig. 1), it is likely that synthesis of chain elongated-desaturated fatty acids may limit maximal postnatal accretion for these components. In this regard, observations reported to date are consistent with the concept that intrauterine accretion of long chain polyenoic fatty acid occurs primarily as a function of mechanisms involving placental transfer. Little quantitative evidence is available to indicate whether $C_{20:4\omega 6}$, $C_{22:4\omega 6}$, $C_{22:5\omega 3}$, and $C_{22:6\omega 3}$ are synthesized in the human fetus or whether the fetus is entirely dependent on mechanisms of placental synthesis and transfer to obtain these very long chain polyunsaturated fatty acids required for the synthesis of essential structural lipids during intrauterine development. Clinical studies suggest that feeding C20 and C22 ω-6 and ω-3 fatty acids is necessary to maintain levels of these fatty acids in plasma phospholipids and thus in lipoprotein phospholipids (data submitted for publication; Table 2). Since recent evidence suggests a relationship between essential fatty acid intake and the development of visual functions (14), it is nutritionally relevant to the feeding of very low birthweight infants to determine whether extrauterine accretion of long chain polyenoic fatty acids requires dietary supply of these fatty acids, perhaps originating as normal constituents of human milk, or arises *in vivo* from chain elongation-desaturation of shorter chain precursors (i.e., $C_{18:2\omega 6}$ and $C_{18:3\omega 3}$).

RELATIONSHIP OF BRAIN DEVELOPMENT TO NUTRITION

It is known in animal models that undernutrition can significantly influence fatty acid profiles of cerebrosides and phospholipids in developing brain, thereby implying relationships between myelination in brain and nutritional stress (15,16). Therefore, it is nutritionally relevant to determine if extrauterine accretion of long chain

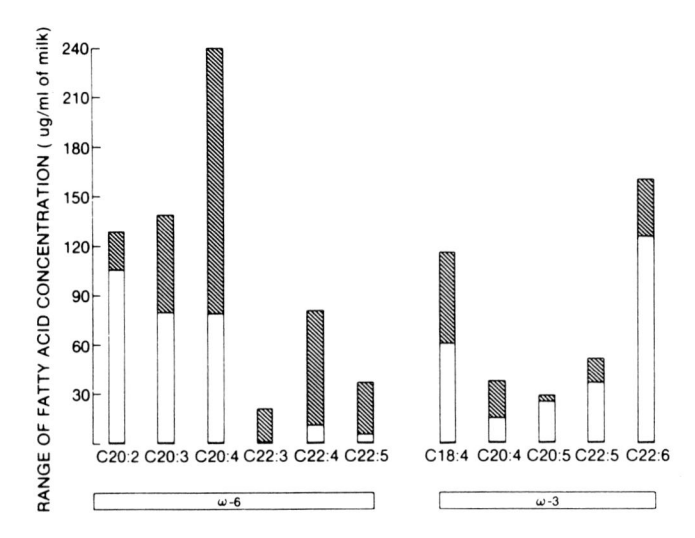

FIG. 2. Long chain polyunsaturated derivatives of 18:2ω6 and 18:3ω3 present in total milk fats. Data represent the range of concentrations of long chain polyenoic fatty acids observed in milk samples obtained at days 4 and 22 of lactation.

polyenoic fatty acids requires dietary supply of these fatty acids, perhaps originating as normal constituents of human milk (Fig. 2), or arises *in vivo* from chain elongation-desaturation of shorter chain precursors, i.e., 18:2ω6 and 18:3ω3. Moreover, in growing animals change in dietary intake of fat alters the composition of specific brain membrane fractions and membrane content of very long chain polyunsaturated fatty acids in a manner that affects the *de novo* synthesis of phosphatidylcholine in the brain (17,18). For example, altering dietary intake of monoenes, 18:2ω6 and 18:3ω3, changes brain content of ω-6 and ω-3 fatty acids in individual phospholipids and may alter the fatty acid content of myelin (18,19). It has also been shown that adding cholesterol to a diet high in ω-3 fatty acid can also markedly increase the 22:6ω3 content of brain phosphatidylethanolamine (19).

BIOSYNTHETIC CAPABILITY

In our laboratory we have defined an animal model exemplifying accretion of long chain homologues of $C_{18:2\omega6}$ and $C_{18:3\omega3}$ in a manner analogous to accretion of these fatty acid components in the human fetal brain. Accretion of fatty acid in the pig brain follows a pattern analogous to the synthesis and accretion of these components in the last trimester of development in the human fetal brain. Accretion of C20 and C22 homologues of the essential fatty acids occurs during the last trimester of development in the brain of the pig, suggesting that the pig would represent a suitable animal model for determining if accretion of long chain polyunsaturated fatty acids in the brain occurs as a function of their synthesis in the fetal tissues or via mechanisms involving placental transport (20). Synthesis of fatty acids elongated from 16:0 is greater at term and at 12 weeks postpartum than during midgestation for the pig brain (21). Liver microsomal synthesis of fatty acids elongated from 16:0 is relatively high midway through gestation relative to this capability after a full term of gestation. Microsomal capability to chain-elongate saturated fatty acids establishes that pig brain and liver are capable of chain-elongating C16 and C18 fatty acids during the intrauterine period.

Synthesis of chain elongation-desaturation products of linoleic acid by liver and brain microsomes during the development of the pig indicates that for fetal piglets midway through gestation, the capability to synthesize trienes, tetraenes, and pentaenes in the brain is relatively limited compared with *in vitro* rates for synthesis of these compounds after a full term gestational period or at 12 weeks postpartum. In pig liver, microsomal synthesis of tetraenes is similarly reduced, but the tetraenes formed from linoleic acid *in vitro* can be converted to pentaenes (22). These observations indicate that in liver and brain capability to chain elongate-desaturate $C_{18:2\omega6}$ (20,23) to longer chain homologues increases significantly during early development in the pig. During gestation activity of the Δ^5-desaturase may limit synthesis of C20 and C22 homologues of linoleic acid. Metabolic conversion to C22 fatty acids by chain elongation of $C_{20:3\omega6}$ does not appear to limit synthesis of very long chain homologues of linoleic acid in fetal liver or brain. When the synthesis of tetraenes and pentaenes from $C_{20:3\omega6}$ by Δ^5-desaturation of this fatty acid by liver and brain microsomes was examined, the capability to synthesize tetraenes dramatically increased during the latter half of gestation when related to microsomal protein (Fig. 3; 23). These observations indicate that in pig liver and brain, the capability to chain elongate-desaturate linoleic acid to longer chain homologues increases during early development, apparently as a function of transitions in activity of the Δ^5-desaturase.

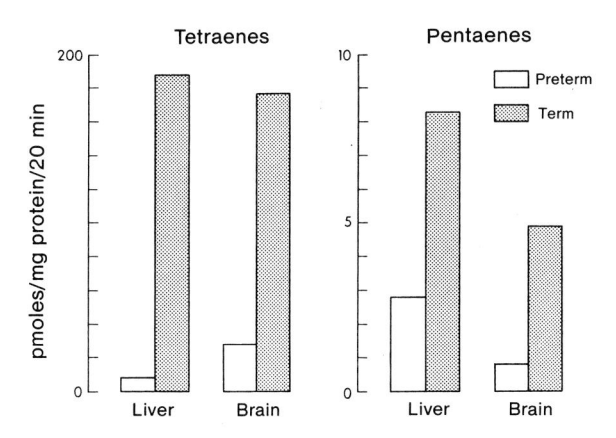

FIG. 3. Synthesis of tetraenes and pentaenes from 20:3(8,11,14) by Δ^5-desaturation in pig liver and brain microsomes. Microsomes were isolated from preterm piglets at 63 days gestation and at 3 days postpartum for term piglets. Microsomal assays were conducted in duplicate, corrected for corresponding control assays, and utilized 20:3 (8,11,14) as the fatty acid substrate. Values for each group represent the mean of four individual animals.

CAN DIET ALTER BRAIN COMPOSITION?

Nutritionally adequate diets containing various dietary fats influence the content and composition of polar lipids in rat brain synaptosomal and microsomal membranes (24,25). These alterations also result in transitions in brain membrane function as evidenced by changes in synaptosomal acetylcholinetransferase and Na^+-K^+ ATPase activity (25). In these experiments, diet altered the phosphatidylcholine and cholesterol content of brain membranes. In brain, many enzymes involved in neurotransmitter metabolism are lipid-dependent, as are functions involved in the synthesis of brain structural lipids. In this regard, phosphatidylcholinetransferase and phosphatidylethanolamine methyltransferase activities in the brain are modulated by diet fat (18) and by diet-induced changes in membrane phospholipid content of long chain polyunsaturated essential fatty acids (19,26) in a manner that is coordinated (18). Therefore, it is logical to postulate a wide variety of potential interactions among dietary lipid, brain lipid, and brain neurotransmitter metabolism and among dietary fatty acid balance, myelin formation, and the function of myelinated brain structures. The cause and effect nature of changes in brain structural constituents remains to be resolved, but it is clear that the brain is sensitive to alteration of dietary lipid intake even in a nutritionally complete diet. It is conceivable that disorders relating to alterations of brain structural lipid may also be responsive to dietary treatment by modulation of brain structural lipid, with subsequent effects on the function of integral membrane proteins.

In humans and animals significant aspects of learning during early development are associated with development of visual acuity. In recent years it has been recognized that dietary ω-3 fatty acids are essential in part because these fatty acids are major constituents of excitable membranes in brain and retina. In the premature infant, research by Dr. Susan Carlson has suggested that development of visual acuity is also associated with dietary intake of very long chain ω-3 fatty acids. It is thus reasonable to anticipate that dietary intake of ω-3 fatty acids may alter the composition of excitable membranes in a manner that alters function.

In this regard we have examined the effect of feeding diets of high or low $C_{20:5\omega 3}$ and $C_{22:6\omega 3}$ fatty acid content on the fatty acid composition of the retina in the growing rat. These studies indicate that dietary intake of ω-3 fatty acid, even in the normally growing animal, alters the 22:6ω3 content of specific phospholipids in retina as well as the biosynthesis of longer chain essential fatty acids of unknown function (unpublished data). Whether or not these diet-induced changes in the retina alter the functional process(es) in the retina remains to be determined.

REFERENCES

1. Gottlieb A, Keidar I, Epstein HT. Rodent brain growth stages: an analytical review. *Biol Neonate* 1977; 32: 166–76.
2. Lebenthal E, Leung YK. Developmental changes of the gastrointestinal tract in the newborn. In: Stern L, ed. *Feeding the sick infant.* (Nestlé Nutrition Workshop Series). New York: Raven Press; 1987: 1–21.

3. Meisami E, Timiras PS. Normal and abnormal biochemical development of the brain after birth. In: Jones CT, ed. *The biochemical development of the fetus and neonate.* New York: Elsevier; 1982: 759–821.
4. Davidson AN. *Biochemical correlates of brain structure and function.* London: Academic Press; 1977: 1.
5. Dobbing J. Undernutrition and the developing brain: the use of animal models to elucidate the human problem. In: Paoletti R, Davidson AN, eds. *Chemistry and brain development.* New York: Plenum Press; 1971: 399–412.
6. McCaman RE, Cook K. Intermediary metabolism of phospholipids in brain tissue. *J Biol Chem* 1966; 241: 3390–9.
7. Feldman M, Van Aerde JE, Clandinin MT. Lipid accretion in the fetus and newborn. In: Polin R, Fox W, eds. *Fetal and neonatal physiology.* Toronto: WB Saunders; 1992:299–314.
8. Timiras PS. *Developmental physiology and aging.* New York: Macmillan; 1972: 129.
9. Clandinin MT, Chappell JE, Leong S, Heim T, Swyer PR, Chance GW. Intrauterine fatty acid accretion rates in human brain: implications for fatty acid requirements. *Early Hum Dev* 1980; 4: 121–9.
10. Clandinin MT, Chappell JE, Heim T. Do low birthweight infants require nutrition with chain elongation-desaturation products of essential fatty acids? *Prog Lipid Res* 1982; 20: 901–4.
11. Clandinin MT, Chappell JE, Leong S, Heim T, Swyer PR, Chance GW. Extrauterine fatty acid accretion in infant brain: implications for fatty acid requirements. *Early Hum Dev* 1980; 4: 131–8.
12. Clandinin MT, Chappell JE, Heim T, Swyer PR, Chance GW. Fatty acid accretion in fetal and neonatal liver: implications for fatty acid requirements. *Early Hum Dev* 1981; 5: 7–14.
13. Clandinin MT, Chappell JE, Heim T, Swyer PR, Chance GW. Fatty acid utilization in perinatal de novo synthesis of tissues. *Early Hum Dev* 1981; 5: 355–66.
14. Uauy R, Treen M, Hoffman DR. Essential fatty acid metabolism and requirements in preterm infants. *Semin Perinatol* 1989; 13: 118.
15. Clandinin MT, Chappell JE, Heim T, et al. Fatty acid accretion in the development of human spinal cord. *Early Hum Dev* 1981; 5: 7–14.
16. Rao SP. Fatty acid composition of cerebrosides and phospholipids in brains of undernourished rats. *Nutr Metab* 1979; 23: 136.
17. Hargreaves K, Clandinin MT. Phosphocholinetransferase activity in plasma membrane: effect of diet. *Biochem Biophys Res Commun* 1987; 145: 309–15.
18. Hargreaves K, Clandinin MT. Co-ordinate control of CDP-choline and phosphatidylethanolamine methyltransferase pathways for phosphatidylcholine biosynthesis occurs in response to change in diet fat. *Biochim Biophys Acta* 1989; 1001: 262–7.
19. Hargreaves K, Clandinin MT. Dietary control of diacylphosphatidylethanolamine species in brain. *Biochim Biophys Acta* 1988; 962: 98–104.
20. Purvis JM, Clandinin MT, Hacker RR. Fatty acid accretion during perinatal brain growth in the pig. A model for fatty acid accretion in human brain. *Comp Biochem Physiol* 1982; 72B: 195–9.
21. Clandinin MT, Wong K, Hacker RR. Synthesis of chain elongated-desaturated fatty acids from palmitic acid by liver and brain microsomes during development of the pig. *Comp Biochem Physiol* 1985; 81B: 53–4.
22. Clandinin MT, Wong K, Hacker RR. Synthesis of chain elongation-desaturation products of linoleic acid by liver and brain microsomes during development of the pig. *Biochem J* 1985; 226: 305–9.
23. Clandinin MT, Wong K, Hacker RR. Delta-5 desaturase activity in liver and brain microsomes during development of the pig. *Biochem J* 1985; 227: 1021–3.
24. Foot M, Cruz TF, Clandinin MT. Influence of dietary fat on the lipid composition of rat brain synaptosomal and microsomal membranes. *Biochem J* 1982; 208: 631–40.
25. Foot M, Cruz TF, Clandinin MT. Effect of dietary lipid on synaptosomal acetylcholinesterase activity. *Biochem J* 1983; 211: 507–9.
26. Hargreaves KM, Clandinin MT. Phosphatidylethanolamine methyltransferase: evidence for influence of diet fat on selectivity of substrate for methylation in rat brain synaptic plasma membranes. *Biochim Biophys Acta* 1987; 918: 97–105.

DISCUSSION

Dr. Koletzko: I was surprised about your data on human milk composition. You showed that Canadian women had an extremely wide range of ω-6 and ω-3 long chain polyunsaturates, ranging from 0.1% to 5.6% and from 0.01% to 3.3% of total fatty acids, respectively. Can you provide additional information on the source of these results? The variations in long chain polyunsaturates seem surprisingly great.

Dr. Clandinin: We needed to know the extreme range found in typical North American milk. For example if a woman ate a salmon steak on the previous evening the level of ω-3 would be raised the next day. I would not expect to find any milk with levels outside this range, which includes all cases.

Dr. Hernell: When you gave formulas differing from breast milk in their cholesteryl esters and phospholipids, the plasma DHA concentration was similar to the breast-fed group but the arachidonic acid was lower. What is the reason for this difference?

Dr. Clandinin: The plasma docosahexaenoic acid (DHA) concentration in infants fed the modified formula is indeed very similar to that of breast milk-fed infants, but it takes only a very small amount of long chain ω-3 (about 0.7%) as an addition to the formula to produce a fairly substantial response in arachidonic acid. In my view ω-3 should not be added without ω-6 because this will reduce arachidonic acid very effectively. Only about one-third of the C20 and C22 ω-6 in the modified formula was arachidonic. This was not as much as we hoped to achieve in the final formula manufacture but that is what we got. The amount is enough to bring the ω-6 to somewhere between the two feeding regimens and closer to breast milk-fed infants than to infants fed without the LCFA ω-6. The important point is that there should be a balance. If you just add fish oil containing ω-3 you disturb that balance.

Dr. Cunnane: You suggested that it makes a big difference whether the arachidonic acid you put in the modified formula is in the phospholipid or the triglyceride form. Could you elaborate on this?

Dr. Clandinin: In terms of the absolute amount that gets into the plasma I'm not sure that it makes much difference. In terms of the practical aspects there are two considerations. First, you can only put a restricted amount of phospholipid into a formula. We would have difficulty in just adding phospholipid of a high arachidonic acid type to provide enough 20:4. Second, some of the sources of high arachidonic phospholipid involve processes that are not acceptable for infant formulas—solvent extraction and so on. The practical solution is to find a triglyceride containing significant amounts of these ω-6 fatty acids.

Dr. Cunnane: What is the biologically acceptable range of a plasma arachidonic acid value and could a significant drop still be within the acceptable range?

Dr. Clandinin: It is a reasonable assumption from some of the experimental data that if the level of arachidonic acid is dropping in the plasma, it is dropping in other tissues as well. However, it is also possible that components may be taken out of the plasma so fast that they are still going into brain at an acceptable level and this depletion is being reflected in the plasma. Whether it is at some critical level is unknown. The quickest way to drive the plasma levels of 20:4, n-6 down and the levels of 20:4, n-6 in other tissues down is to add enough ω-3 fatty acid.

Dr. Deckelbaum: In the American population there are many children with disorders such as abetalipoproteinemia and intestinal lymphangiectasia in whom part of the therapy, beginning as early as the 1st month of life, is to limit the fat intake to no more than 5–10% of total energy. Assuming they receive the right amounts of EFA, will they be at risk of defects in neurological development? And do you think there is any danger in feeding all children over the age of 6 months on the American Heart Association step 1 diet (total fat intake not exceeding 30% of energy and saturated fat not exceeding 10%)?

Dr. Clandinin: In answer to your first question, yes, I think this group is of potential concern. As to your second question, the important issue seems to me to be whether ω-3 fatty acids are more effective in terms of any hypolipidemic effect if they are fed against a background of a diet high in saturated fats. If ω-3 fatty acids are fed in competition with an intake that is higher in ω-6, the ω-3 is relatively much less effective in causing a reduction in plasma lipids. If one could demonstrate that some of the same benefits could be achieved with the addition of ω-3 alone there might be a much more effective way to reach the desired goal, since it takes a relatively small amount of ω-3 in the diet and a relatively small dietary change to be effective. The overall approach of increasing ω-6 intake is questionable.

Dr. Crawford: The brain at birth uses 60% of the energy consumed by the baby and to achieve that requires a superb respiratory system and vascular supply. The cardiovascular system is developing at the same time as the central nervous system so the two go together. Any principles that apply to the prevention of cardiovascular disease would in my opinion have to be applied to fetal growth and early postnatal development as well.

Dr. Small: What is your source of arachidonic-rich triglyceride oils?

Dr. Clandinin: Catfish oil. When this oil is cleaned up and redistilled it is a useful peroxide-free product containing some ω-6 fatty acid. You can get it without having to resort to solvent extraction.

Supply, Uptake, and Utilization of Docosahexaenoic Acid During Photoreceptor Cell Differentiation

Nicolas G. Bazan

Department of Ophthalmology and Neuroscience Center, Louisiana State University Medical Center, New Orleans, Louisiana, 70112-2234, USA

During the perinatal development of brain and retina profound changes in cell structure, organization, and function occur. The events underlying these changes which are a part of neural cell differentiation, including synaptogenesis, ultimately lead then to neuron-neuron communication, neuron-glia interrelationships, and the formation of synaptic circuitry. The establishment of synapses is preceded by growth cone formation, path finding, and axonal guidance. In the retina, photoreceptor cells evolve rapidly from round, somewhat elongated cells into bipolar structures having a distal outer segment and a proximal synaptic ending (Fig. 1).

Many of the perinatal cell differentiation events are related to the rapid expansion and specialization of neural plasma membranes, which then become excitable membranes, displaying by far the largest surface area of all cells. Since these membranes are rich in phospholipids, neural cells undergo active phospholipid biosynthesis concomitant with membrane biogenesis during the perinatal period. The membrane phospholipids that need to be synthesized for neural and photoreceptor cells are uniquely enriched in docosahexaenoic acid (DHA), the major derivative of the essential fatty acid, linolenic acid. Therefore, the perinatal period creates large nutritional requirements for essential fatty acids.

In the present contribution, features of the metabolic routes and interorgan mechanisms underlying these requirements are addressed. First, differences in the accumulation of the major end-products of linoleic and linolenic acids in photoreceptor cells during perinatal development are shown. Second, studies revealing that DHA, and not linolenic acid, is the preferred n-3 fatty acid utilized by retina and brain are summarized. Third, it is emphasized that the liver plays a central role in the supply of DHA synthesized from dietary linolenic acid to retina and brain during postnatal development.

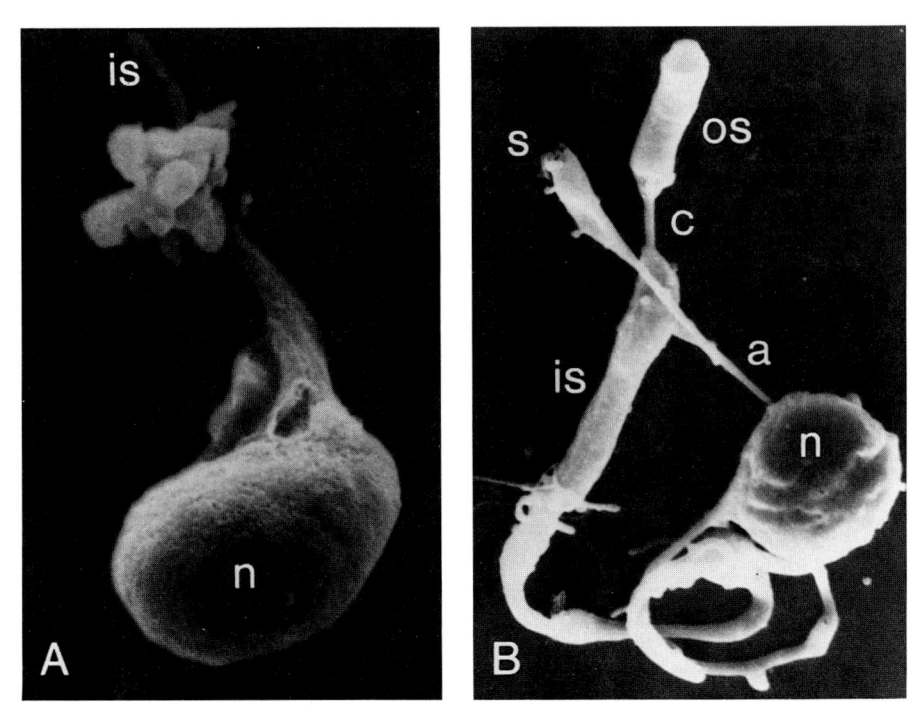

FIG. 1. Dissociated, isolated photoreceptor cells from the postnatal developing mouse retina. Scanning electron micrographs were obtained from cells isolated from 5 **(A)** and 11 day old **(B)** mice. a, axon; c, connecting cilium; is, inner segment; n, nucleus; os, outer segment; s, synaptic terminal. From Scott BL, et al. (1).

ACCUMULATION OF DOCOSAHEXAENOIC ACID IN PHOTORECEPTOR CELLS DURING POSTNATAL DEVELOPMENT

Until recently it was thought that DHA was the only end-product of the linolenic fatty acid family. However, several longer chain fatty acids (up to 36 carbon atoms) are now known to be formed by successive elongation reactions (1). Nevertheless, DHA is by far the most prevalent linolenic acid product present in cells. In the outer segments of photoreceptor cells up to 15% of the total n-3 fatty acid pool is made up of very long chain polyunsaturated fatty acids (2). The retina also contains molecular species of phospholipids with two DHA moieties, which are called supraenoic molecular species (3–5). The physiological significance and pathological implications of these very long chain polyunsaturated fatty acids and supraenoic molecular species represent an interesting area for the further investigation of DHA biology.

A striking accumulation of DHA occurs in phospholipids of photoreceptor cells during the postnatal development of the mouse. Figure 2 shows that the content of docosahexaenoyl chains in the major membrane phospholipids, phosphatidylcholine, and phosphatidylethanolamine of isolated cells more than doubles between 5–6 days

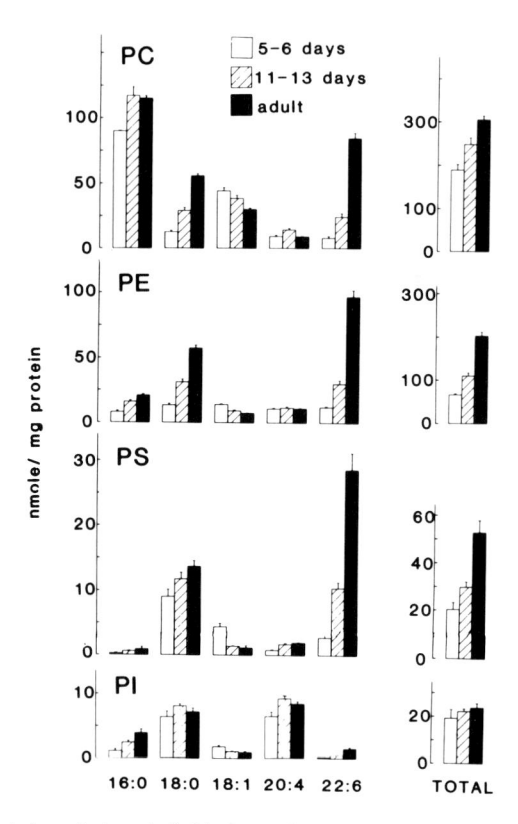

FIG. 2. Fatty acyl chains of phospholipids from photoreceptor cells isolated from 5–6 day old, 11–13 day old, and adult C57BL/6J mice. PC, phosphatidylcholine; PE, phosphatidylethanolamine; PS, phosphatidylserine; PI, phosphatidylinositol. From Bazan NG (6).

and 11–13 days after birth. In phosphatidylserine the enrichment in DHA almost triples in these two periods. An increase in DHA can also be seen in phosphatidylinositol, although this phospholipid contains lower overall amounts of DHA than the other two species. The content of DHA is also greatly enhanced in all these phospholipids between 11–13 days after birth and adulthood (Fig. 2). If fact, most of the total increase in the mass of phospholipids in photoreceptor cells during these periods is the result of increases in DHA in each lipid class. Figure 2 shows that the total increase is far lower than the net increase of DHA in phospholipids. No other fatty acyl chain is enriched in any phospholipid at a rate comparable to that of DHA.

These findings indicate that the bulk of DHA is introduced into membrane phospholipids of photoreceptor cells during the postnatal period of development of the mouse preceding biogenesis of photoreceptor outer segments, which contain rhodopsin. Therefore the dietary supply of n-3 fatty acids during this period is crucial to support photoreceptor cell differentiation and function. Although these studies were conducted in mice, recent data obtained in nonhuman primates (rhesus monkeys) demonstrate that dietary deprivation of linolenic acid for prolonged periods of time, including the early perinatal period, results in impairment of retinal function, including decreased visual acuity (7).

In the rat, DHA is known to accumulate in brain phospholipids most actively between birth and 20 days of age, which correlates well with neural cell differentiation and synaptogenesis. In humans, DHA accumulates in brain before birth and for up to 12 weeks thereafter (8). During embryonic development DHA seems to be derived from n-3 fatty acids from the maternal blood stream delivered by the placenta, and in the human neonate DHA is derived from n-3 fatty acids from maternal milk (9).

DEPOSITION OF ARACHIDONIC ACID IN DEVELOPING PHOTORECEPTOR CELLS

One striking observation emerging from the study of phospholipids of dissociated developing photoreceptor cells from the neonatal mouse is that the other essential fatty acid family, the n-6 series of linoleic and arachidonic acid, displays a pattern completely different from that of DHA. Thus, in phosphatidylethanolamine no net increase in arachidonoyl chains was measurable from 5 days after birth to adulthood. There is an increase in arachidonoyl chains in phosphatidylcholine, phosphatidylserine, and phosphatidylinositol between 5 and 11 days. It is clear that stearoyl and arachidonoyl chains are the major components of phosphatidylinositol. Stearoyl-arachidonoyl-*sn*-glycerophosphorylinositol is the prevailing molecular species of this lipid in all cells explored to date. This compound is actively engaged in cell signaling, subsequently giving rise to synthesis of phosphatidylinositol phosphate and phosphatidylinositol 4′,5′-bisphosphate. Photoreceptor cells seem to have the machinery to synthesize stearoyl-arachidonoyl molecular species during early postnatal development at a time which precedes the endowment of phospholipids with DHA. This disparity between the rates of acquisition of arachidonoyl and docosahexaenoyl chains in membrane phospholipids may be related to "windows" of requirements for the essential fatty acid families during perinatal development.

CENTRAL ROLE OF LIVER IN SUPPLY OF DHA TO RETINA AND BRAIN

The metabolic pathways and interorgan relationships that lead to an enriched content of DHA in neural cells during development involve the liver (10). Dietary linolenic acid (18:3) is elongated and desaturated primarily in the liver. In the mouse, the stomach contents during the first 3 weeks after birth contain far more 18:3 than DHA (Fig. 3). In serum, on the other hand, the opposite is true. This suggests that

FIG. 3. Endogenous content of linolenic acid and DHA in total lipids of stomach **(A)** and serum **(B)** of developing mouse pups. Data recalculated from Scott BL and Bazan NG (11).

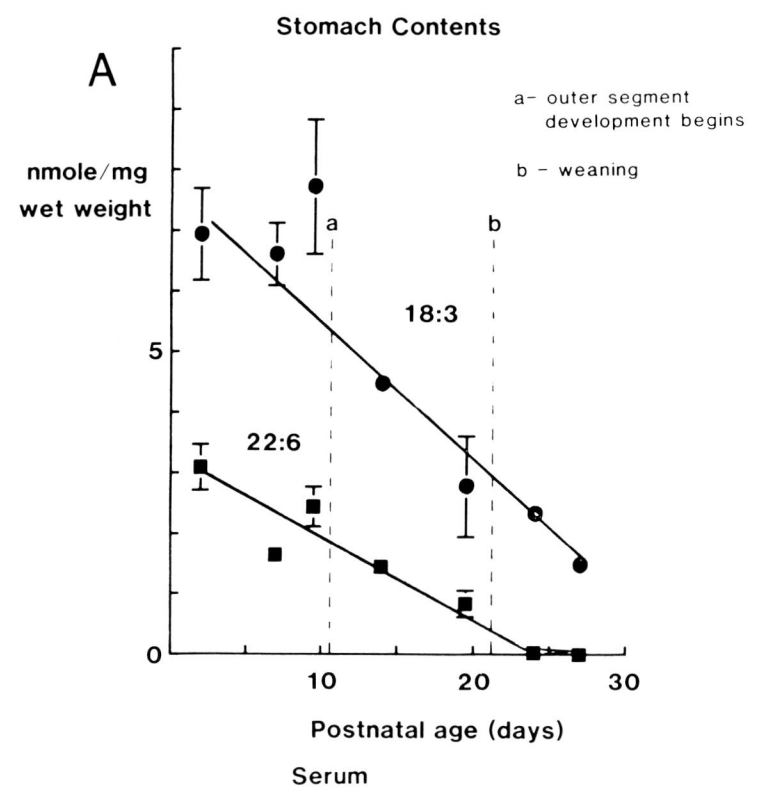

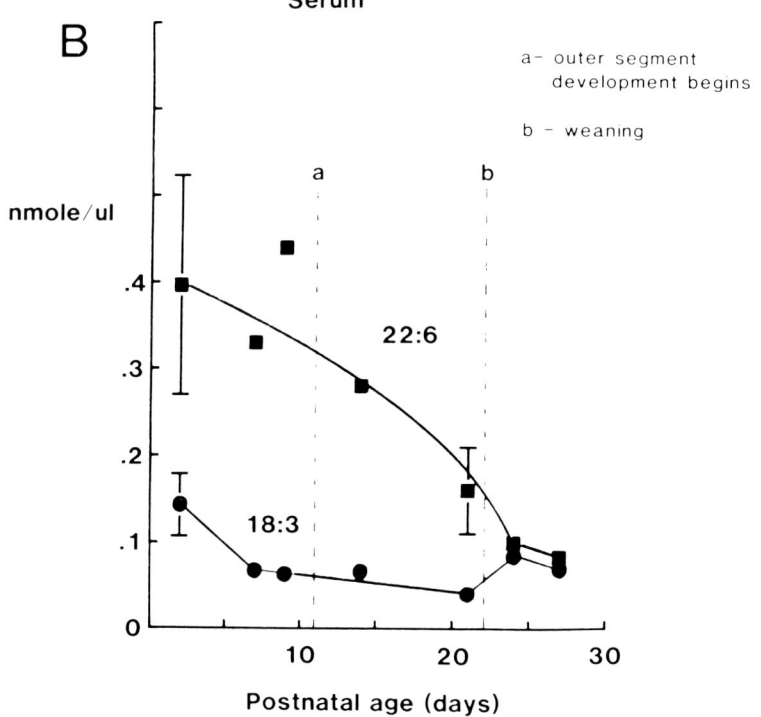

Stomach Contents

A

nmole/mg wet weight

a – outer segment development begins
b – weaning

18:3

22:6

Postnatal age (days)

Serum

B

nmole/ul

a – outer segment development begins
b – weaning

22:6

18:3

Postnatal age (days)

an elongating and desaturating system is very active, and at the same time, that the end-product, DHA, is secreted into the blood stream. The content of DHA decreases in serum as a function of postnatal development in an inverse correlation with synaptogenesis and photoreceptor membrane biogenesis (Fig. 3).

To trace the interorgan pathways of n-3 fatty acids, 3 day old mouse pups were injected with radiolabeled 18:3. An initial build-up of radioactivity was observed in the liver, followed by rapid DHA synthesis. In Fig. 4, it is shown that no labeled 18:3 is detected in brain and retina, and the conversion of 18:3 to DHA in liver is illustrated as a function of time. From 24 to 72 hours after injection, increased amounts of newly synthesized DHA appeared esterified in phospholipids, amounting to more than 50% of the total radioactivity (this also includes some 22:5, but no 18:3). Labeling in the liver and serum declined simultaneously, with a well-defined shift from 18:3 to DHA. Therefore, the liver, after elongation and desaturation of 18:3, utilizes DHA for the synthesis of phospholipids, which in turn are secreted into the blood stream in the form of lipoproteins. Triacylglycerols containing radiolabeled DHA are also made in the liver and appear in the blood stream (11). These

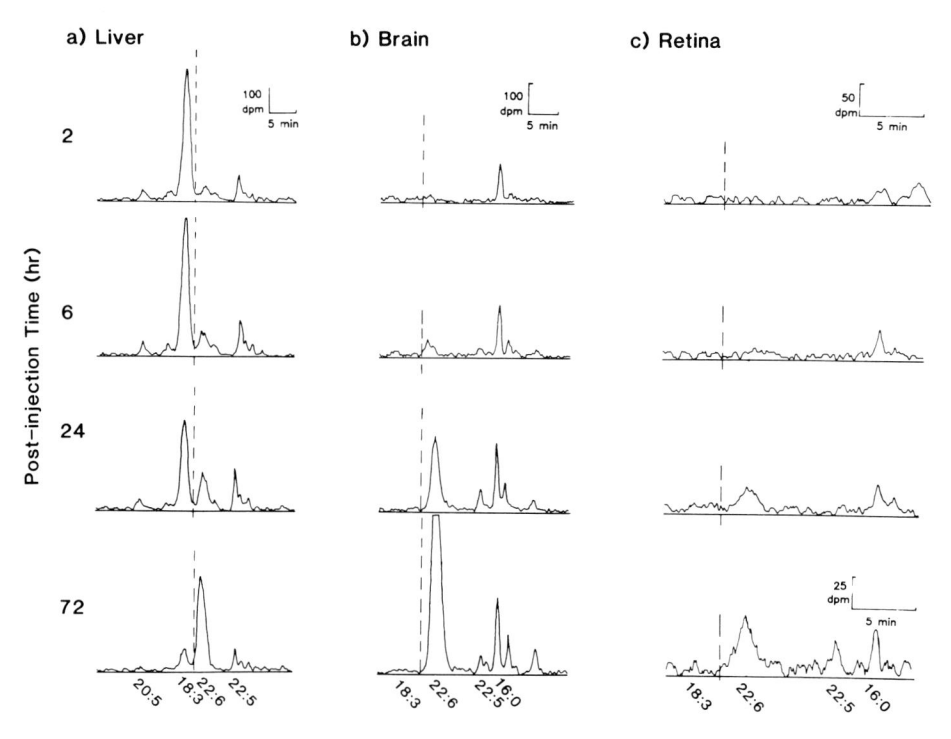

FIG. 4. *In vivo* metabolism and uptake of n-3 fatty acids in liver, brain, and retina of 3 day old mouse pups. Reverse-phase HPLC of radiolabeled fatty acids was performed at different times after intraperitoneal injection of 1-^{14}C-18:3. The total dpm of fatty acids injected into the HPLC column ranged from 12,000 to 17,500 for liver, 3,300 to 22,000 for brain, and 810 to 4,020 for retina. From Scott BL and Bazan NG (11).

carriers of DHA are likely to be the ones that finally provide DHA to brain and retina, since most of the injected radiolabeled 18:3 does not go directly to these tissues. Therefore, during early development, carrier molecules containing DHA are present in the blood stream.

Since most of the circulating DHA-containing molecules are taken up by brain and retina, a trapping mechanism or receptor system may operate in those tissues. In fact, an apolipoprotein E low density lipoprotein (LDL) receptor has been found in developing photoreceptor cells, apparently for the binding and internalization of lipoproteins carrying DHA-containing phospholipids (12). The neural microvasculature and glial cells, such as Müller cells in the retina, may also participate in the uptake of DHA (13). Once the DHA-containing lipid has been internalized, any free DHA generated by subsequent degradation within the cell is retained by an active, low-K_m docosahexaenoyl-coenzyme A synthetase. The product of this enzyme's activity in turn proceeds to an acyltransferase that incorporates the fatty acid into a phospholipid. Docosahexaenoyl-coenzyme A synthetase may therefore function as an intracellular trapping mechanism for DHA, just as sugar phosphorylation by hexokinase retains monosaccharides within cells. Docosahexaenoyl-coenzyme A synthetase also shows a developmental pattern coincident with the arrival and utilization of DHA (14). Moreover, synaptic membranes (15), retinal pigment epithelial cells, and retinas from experimental animals and humans (16) display this enzyme activity. A very high avidity for the uptake of DHA by photoreceptor cells has also been shown in adults of several animal species. Fig. 5 illustrates the cellular distribution in frog and human retinas.

DIETARY SUPPLY OF DHA: INTERORGAN METABOLISM AND CELLULAR UPTAKE AND TRAFFICKING

The requirements for n-3 polyunsaturated fatty acids of the central nervous system have been highlighted by recent studies showing functional impairment of visual acuity in nonhuman primates when dietary deprivation occurs during intrauterine life and after birth (7,17–19). Therefore the selective accumulation of DHA in photoreceptor membranes during development must have an important physiological significance in primates. Although the relationship between brain function and the DHA of neural membranes, such as synaptic membranes, is not as clear as in retina, the work of Lamptey and Walker (20) suggests that learning impairments do occur in 18:3 deficiencies.

Our own work discussed in this chapter aims to understand the dietary supply of essential polyunsaturated fatty acids to the developing retina and, more specifically, to the developing photoreceptor cells. After ingestion, most of the 18:3 is taken up by the liver and rapidly elongated and desaturated. During the postnatal development of the mouse the DHA content is far higher than the 18:3 content in blood serum whereas the opposite is true for stomach contents (Fig. 3), supporting the suggestion that a massive activation of the 18:3 pathway toward DHA synthesis takes place

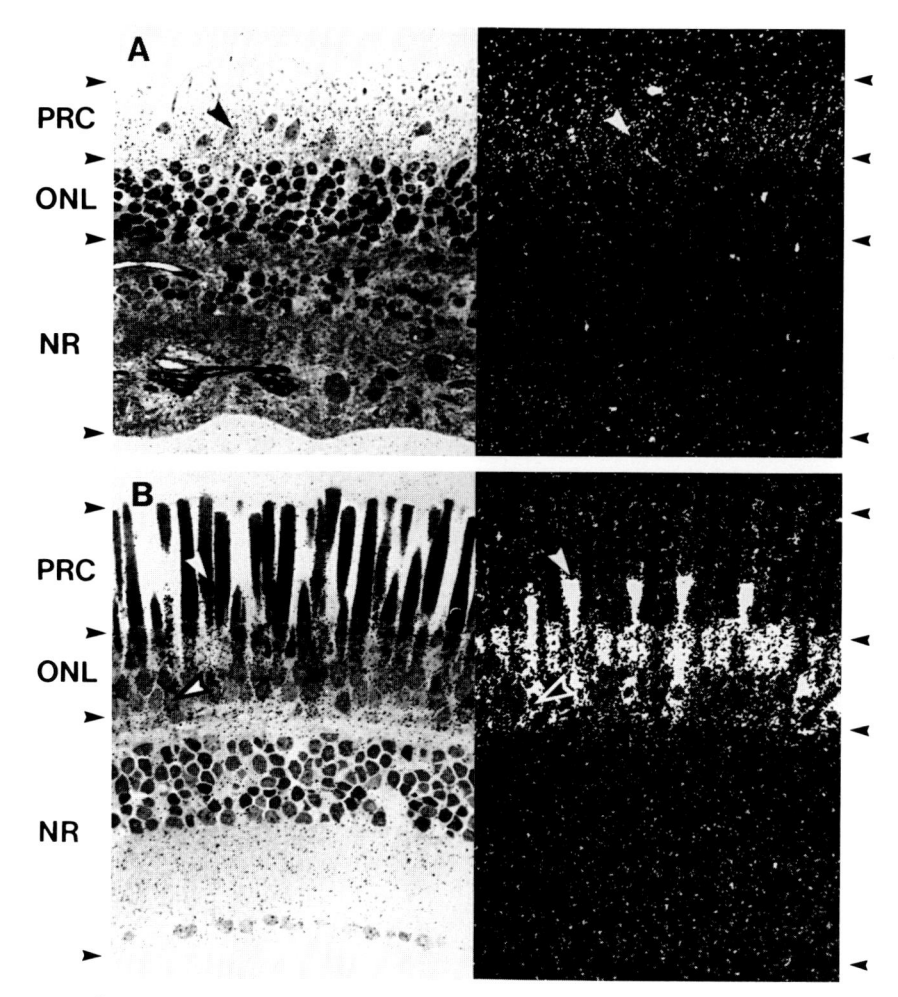

FIG. 5. ^{3}H-DHA autoradiography of retinas showing preferential uptake in photoreceptor cells. *Left,* bright-field microscopy; *right,* dark-field microscopy of the same section. **A:** Autoradiography of a human retina biopsy tissue showing selective uptake of ^{3}H-DHA in inner segments of photoreceptor cells. **B:** Autoradiography of a frog (*Rana pipiens*) retina showing the high avidity of fatty acid uptake by photoreceptor cells. Solid arrow in A indicates a cone photoreceptor inner segment. Solid arrow in B indicates a heavily labeled 435-rod cell inner segment. Outlined arrow in B indicates a 435-rod cell nucleus with well-labeled perinuclear cytoplasm. NR, neural retina; ONL, outer nuclear layer; PRC, photoreceptor cells.

and that most of this end-product is available in the blood stream. Figure 6 presents an outline of the supply, interorgan relationship, and interstitial and cellular trafficking of DHA. The supply seems to be linked to an interorgan distribution in which the liver plays a central role (11). It is likely that the liver acylates DHA, predominantly in phospholipids, and assembles lipoproteins, which, once secreted, are

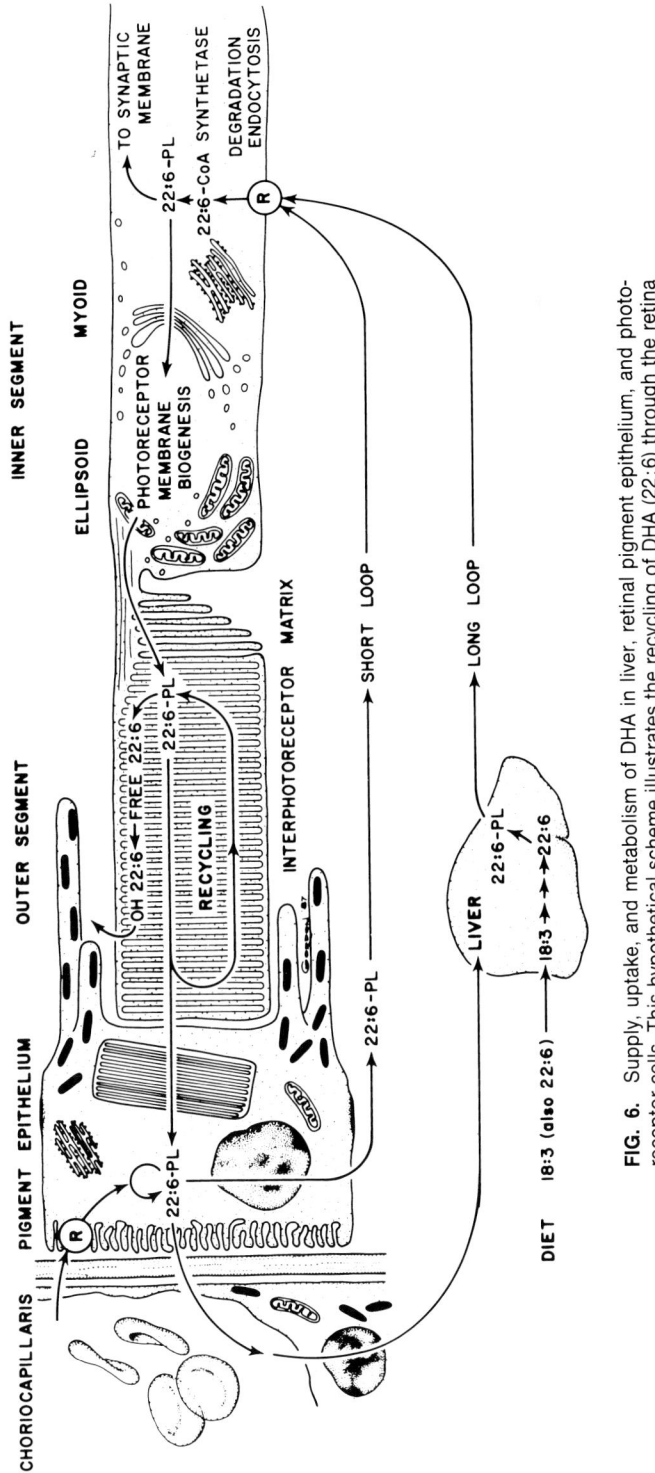

FIG. 6. Supply, uptake, and metabolism of DHA in liver, retinal pigment epithelium, and photoreceptor cells. This hypothetical scheme illustrates the recycling of DHA (22:6) through the retina during photoreceptor renewal, both by way of a short loop through the inner segment, as well as by a long loop through the liver. From Bazan NG (21).

distributed through the blood stream. Some DHA may be formed by retina and brain by direct uptake of precursors (e.g., 18:3).

This brings us to the issue of DHA uptake by different tissues. Since there is an uneven distribution in the content of DHA among different tissues, it is conceivable that some of them express relatively more abundant mechanisms for DHA uptake. The organ and cellular uptake mechanisms are not well understood. Glial cells, such as the Müller cells in the retina, may be involved in transient retention during DHA handling in the interstitial space (13). In the space surrounding photoreceptor cells (interphotoreceptor matrix) interphotoreceptor retinoid-binding protein and other as-yet-unidentified proteins contain endogenous noncovalently bound DHA (22). Intercellular trafficking of molecules occurs through this interstitial space, particularly nutrients arriving through the choriocapillaris beneath the retinal pigment epithelium. In frogs *in vivo* DHA arrives by this route at the photoreceptor cells (13). The retinal pigment epithelial cells, along with the photoreceptors, form a boundary that takes up DHA preferentially from the bloodstream (6,13,21) (Fig. 6).

The chemical form of the fatty acid arriving at the retina and brain is not clearly defined. Most of the DHA seems to be esterified as phospholipids in the blood stream (11). However, once it arrives at the interphotoreceptor space it is unknown whether the DHA is released from the phospholipids by the retinal pigment epithelial cells or whether other cells (e.g., the Müller cells) take up DHA or the DHA-containing lipid and assemble it into a lipoprotein form to be released into the interstitial space prior to its uptake by the inner segments of the photoreceptor cells (12). Apolipoprotein E is synthesized in glial cells (23), is a component of the interstitial space (24), and has been detected in cerebrospinal fluid (25,26). Therefore, apolipoprotein E may be secreted to the interphotoreceptor matrix as a lipoprotein containing DHA-bearing lipids, with the purpose of efficient cellular uptake through an LDL receptor-mediated process (12).

Because the photoreceptor cells undergo an active daily renewal process of their outer segments (membrane discs enriched in DHA-containing phospholipids) through shedding and phagocytosis by the retinal pigment epithelium (27), certain routes for the retrieval of DHA may operate. Two possible retrieval routes, a short and a long loop, are depicted in Fig. 6. The short loop involves the components of the interstitial space described above. The long loop illustrates the possibility that DHA is recycled back into the retina through the blood stream.

In conclusion, the interorgan relationship, the interstitial DHA handling, and the cellular uptake and trafficking provide the basis for the efficient supply of n-3 fatty acids during critical periods of development. DHA is accumulated during photoreceptor cell differentiation and synaptogenesis subsequent to the deposition of arachidonic acid (from the n-6 fatty acid family). DHA, and not 18:3, is preferentially taken up by the developing retina. Moreover, the liver plays a central role in supporting the biogenesis of visual cells and synaptic activity in brain and retina. The interorgan metabolism and uptake of DHA are likely also to operate throughout life, ensuring the supply of this essential fatty acid. Diseases that disrupt these cycles may be involved in the pathogenesis of disorders such as retinal degenerations (28).

ACKNOWLEDGMENTS

The work described in this paper that was performed in the author's laboratory was supported by United States Public Health Service Grant EY04428 from the National Eye Institute, National Institutes of Health, Bethesda, Maryland. The author is the Ernest C. and Yvette C. Villere Professor of Ophthalmology, and holds a Jacob Javits Neuroscience Investigator Award (NS23002) from the National Institute of Neurological Diseases and Stroke.

REFERENCES

1. Aveldaño MI. A novel group of very long chain polyenoic fatty acids in dipolyunsaturated phosphatidylcholines from vertebrate retina. *J Biol Chem* 1987; 262: 1172–9.
2. Aveldaño MI. Phospholipid species containing long and very long polyenoic fatty acids remain with rhodopsin after hexane extraction of photoreceptor membranes. *Biochemistry* 1988; 27: 1229–39.
3. Aveldaño de Caldironi MI, Bazan NG. Acyl groups, molecular species, and labeling by ^{14}C-glycerol and ^{3}H-arachidonic acid of vertebrate retina glycerolipids. *Adv Exp Med Biol* 1977; 83: 397–404.
4. Aveldaño de Caldironi MI, Bazan NG. Composition and biosynthesis of molecular species of retina phosphoglycerides. *Neurochem Int* 1980; 1: 381–92.
5. Aveldaño MI, Pasquare de Garcia SJ, Bazan NG. Biosynthesis of molecular species of inositol, choline, serine, and ethanolamine glycerophospholipids in the bovine retina. *J Lipid Res* 1983; 24: 628–38.
6. Bazan NG. Supply of n-3 polyunsaturated fatty acids and their significance in the central nervous system. In: Wurtman RJ, Wurtman JJ, eds. *Nutrition and the brain*, vol 8. New York: Raven Press Ltd; 1990: 1–24.
7. Neuringer M, Connor WE, Van Petten C, Barstad L. Dietary omega-3 fatty acid deficiency and visual loss in infant rhesus monkeys. *J Clin Invest* 1984; 73: 272–6.
8. Clandinin MT, Chappell JE, Heim T, Swyer PR, Chance GW. Fatty acid accretion in fetal and neonatal liver: implications for fatty acid requirements. *Early Hum Dev* 1981; 5: 1–6.
9. Galli C, Simopoulos AP, eds. *Dietary ω3 and ω6 fatty acids: biological effects and nutritional essentiality*. New York: Plenum; 1989.
10. Scott BL, Racz E, Lolley RN, Bazan NG. Developing rod photoreceptors from normal and mutant rd mouse retinas: altered fatty acid composition early in development of the mutant. *J Neurosci Res* 1988; 20: 202–11.
11. Scott BL, Bazan NG. Membrane docosahexaenoate is supplied to the developing brain and retina by the liver. *Proc Natl Acad Sci USA* 1989; 86: 2903–7.
12. Bazan NG, Cai F. Internalization of apolipoprotein E (APO E) in rod photoreceptor cells by a low-density lipoprotein receptor. *Suppl Invest Ophthalmol Vis Sci* 1990; 31: 471.
13. Gordon WC, Bazan NG. Docosahexaenoic acid utilization during rod photoreceptor cell renewal. *J Neurosci* 1990; 10: 2190–204.
14. Reddy TS, Bazan NG. Long-chain acyl coenzyme A synthetase activity during the postnatal development of the mouse brain. *Int J Dev Neurosci* 1984; 2: 447–50.
15. Reddy TS, Bazan NG. Synthesis of arachidonoyl coenzyme A and docosahexaenoyl coenzyme A in synaptic plasma membranes of cerebrum, cerebellum, and brain stem of rat brain. *J Neurosci Res* 1985; 13: 381–90.
16. Reddy TS, Bazan NG. Synthesis of docosahexaenoyl-, arachidonoyl-, and palmitoyl-coenzyme A in ocular tissues. *Exp Eye Res* 1985; 41: 87–95.
17. Neuringer M, Connor WE, Luck SJ. Suppression of ERG amplitude by repetitive stimulation in rhesus monkeys deficient in retinal docosahexaenoic acid. *Suppl Invest Ophthalmol Vis Sci* 1985; 26: 31.
18. Neuringer M, Connor WE. N-3 fatty acids in the brain and retina: evidence for their essentiality. *Nutr Rev* 1986; 44: 285–94.
19. Neuringer M, Connor WE, Lin DS, Barstad L, Luck SJ. Biochemical and functional effects of prenatal

and postnatal omega-3 fatty acid deficiency on retina and brain in rhesus monkeys. *Proc Natl Acad Sci USA* 1986; 83: 4021–5.
20. Lamptey MS, Walker BL. A possible essential role for dietary linolenic acid in the development of the young rat. *J Nutr* 1976; 10: 86–93.
21. Bazan NG. The identification of a new biochemical alteration early in the differentiation of visual cells in inherited retinal degeneration. In: Hollyfield J *et al.*, eds. *Inherited and environmentally induced retinal degenerations*. New York: Alan R. Liss; 1989: 191–215.
22. Bazan NG, Reddy TS, Redmond TM, Wiggert B, Chader GJ. Endogenous fatty acids are covalently and noncovalently bound to interphotoreceptor retinoid-binding protein in the monkey retina. *J Biol Chem* 1985; 260: 13677–80.
23. Pitas RE, Boyles JK, Lee SH, Foss D, Mahley RW. Astrocytes synthesize apolipoprotein E and metabolize apolipoprotein E-containing lipoproteins. *Biochim Biophys Acta* 1987; 917: 148–61.
24. Sloop CH, Dory L, Roheim PS. Interstitial fluid lipoproteins. *J Lipid Res* 1987; 28: 225–37.
25. Roheim P, Carey M, Forte T, Vega G. Apolipoprotein in human cerebrospinal fluid. *Proc Natl Acad Sci USA* 1979; 76: 4646–9.
26. Pitas RE, Boyles JK, Lee SH, Hui D, Weisgraber KH. Lipoproteins and their receptors in the central nervous system. *J Biol Chem* 1987; 262: 14352–60.
27. Bok D. Retinal photoreceptor-pigment epithelium interactions. *Invest Ophthalmol Vis Sci* 1985; 26: 1659–94.
28. Bazan NG, Scott BL, Reddy TS, Pelias MZ. Decreased content of docosahexaenoate and arachidonate in plasma phospholipids in Usher's syndrome. *Biochem Biophys Res Commun* 1986; 141: 600–4.

DISCUSSION

Dr. Deckelbaum: Vitamin E deficiency is associated with irreversible changes in retinal function and retinal degeneration. Is there any interaction between vitamin E and DHA in this process, and is DHA deficiency reversible in terms of restoring function?

Dr. Bazan: There is an important role for vitamin E, particularly in photoreceptor cells and in the synapses. There are high concentrations of vitamin E in photoreceptor membranes and we understand little about how they are maintained and how these concentrations protect DHA. It is likely that the protection is through antioxidation. It has been shown that vitamin E exerts well-defined protective effects on light-induced retinal damage.

Dr. Heim: You mentioned a close relationship between β receptor function in the retinal rhodopsin and DHA metabolism. Could you elaborate on this?

Dr. Bazan: Rhodopsin belongs to the same superfamily as the β adrenergic receptor. It is surrounded by docosahexaenoyl phospholipids in a unique environment. During rod outer segment renewal newly synthesized rhodopsin moves along with these phospholipids. Although DHA is mainly in the central nervous system it is also present in other plasma membranes in much smaller concentrations. Perhaps it has unique interactions with certain receptors.

Dr. Jeremy: You mentioned that DHA accumulates in the testes. Why is this?

Dr. Bazan: The concentrations in the testes are far higher than in other nonneuronal tissues, far lower than in brain and retina. In Usher syndrome there is decreased sperm mobility as well as abnormalities in the connecting cilium. Photoreceptor cells and hair cells in the inner ear degenerate. These cells also contain a connecting cilium. Usher's patients are deaf at birth and become blind early in life due to retinitis pigmentosa. Therefore at least three types of ciliated cells are affected in that disease. The function of DHA in the testis is not known.

Dr. Cunnane: Space-occupying models suggest that phosphatidylcholines with 16:0 and 16:1 occupy the same amount of space as those with 16:0 and 22:6. Why then does 22:6

have a unique role in the rat? What is it doing if it occupies the same space as a fairly easily synthesized phosphatidylcholine?

Dr. Bazan: Phosphatidylcholine with 22:6 interacts intimately with rhodopsin and these highly unsaturated phosphatidylcholines move along with rhodopsin during photoreceptor cell renewal, traveling along the outer segment of the visual cells. These experiments were done by autoradiography, comparing ^{3}H-leucine with ^{3}H-DHA in frogs. From a biophysical point of view it is an interesting question how DHA may be distributed and what might be the consequences for rhodopsin behavior.

Dr. Deckelbaum: What is the evidence that lipid uptake in the retina is by an apolipoprotein E (apo E) receptor?

Dr. Bazan: A receptor-mediated uptake of lipids by photoreceptor cells and retina does operate and apo E is a specific ligand for internalization; 22:6 phospholipids can be internalized by such a route. We performed binding, internalization, and degradation assays in 10 day old mouse retina, as well as in photoreceptor cells dissociated from retinas of the same age. We did saturation curves as well as competition studies with high-density lipoprotein (HDL) and LDL and they don't compete for iodinated apo E/DMPC internalization. However, apo E/DMPC competes with the uptake. The reason that most of the data are for internalization is that intact retinas are incubated and then at the end of the experiment photoreceptor cells are dissociated with pronase. This proteolytic enzyme may hydrolyze surface receptors and therefore under these conditions we cannot deal with specific binding. Our data for binding are only for intact retinas. In subsequent experiments we loaded ^{3}H-labeled 22:6-containing phospholipids instead of apo E and we showed that most of them end up in the photoreceptors. Proteins of the interphotoreceptor matrix in monkey retinas contain DHA bound to interphotoreceptor retinoid-binding protein. The delivery of free fatty acid to the photoreceptor cell may be mediated through proteins of this kind. So endocytosis of lipids by retinal cells may be through an apo E mechanism, and perhaps this mechanism is also involved in delivery of cholesterol.

Long Chain Polyunsaturated Fatty Acids in the Diets of Premature Infants

Berthold Koletzko

Kinderpoliklinik der Ludwig-Maximilians-Universität, D-W-8000 Munich 2, Germany

In the past, guidelines on the feeding of premature infants have recommended a dietary supply of linoleic and partly also of α linolenic acid but not of any other essential fatty acids (1–3). These recommendations are based on the assumption that preterm infants can effectively transform linoleic and α linolenic acids into long chain polyunsaturated fatty acids (LCPUFA) by microsomal desaturation and chain elongation (Fig. 1), and that the activity of this metabolic pathway is sufficient to meet their LCPUFA requirements fully. However, results of more recent investigation raise questions as to the validity of this concept.

During perinatal development, the fetus and newborn infant require relatively large amounts of LCPUFA with 20–22 carbon atoms and two to six double bonds, such as arachidonic (20:4n-6) and docosahexaenoic (22:6n-3) acids. LCPUFA both of the Ω-6 (n-6) and of the Ω-3 (n-3) series are essential precursors for the synthesis of prostaglandins and other eicosanoids which are potent regulators of various physiological processes during early life. Moreover, LCPUFA are indispensable components of structural lipids in membrane systems of all organs. The extent of LCPUFA incorporation into membrane phospholipids in growing tissues is of great importance for a number of membrane functions, such as their fluidity and permeability, the activity of membrane-bound receptors and enzymes, and the electrical response to excitation (4).

Brain and retina lipids of the newborn infant are particularly rich in LCPUFA, primarily arachidonic and docosahexaenoic acids, whereas they contain only very minor concentrations of linoleic and α linolenic acids (5,6). During intrauterine development, significant amounts of n-6 and n-3 LCPUFA have to be incorporated into the lipid-rich brain, the weight of which increases more than fivefold between the 24th and the 40th week of gestation. The extent of early n-3 LCPUFA accretion in neural tissues is closely related to the development of visual acuity, and possibly also of discrimination learning, in infant rats and rhesus monkeys (7–9). Similar functional effects can be documented in man. The development of visual function in premature infants correlates with n-3 LCPUFA content in plasma and red blood cell lipids (10,11). Although the significance of n-3 LCPUFA accretion must be

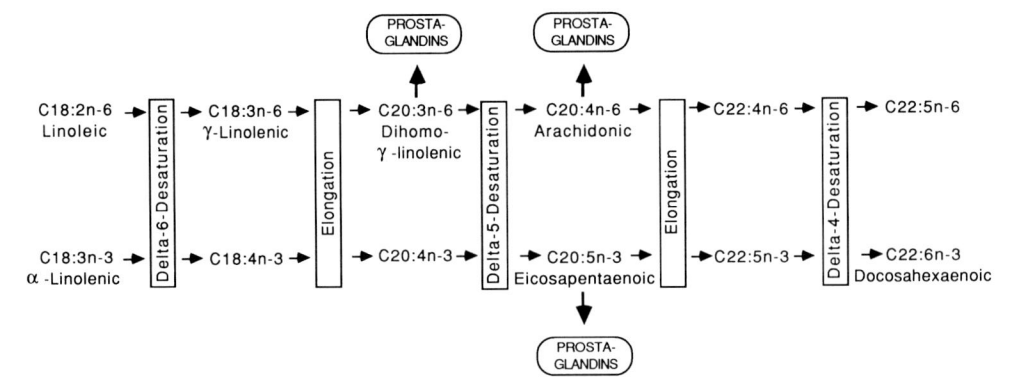

```
C18:2n-6  →[Δ6-Desat]→ C18:3n-6  →[Elong]→ C20:3n-6  →[Δ5-Desat]→ C20:4n-6  →[Elong]→ C22:4n-6  →[Δ4-Desat]→ C22:5n-6
Linoleic              γ-Linolenic           Dihomo-                Arachidonic
                                            γ-linolenic
                                                      ↑PROSTAGLANDINS   ↑PROSTAGLANDINS

C18:3n-3  →[Δ6-Desat]→ C18:4n-3  →[Elong]→ C20:4n-3  →[Δ5-Desat]→ C20:5n-3  →[Elong]→ C22:5n-3  →[Δ4-Desat]→ C22:6n-3
α-Linolenic                                                       Eicosapentaenoic                          Docosahexaenoic
                                                                            ↓PROSTAGLANDINS
```

FIG. 1. Major pathways for the synthesis of long chain polyunsaturated fatty acids from linoleic (Ω-6 series) and α linolenic (Ω-3 series) acids. Fatty acids from both series compete for the same microsomal enzyme system. From Koletzko B, et al. (32).

emphasized, it should be remembered that in newborn infants the concentration of n-6 LCPUFA is twofold higher than that of n-3 LCPUFA in brain (5) and 1.3-fold higher in retina (12). The functional roles of n-6 LCPUFA have not yet been fully elucidated but there are indications that their availability is related to tissue growth. We found a significant positive correlation ($r = 0.47$, $p = 0.01$) of arachidonic acid status, but not of linoleic or any Ω-3 fatty acid, with body weight in a group of premature infants (13). Arachidonic acid may have a growth-promoting activity in the human fetus and infant, and its reduction in infants with essential fatty acid deficiency might actually be the causative factor for the growth failure developing in those infants (14).

IS THE CAPACITY FOR LCP BIOSYNTHESIS LOW IN THE HUMAN NEONATE?

The ability to synthesize the physiologically important LCPUFA from the precursors seems to be rather limited in the human neonate, as is apparent from investigations on the essential fatty acid metabolism in parenterally fed infants. In a study performed in collaboration with Dr. R. Filler and Dr. T. Heim at the Hospital for Sick Children, Toronto, the composition of plasma lipoproteins was analyzed in 17 newborn infants with a mean birthweight of 3,126 g and a mean gestational age of 39.4 weeks who required parenteral feeding after neonatal surgery (15,16). All infants were studied first after 4.9 ± 1.6 days (mean $\pm$ SD) of intravenous administration of glucose and amino acids (mean doses 10.9 and 1.5 g/kg·day, respectively) and again after 5.5 ± 2.5 days of total parenteral nutrition with glucose, amino acids, and a soybean oil emulsion (mean doses 13.5, 2.8, and 2.2 g/kg·day, respectively). The lipid emulsion used contained 52% linoleic and 7% α linolenic acids but only minor amounts of LCPUFA. During parenteral feeding, conclusions on the infantile hepatic metabolism of infused essential fatty acids can be drawn from the study of high density lipoprotein (HDL) composition. Therefore, Fig. 2 shows the proportions of the major Ω-6 and Ω-3 fatty acids in the HDL lipid classes of the infants studied. We found that absolute concentrations of HDL lipids did not differ between the two phases of the study, but their fatty acid pattern changed markedly. After lipid infusion, linoleic and α linolenic acids showed a striking increase in all lipid classes, which demonstrates the avid incorporation of infused essential fatty acids into HDL lipids. In contrast, arachidonic acid as the principal linoleic acid metabolite did not increase but showed a decreasing trend, with a significant reduction in HDL phospholipids (Fig. 2). Similarly, there was no increase of HDL docosahexaenoic acid, which was also supplied in small amounts with the infusate. The infants obviously had a quite limited capacity to convert the infused precursor fatty acids to LCP.

INTRAUTERINE LCP SUPPLY

When considering different options for the feeding of premature infants, it is worthwhile to recapitulate the biological models of perinatal nutrient supply. During intrauterine life, the human fetus apparently does not require an active synthesis pathway for LCP, because they are supplied by the placenta. We studied the plasma lipid composition of 30 pairs of neonates born at term (gestational age 40.1 ± 1.2 weeks, birthweight 3,501 ± 326 g; mean ± SD) and their mothers at the time of delivery (17). Mean percentage levels of both linoleic and α linolenic acids in cord plasma lipids were less than half of the maternal ones (Table 1). In contrast, LCP such as dihomo-γ-linolenic, arachidonic, and docosahexaenoic acids contributed a much larger proportion to cord than to maternal plasma lipids. Although the

TABLE 1. *Major essential fatty acids in plasma lipids of 30 pairs of mothers and their newborn infants at the time of birth (% wt/wt, mean ± SE)*

	Maternal plasma	Cord plasma	p
Ω-6 fatty acids			
Linoleic (18:2n-6)	23.6 ± 0.6	10.0 ± 0.4	<0.0001
Dihomo-γ-linolenic (20:3n-6)	1.6 ± 0.1	2.7 ± 0.1	<0.0001
Arachidonic (20:4n-6)	5.7 ± 0.2	12.1 ± 0.4	<0.0001
Total n-6 LCP	7.8 ± 0.3	15.6 ± 0.5	<0.0001
Ω-3 fatty acids			
α-Linolenic (18:3n-3)	0.6 ± 0.1	0.3 ± 0.1	<0.05
Docosahexaenoic (22:6n-3)	2.4 ± 0.1	3.6 ± 0.2	<0.0001
Total n-3 LCP	2.7 ± 0.1	3.8 ± 0.2	<0.0001
Sums and ratios			
Total essential fatty acids	34.8 ± 0.6	29.9 ± 0.6	<0.0001
Total LCPUFA	10.5 ± 0.4	19.4 ± 0.6	<0.0001
Ratio n-6/n-3 LCP	3.0 ± 0.1	4.3 ± 0.2	<0.0001

Adapted from Koletzko B and Müller J (17).

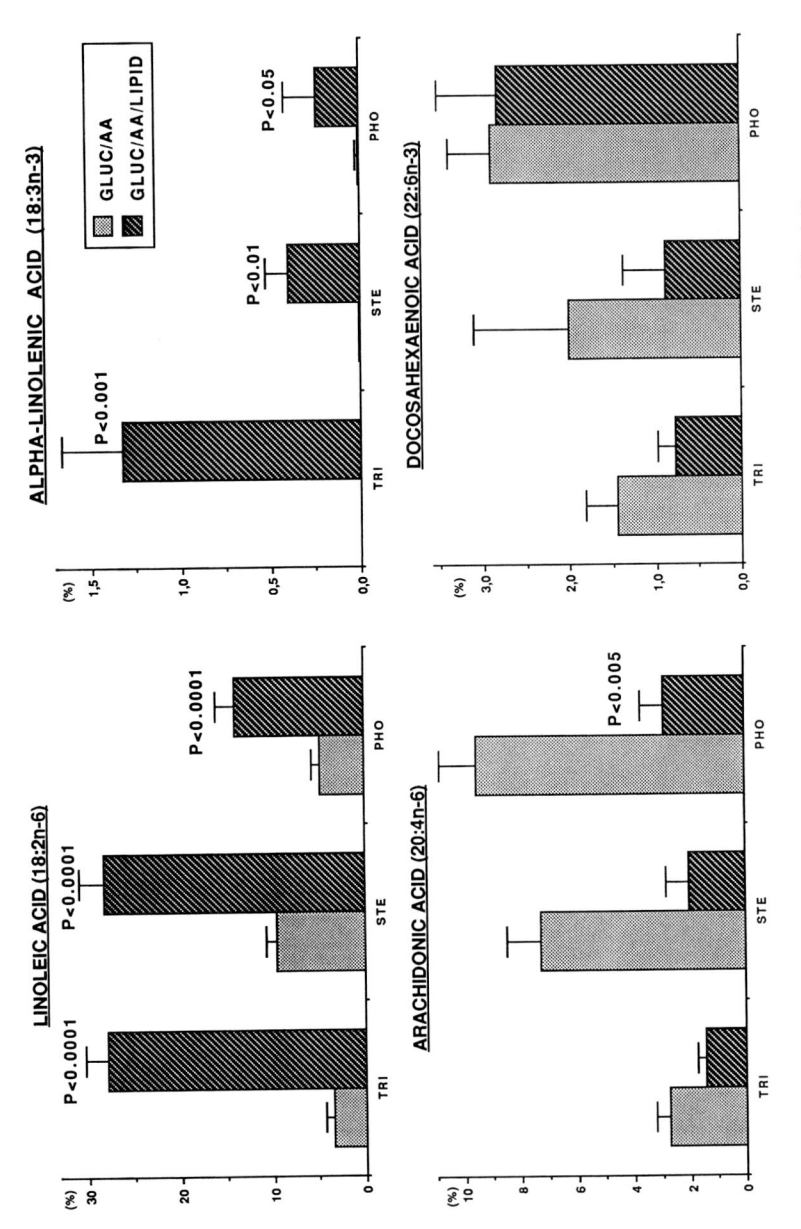

FIG. 2. Major essential fatty acids in high density lipoprotein lipids (% wt/wt, means ± SE) of 17 newborn infants during parenteral nutrition with glucose/amino acids (GLUC/AA) and after the addition of an intravenous lipid emulsion (GLUC/AA/LIPID). The addition of lipids to the infusate led to a marked increase of linoleic and α linolenic acids, indicating the avid incorporation of the infused essential fatty acids into endogenously synthesized lipids. In contrast, their major LCP metabolites did not increase as a result of a limited capacity for LCP biosynthesis (for details see text).

proportion of total essential fatty acids was lower in the infants, the contribution of total LCP was almost twice as high as in the mothers. These data suggest a selective and preferential maternofetal transfer of LCP. It appears possible that the transfer mechanisms involved discriminate between n-6 and n-3 LCP and, thereby cause the significant increase of the n-6/n-3 LCP ratio from maternal to cord plasma lipids found in our study (Table 1).

POSTNATAL LCP INTAKE OF THE BREAST-FED AND THE FORMULA-FED INFANT

Even after birth, infants fed human milk seem not to require an active synthesis pathway. Human milk contains significant amounts of LCP and provides a generous supply as compared to the calculated LCP requirements for postnatal tissue accretion (18). A breast-fed infant consuming 175 ml milk/kg bodyweight per day with a mean fat content of 35 g/l and an average fatty acid composition (19) gets not only 660 mg linoleic and 50 mg α linolenic acid per kg bodyweight per day, but also 70 mg n-6 LCP and 33 mg n-3 LCP (20). It is of interest that the n-6/n-3 LCP ratio in human milk of about 2 is similar to that in neonatal brain lipids. Moreover, there is a correlation of n-6 and n-3 LCP in human milk lipids (Fig. 3) which provides the infant with a relatively constant dietary n-6/n-3 LCP ratio and may represent a protective mechanism to prevent an unbalanced ratio of these biologically potent compounds in infantile tissues (19).

Unlike human milk, currently available infant formulas are devoid of LCP if their fat body is composed solely of vegetable oils, or they contain only very minor amounts of LCP if butterfat is used for their production. We could not detect any docosahexaenoic acid in 25 infant formulas sold in Germany, while nine products contained very small concentrations of arachidonic acid (median value 0.06% of total fatty acids in these nine formulas) (21).

When such conventional formulas supplying linoleic and α linolenic acids as the only essential fatty acids are fed to premature infants, n-6 and n-3 LCP content of plasma and membrane phospholipids decrease rapidly to levels significantly lower than in babies fed human milk (22–25). In view of the important structural and functional roles of LCP, a dietary supplementation with metabolites of the classical essential fatty acids appears desirable for these babies.

SHOULD WE SUPPLEMENT FISH OILS TO FORMULA-FED PREMATURE INFANTS?

It has been proposed that the essential fatty acid status of formula-fed premature infants could be improved by adding fish oils to the diet (10,26). This strategy is effective with respect to increasing the content of docosahexaenoic acids in phospholipids and improving visual function (10,11,26). However, its reported side effects are a concomitant marked increase of eicosapentaenoic acid, which is usually found

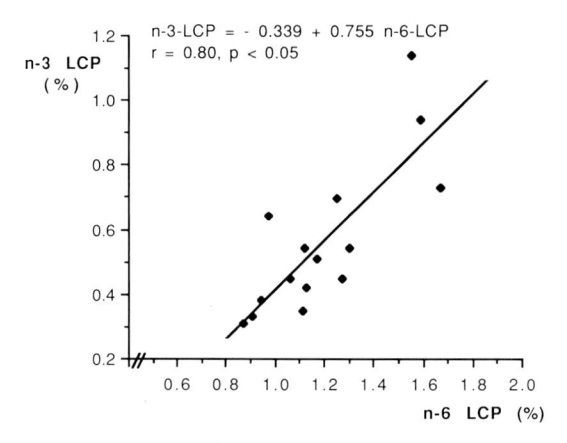

FIG. 3. Correlation of n-6 and n-3 LCP in lipids of mature human milk, resulting in a relatively constant dietary n-6/n-3 LCP ratio for the breast-fed infant. Reproduced in modified form from Koletzko B, et al. (19).

only at very minor concentrations in human milk and infantile tissues, and a significant reduction of n-6 LCP values (10,11,26). Fatty acids of the n-3 and n-6 series compete for binding to microsomal enzymes and incorporation into structural lipids, differ in biological effects, and are certainly not interchangeable. In a number of cases, n-6 and n-3 LCP are physiologic antagonists; therefore an unbalanced ratio may have untoward effects for the preterm infant. For example, arachidonic acid (20:4n-6) enhances platelet aggregation and vasoconstriction in man, while eicosapentaenoic acid (20:5n-3) has the opposite effects (27). An excess of eicosapentaenoic acid over arachidonic acid can cause bleeding in children, as recently observed in eight of 11 pediatric patients treated with fish oil capsules for hyperlipidemia (28), and it might carry very serious risks for low birthweight infants that are already prone to intracranial hemorrhage. Moreover, a high n-3/n-6 LCP ratio impairs the synthesis of prostaglandin E (29) and also has strong anti-inflammatory effects with a suppression of neutrophil functions such as chemotaxis (30,31); thereby it might increase the risk for infections, which is already extremely high in premature babies.

ENRICHMENT OF THE PREMATURE INFANT DIET WITH BOTH Ω-6 AND Ω-3 LCP

As a novel and in our opinion more physiologic approach to improve the essential fatty acid status of premature infants, we chose to try for the first time a formula enriched with LCP both of the n-6 and the n-3 series. The effects of this experimental formula on plasma lipid composition were compared with those of human milk and a conventional formula without LCP in a controlled feeding trial (32). Twenty-nine premature babies with a birthweight $\geq$1,300 g (1,700 $\pm$ 127 g; mean $\pm$ SD) and a gestational age of 33.6 $\pm$ 1.4 weeks were enrolled. All patients were in good clinical

TABLE 2. *Essential fatty acid composition (% wt/wt) of human milk, conventional infant formula, and an experimental LCP-enriched formula used for our feeding trial in premature infants*

	Human milk	Formula	Enriched formula
Ω-6 fatty acids			
Linoleic (18:2n-6)	10.8	13.2	11.8
γ-Linolenic (18:3n-6)	0.2	0.1	0.1
Arachidonic (20:4n-6)	0.4	n.d.	0.2
Total n-6 LCPUFA	1.1	0.1	0.4
Ω-3 fatty acids			
α-Linolenic (18:3n-3)	0.8	1.0	0.7
Docoshexaenoic (22:6n-3)	0.2	n.d.	0.1
Total n-3 LCPUFA	0.5	n.d.	0.1

n.d., not detectable.

condition, did not require respiratory support after day 2 of life, tolerated full enteral feeding, and were free of serious congenital anomalies or metabolic disorders. No patient had received intravenous lipid emulsions.

During the study period from day 4 to day 21 of life, the infants were either fed exclusively human milk if the mother decided to breast feed, or they were randomly assigned to receive exclusively one of the two formulas. The conventional and the LCP-enriched formulas were similar to human milk in their contents of protein (15, 16, and 13 g/l respectively), carbohydrate (70, 7, and 72 g/l), and fat (all 35 g/l) but differed in their fatty acid composition (Table 2). Linoleic and α and γ linolenic acid contents of both formulae were similar to human milk. The conventional formula did not contain n-3 LCP and only traces of n-6 LCP. The experimental formula was enriched with arachidonic and docosahexaenoic acids in a ratio of 2:1, which is equal to that in human milk, but their absolute concentrations were only about half of average human milk values. In addition, there were small amounts of other LCP.

Blood samples were obtained from all patients on both days 4 and 21 of life, and plasma phospholipid composition was measured by high-resolution capillary gas-liquid chromatography. Phospholipid fatty acids were not different among the three feeding groups at the start of the study. By day 21, linoleic acid was markedly increased in all feeding groups, with a somewhat more pronounced increase in formula-fed babies (Table 3). In infants fed human milk, n-6 and n-3 LCP were maintained at fairly stable levels throughout the study period. In contrast, infants fed the conventional formula developed a severe depletion of n-6 and n-3 LCP in phospholipids in spite of high precursor levels. This finding confirms the fact that premature infants have a limited capacity for endogenous LCP biosynthesis from the classical essential fatty acids, which is lower than the plasma clearance of LCP, i.e. uptake for tissue deposition and eicosanoid synthesis, and oxidation. Therefore, for this group of patients LCP seem to be essential nutrients that have to be supplied with the diet for optimal tissue growth and development.

TABLE 3. *Plasma phospholipid fatty acids (% wt/wt, mean ± SE) of premature infants fed human milk, conventional infant formula, or a formula enriched with both n-6 and n-3 LCP*[a]

	Day 4: all infants	Day 21: human milk	Formula	LCP formula
Ω-6 fatty acids				
Linoleic (18:2n-6)	12.8 ± 0.5	18.6 ± 0.6*	23.6 ± 1.0*[,b]	22.1 ± 0.8*[,b]
Dihomo-γ-linolenic (20:3n-6)	2.2 ± 0.1	3.0 ± 0.2	2.3 ± 0.1[b]	2.2 ± 0.2[b]
Arachidonic (20:4n-6)	12.5 ± 0.5	11.5 ± 0.5	6.3 ± 0.4*[,b]	8.4 ± 0.4*[,b,c]
Total n-6 LCP	15.7 ± 0.6	15.7 ± 0.6	9.6 ± 0.6*[,b]	11.5 ± 0.6*[,b,c]
Ω-3 fatty acids				
α-Linolenic (18:3n-3)	0.1 ± 0.01	0.1 ± 0.01	0.1 ± 0.01	0.1 ± 0.01
Docosapentaenoic (22:5n-3)	0.2 ± 0.03	0.6 ± 0.04*	0.3 ± 0.04	0.4 ± 0.1*[,b]
Docosahexaenoic (22:6n-3)	2.7 ± 0.2	3.1 ± 0.1	1.8 ± 0.2*[,b]	2.1 ± 0.1*
Total n-3 LCP	3.2 ± 0.2	4.1 ± 0.1	2.3 ± 0.8*[,b]	2.8 ± 0.1*[,b]

[a] Results are shown on day 4 for all infants and on day 21 for the three feeding groups. Symbols indicate significant differences ($p < 0.05$) of values on day 21 vs. day 4 within the same feeding group (*; paired t test) and between results of different feeding groups on day 21 of life ([b]vs. human milk, [c]vs. conventional formula; unpaired t test corrected after Bonferroni for multiple group comparison).

The results in the infants fed the LCP-enriched formula demonstrated a significantly improved essential fatty acid status, as compared to the conventional formula group, although the LCP content in phospholipids did not equal that of infants fed human milk, who received a threefold higher dietary LCP supply.

It is striking that seemingly low LCP proportions in milk lipids have pronounced effects on plasma phospholipid composition. A dietary LCP supply of only 1.7% and 0.5%, respectively, with human milk and the experimental formula, increased phospholipid LCP at 3 weeks of age by about 8% and 3%, respectively, over those of infants fed a formula without LCP. Apparently, the infant preferentially channels dietary LCP into structural lipids and spares them from other pathways such as oxidation, which is similar to findings in animal models (33,34).

CONCLUSION

In conclusion, this study clearly demonstrates that the essential fatty acid status of formula-fed premature infants can be effectively improved by enrichment of their diet with a balanced ratio of both linoleic and α linolenic acid metabolites. These results should encourage further investigation on the practicability, physiological effects, and safety of such dietary enrichments.

ACKNOWLEDGMENT

This work was financially supported by the Deutsche Forschungsgemeinschaft, Bonn, Germany [Ko 912/2-1 and Ko 912/4-1].

REFERENCES

1. Nutrition Committee, Canadian Paediatric Society. Feeding the low-birthweight infant. *Can Med Assoc J* 1981; 15: 1301–11.
2. American Academy of Pediatrics, Committee on Nutrition. Nutritional needs for low-birth-weight infants. *Pediatrics* 1985; 75: 976–86.
3. ESPGAN Committee on Nutrition of the Preterm Infant. Nutrition and feeding of preterm infants. *Acta Paediatr Scand (Suppl)* 1987; 336: 1–14.
4. Koletzko B. Essentielle Fettsäuren: Bedeutung für Medizin und Ernährung. *Aktuel Endokr Stoffw* 1986; 7: 18–27.
5. Svennerholm L. Distribution and fatty acid composition of phosphoglycerides in normal human brain. *J Lipid Res* 1968; 9: 570–9.
6. Ballabriga A, Martinez M. A chemical study on the development of the human forebrain and cerebellum during the brain "growth spurt" period. II. Phosphoglyceride fatty acids. *Brain Res* 1978; 159: 363–70.
7. Lamptey MS, Walker BL. A possible essential role for dietary linolenic acid in the development of the young rat. *J Nutr* 1976; 102: 86–93.
8. Neuringer M, Connor WE, Van Petten C, Barstd L. Dietary omega-3 fatty acid deficiency and visual loss in infant rhesus monkeys. *J Clin Invest* 1984; 73: 272–6.
9. Yamamoto N, Saitoh M, Moiruchi A, Nomura M, Okuyama H. Effect of dietary a-linolenate/linoleate balance on brain lipid compositions and learning ability of rats. *J Lipid Res* 1987; 28: 144–51.
10. Uauy R, Birch D, Birch E, Tyson J, Hoffman D. Effect of dietary omega-3 fatty acids on retinal function of very-low-birth-weight neonates. *Pediatr Res* 1990; 28: 485–92.
11. Carlson SE, Werkman SH, Peeples JM, Cooke RJ, Wilson WM. Plasma phospholipid arachidonic acid and growth and development of preterm infants. In: van Biervielt JP, Koletzko B, Okken A, Rey J, Salle B, eds. *Recent advances in infant feeding.* Stuttgart: Thieme Verlag [in press].
12. Martinez M, Ballabriga A, Gil-Gibernmau JJ. Lipids of the developing human retina: I. Total fatty acids, plasmalogens, and fatty acid composition of ethanolamine and choline phosphoglycerides. *J Neurosci Res* 1988; 20: 484–90.
13. Koletzko B, Braun M. Arachidonic acid and early human growth: Is there a relation? *Ann Nutr Metab* 1991; 35: 128–131.
14. Hansen AE, Wiese HF, Boelsche AN, Haggard ME, Adam DJD, Davis H. Role of linoleic acid in infant nutrition. *Pediatrics* 1963; 31: 171–92.
15. Koletzko B, Whitelaw A, Takeda J, Filler RM, Heim T. Linoleic acid metabolism in parenterally fed infants. *Pediatr Res* 1987; 22: 232.
16. Koletzko B, Filler R, Heim T. Stoffwechsel einer Lipidemulsion bei parenteral ernährten Neugeborenen: Analyse der Plasma-Lipoproteine. In: Grünert A, Reinauer H, eds. *Das Problem "Fett" in der Ernährungstherapie.* Basel: Karger Verlag [in press].
17. Koletzko B, Müller J. Cis- and trans-isomeric fatty acids in plasma lipids of newborn infants and their mothers. *Biol Neonate* 1990; 57: 172–8.
18. Clandinin MT, Chappell JE, Leong S, Heim T, Swyer PR, Chance GW. Extrauterine fatty acid accretion in infant brain: implications for fatty acid requirements. *Early Hum Dev* 1980; 4: 131–8.
19. Koletzko B, Mrotzek M, Bremer HJ. Fatty acid composition of mature human milk in Germany. *Am J Clin Nutr* 1988; 47: 954–9.
20. Koletzko B. Improved essential fatty acid status of premature infants by dietary supplementation of both omega-6 and omega-3 long-chain polyunsaturates. In: van Biervielt JP, Koletzko B, Okken A, Rey J, Salle B, eds. *Recent advances in infant feeding.* Stuttgart: Thieme Verlag [in press].
21. Koletzko B, Bremer HJ. Fat content and fatty acid composition of infant formulas. *Acta Paediatr Scand* 1989; 78: 513–21.
22. Ballabriga A, Martinez M. Changes in erythrocyte lipid stroma in the premature infant according to dietary fat composition. *Acta Paediatr Scand* 1976; 65: 705–9.

23. Carlson SE, Rhodes PG, Ferguson MG. Docosahexaenoic acid status of preterm infants at birth and following feeding with human milk or formula. *Am J Clin Nutr* 1986; 44: 798–804.
24. Koletzko B, Schmidt E, Bremer HJ. Long-chain polyunsaturated fatty acids in human milk: small but beautiful. In: Atkinson SA, Hanson LA, Chandra RK, eds. *Breastfeeding, nutrition, infection and infant growth in developed and emerging countries*. St. Johns, Newfoundland: ARTS Biomedical Publishers & Distributors; 1990: 495–7.
25. Innis SM, Arbuckle LD, Phang M. N-3 fatty acid requirements: effect of formula feeding and early parenteral nutrition. In: van Biervielt JP, Koletzko B, Okken A, Rey J, Salle B, eds. *Recent advances in infant feeding*. Stuttgart: Thieme Verlag [in press].
26. Liu CCF, Carlson SE, Rhodes PG, Rao VS, Meydrech EF. Increase in plasma phospholipid docosahexaenoic and eicosapentaenoic acids as a reflection of their intake and mode of administration. *Pediatr Res* 1987; 22: 292–6.
27. Needleman P, Raz A, Minkes MS, Ferrendelli JA, Sprecher H. Triene prostaglandins: prostacyclin and thromboxane synthesis and unique biological properties. *Proc Natl Acad Sci USA* 1979; 76: 944–8.
28. Clarke JTR, Cullen-Dean, Regelink E, Chan L, Rose V. Increased incidence of epistaxis in adolescents with familial hypercholesterolemia treated with fish oil. *J Pediatr* 1990; 116: 139–41.
29. Ferretti A, Flanagan VP. Modification of prostaglandin metabolism in vivo by long-chain omega-3 polyunsaturates. *Biochim Biophys Acta* 1990; 1045: 299–301.
30. Lee TH, Hoover RL, Williams JD, et al. Effect of dietary enrichment with eicosapentaenoic and docosahexaenoic acids on in vitro neutrophil and monocyte leukotriene generation and neutrophil function. *N Engl J Med* 1985; 312: 1217–24.
31. Endres S, Ghorbani R, Kelley VE, et al. The effect of dietary supplementation with n-3 polyunsaturated fatty acids on the synthesis of interleukin-1 and tumor necrosis factor by mononuclear cells. *N Engl J Med* 1989; 320: 265–71.
32. Koletzko B, Schmidt E, Bremer HJ, Haug M, Harzer G. Effects of dietary long-chain polyunsaturated fatty acids on the essential fatty acid status of premature infants. *Eur J Pediatr* 1989; 148: 669–75.
33. Sinclair AJ. Incorporation of radioactive polyunsaturated fatty acids into liver and brain of developing rat. *Lipids* 1975; 10: 175–84.
34. Leyton J, Drury PJ, Crawford MA. Differential oxidation of saturated and unsaturated fatty acids in vivo in the rat. *Br J Nutr* 1987; 57: 383–93.

DISCUSSION

Dr. Clandinin: In the ω-3 fatty acid feeding study you mentioned, how much long chain ω-3 were the children being fed when they developed nose bleeds?

Dr. Koletzko: This was a study by Joe Clarke and coworkers. Eleven young people with hyperlipidemia were studied, aged 11–21 years. They were given fish oil capsules, providing an estimated intake of ω-3 long chain polyunsaturates of about 100–200 mg/kg daily. Eight of them developed nose bleeds, so the study had to be stopped prematurely.

Dr. Clandinin: This is quite a high level of ω-3 intake—about five times the quantity that would be considered effective in altering platelet function.

Dr. Koletzko: I agree, but on a by-weight-basis such doses have in fact been given to premature infants in feeding studies. If such side effects can occur in relatively stable individuals of adolescent age, one must be very careful about the possible effects in premature infants.

Dr. Cunnane: Sue Carlson has suggested that weight gain in fish oil-supplemented infants is less than normal. This is another contraindication to add to your list.

Dr. Koletzko: I have seen these data which show an adverse effect on growth of high doses of ω-3 long chain polyunsaturates, and also a somewhat weak but significant association between arachidonic acid and neurodevelopmental outcome. These observations fit very well with our view that the ratio of arachidonic and docosahexaenoic acids may be important.

Dr. Widhalm: You say that we should supplement premature infants with ω-3 fatty acids.

I should like to add cholesterol. This has been confirmed by Clandinin's studies, where it was clearly shown that an increase in cholesterol intake of only 1% increases the ω-3 fatty acids twofold.

Dr. Koletzko: In a short-term study we did, we did not find any effect of cholesterol supplementation. On the other hand, van Biervliet has recently shown in term infants followed for a longer period that cholesterol supplementation does in fact alter plasma lipoprotein composition.

Dr. Small: On the subject of cholesterol, I remember reading that increasing the cholesterol in the diets of children can lead to increased cholesterol in later life. Is this true?

Dr. Koletzko: The contrary hypothesis has also been proposed. This is based on animal data and suggests that high cholesterol intake in early life may enable the individual to handle cholesterol better in later life. There are more recent data that point to exactly the opposite. These data are very controversial and we don't have the final answer as yet.

Dr. Spielmann: You said there is no relation between linoleic acid intake and arachidonic acid composition in human milk, but couldn't this be explained by substrate inhibition at high levels of linoleic acid intake?

Dr. Koletzko: Your question is what level of linoleic acid intake in maternal diet suppresses arachidonic acid in human milk. Before answering that, one first has to prove that dietary linoleic acid does in fact reduce milk arachidonate. I think the available studies do not document such an effect. For example, Clandinin has given highly different amounts of linoleic acid in his trials by changing margarine brands used by lactating women, and there was no effect on arachidonic acid. Other studies have shown no clear reduction in arachidonic acid content in milk lipids in vegetarian mothers with a high linoleic acid intake. I therefore question whether inhibition of arachidonic acid secretion in human milk does happen at all at reasonable levels of dietary linoleic acid.

Dr. Small: There seems to be a great deal of concern about making appropriate supplementation of the diet. I wonder whether anyone has considered different routes of administration, for example cholesterol arachidonate injected into adipose tissue.

Dr. Koletzko: One noninvasive approach to supplementation is the application of fatty acids to the skin. We have used this method to supply EFA to infants who do not tolerate enteral lipids. Dermal application can be effective and has been shown to result in increases of EFA in plasma lipids. However, in our experience the response is extremely variable and unreliable.

Dr. Heim: Before we recommend supplementation of the long chain derivatives of ω-6 and ω-3 fatty acids could you briefly cite the evidence that preterm and full-term infants are unable to chain elongate and desaturate EFA to LCP? Could you also elaborate on the metabolism of LCP? I would like to see really good data on this complex issue before accepting your conclusions.

Dr. Koletzko: I certainly agree that we should try to gather more information. However, I don't think we can conclude that premature infants are entirely unable to synthesize LCP. We can only conclude from measurements of plasma and tissue lipids that infants supplied with a diet devoid of LCP develop a marked depletion of these EFA metabolites in plasma and tissue lipids. Thus the capacity of these infants to synthesize LCP from the precursors is insufficient to maintain the levels they would have had *in utero* or during human milk feeding. We now have accumulating evidence that such depletion of LCP has untoward functional effects, both in newborn animals and in human premature infants. I think the time has come to call the long chain polyunsaturates semiessential nutrients during this period of life.

It is interesting to recall Alan Lucas's studies comparing premature infants fed on pooled breast milk *vs.* a formula designed for full-term infants, both having similar amounts of protein and energy. Neurodevelopmental follow-up showed worse performance at 18 months in those fed the formula. Since energy and protein intakes were the same, this supports the view that the qualitative supply of lipid in human milk may be relevant to long-term development.

Dr. Crawford: The very low birthweight babies are born with significant built-in deficits of arachidonic acid already and so it is not just a question of trying to consider what you do to maintain postnatal levels of arachidonic acid. We need to start thinking about how we make up for prenatal deficits because those prenatal deficits as determined by plasma levels are bound to show up in other tissues in fat stores. The point I would emphasize to those who are not involved in this particular area is that when you are talking about these very low birthweight babies you are talking about a group of babies who are at very high risk of neural development damage. The incidence of neural development damage in the 3,500–4,500 g birthweight is about 1.6/1,000 births. In these very low birthweight babies it goes up to 260 and that is really a very serious concern. The arachidonic acid is not just a major component in the central nervous system, it is also quantitatively the most important essential fatty acid in the inner membrane.

Dr. Bazan: Following up on the comment of Dr. Crawford we should keep in mind the possibility of other cell-specific functions of essential polyunsaturated fatty acids, i.e., cell signal transduction events whereby inositol lipids and arachidonic acid play important roles in cell-to-cell communication. We have been dealing recently with cell signal transduction genes (immediate-early genes) and we have found that lipid mediators may play a role in cell growth and differentiation. For the future we have to expand our thinking in terms of cell signal transduction events taking place in the plasma membrane and how those events may be coupled to cell signal transduction genes.

Dr. Koletzko: The point raised by Dr. Crawford on differences among infants at the time of birth, and the potential of deficits developing already prenatally, appears quite important. We should keep in mind that premature birth is not a physiological event, and that it is often associated with placental dysfunction and disturbed nutrient supply. Essential fatty acids status may also be affected, and in this respect Dr. Bazan's perspective on future research into the possible functional effects of such differences is very exciting.

Polyunsaturated Fatty Acids in Human Nutrition,
edited by U. Bracco and R. J. Deckelbaum.
Nestlé Nutrition Workshop Series, Vol. 28.
Nestec Ltd., Vevey/Raven Press, Ltd., New York © 1992.

Dietary Long Chain Polyunsaturated Fatty Acids: Sources, Problems, and Uses

Umberto Bracco

Nestlé Research Centre, Nestec Ltd., Vers-chez-les-Blanc, 1000 Lausanne 26, Switzerland

Infant formulas generally derive their lipid composition from vegetable and animal oils and thus do not contain polyunsaturated fatty acids with chain lengths more than 18 carbon atoms. It is assumed that under normal conditions a series of chain desaturations and elongations at the carboxyl terminus occurs, yielding more unsaturated lipids that are physiologically and structurally active.

However, this compositional difference *versus* breast milk could be translated over time into differences in membrane composition *in vivo*, in particular in the red blood cells. This suggests that the presence of parent fatty acids of n-6 and n-3 series (i.e., linoleic and linolenic acids) is not always sufficient for optimal nutrition in early life: in fact, the *in vivo* biosynthesis of long chain fatty acids may be a limiting factor in newborns (1).

Recent discoveries on essential fatty acid metabolism and requirements during the developmental stage have promoted nutritional recommendations for the introduction of n-3, n-6 long chain fatty acids (LCFA) in infant formula, which constitute a new challenge for the food industry. The purpose of this paper is to examine the opportunities and the problems of incorporating such materials into foods. In particular we shall discuss potential sources of n-3 and n-6 long chain fatty acids and problems related to structure/bioavailability and reactivity/nutritional value interactions, with a view to formulating products better suited to meet the lipid requirements in early life.

THE LONG CHAIN "n-6"–"n-3" WORLD

The target fatty acids are the final products of the elongation and desaturation of the C18 linoleic acids (LA) and α-linolenic acids (ALNA). These are γ-linolenic (GLA), dihomo-γ-linolenic (DGLA), arachidonic (AA), eicosapentaenoic (EPA), and docosahexaenoic (DHA) acids. In particular, a major concern appears to be the adequate supply of AA and DHA to membranes in developing tissues. Table 1 shows the potential natural sources of C > 18 fatty acids, and Table 2 shows alternative sources for these active fatty acids.

TABLE 1. *PUFA (C > 18): animal and vegetable source*

Origin	Type of fatty acid	Description	References
Marine oils	EPA/DHA	RBD fish oil Fish oil fractions Esters	(2,3)
Blackcurrant seed	GLA/SA	RBD from seeds Fractions	(4,5)
Evening primrose	GLA	RBD from seeds	(6)
Egg lecithin	AA	Phospholipid-bound fatty acids	(7)
Human placenta	AA/DHA/DGLA	Alcohol extract	(8)
Human milk	GLA/DGLA/AA/DHA	—	(9)

SA, stearidonic acid; RBD, refined.

The fatty acid composition of lipids, particularly those originating in microorganisms, is influenced both qualitatively and quantitatively by environmental conditions and by technological variables such as aeration, light intensity, light-dark cycle, and culture age.

In contrast to oil-bearing vegetable material, marine oils, the logical carriers of DHA, also possess highly variable levels of fatty acids: environmental factors such as diet, season, temperature, and biological differences (sex, age) affect both the lipid content and the fatty acid composition.

LONG CHAIN FATTY ACIDS: STRUCTURE AND BIOLOGICAL VALUE

The biological and clinical efficacy of oils cannot be determined on the basis of their fatty acid composition alone. However, and particularly for the long chain series, the triacylglycerol structure and the polarity of the carrier lipids (amphiphatic lipids) play a key role in absorption, intracellular lipoprotein formation, and intravascular lipoprotein metabolism. Thus structural analyses of plant (18), fungal, and marine oils have been performed to identify the distribution of fatty acids affecting the stereospecificity of digestive enzymes and fat absorption.

TABLE 2. *PUFA (C > 18): alternative sources*

Origin	Type of fatty acid	Description	References
Algae (spirulina)	EPA/DHA GLA	Blue greeen algae (autotrophic)	(10)
Microalgae	DHA	Heterotrophic algae	(11)
Molds	GLA/AA	Mycelia (*Mortierella*)	(12–14)
Mosses	DGLA/AA	Moss cell fermentation	(15)
Microorganisms	DGLA/AA	*Penicillium*	(16,17)

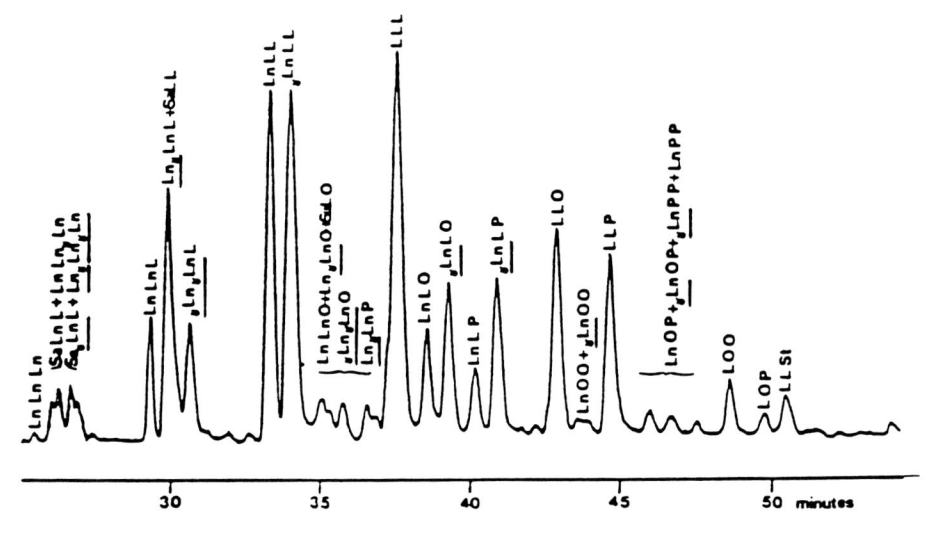

FIG. 1. HPLC of blackcurrant seed oil with a laser light scattering detector.

We developed a reverse phase high-performance liquid chromatography (HPLC) analysis coupled to a laser light scattering detector to check the distribution of γ linolenic acid in blackcurrant oil (19). Figure 1 shows the triglyceride composition obtained by gradient elution, which is absolutely necessary considering the complexity of the sample. As γ linolenic acid, although not α linolenic acid, resists pancreatic hydrolysis, it is also possible to have triacylglycerol-stereospecific analysis by coupling phospholipase C, which generates 1,2 diglycerides, and phospholipase A_2, which generates lysophosphatidylcholine.

It is interesting to note that long chain fatty acids in blackcurrant oil seem preferentially to concentrate in position 3 of the triacylglycerol (Table 3), which has also been reported for linoleic and α-linolenic acid in human but not in bovine milk (20). We know that the sn-3 position of the triglyceride is the preferred site of attack by lingual lipase (21,22), which governs the lipolytic splitting of fats in the stomach jointly with gastric lipase. The degree of splitting of the fatty acid from triglyceride is also dependent on the positional distribution of the double bonds in the fatty acid: as an example, docosahexaenoyl glycerides are hydrolyzed at a slower rate than

TABLE 3. *Triacylglycerol stereospecific analysis of blackcurrant oil*

Position	16:0	18:0	18:1	18:2 n-6	18:3 n-6	18:4 n-3
All	6.9	1.3	10.8	46.7	15.9	2.9
1	14.2 ± 2.7	4.9 ± 0.7	12.6 ± 1.4	42.7 ± 1.2	4.1 ± 0.7	0.7 ± 0.2
2	2.0 ± 1.0	1.5 ± 1.7	14.1 ± 1.1	53.1 ± 0.9	17.4 ± 1.7	2.6 ± 0.6
3	4.4 ± 1.1	0	5.1 ± 1.1	43.8 ± 1.6	25.8 ± 1.7	5.6 ± 0.4

oleoylglycerides (23), even when these fatty acids are in position sn-3 on the triacylglycerol. This seems to be related to the proximity of the first double bond to the carboxyl group.

In view also of the nonstereospecificity of the bile-salt-stimulated lipase in the small intestine, and the specificity of pancreatic lipase for 1,3 esters in the duodenum, one could also engineer structured triacylglycerols, where the 2-position is occupied preferentially by long chain fatty acids.

Jandacek et al. reported recently (24) that rapid hydrolysis and efficient absorption of triglycerides occurred with octanoic acid in the 1- and 3-positions and C_{18} fatty acids in the 2-position, while Hamosh et al. (25) have shown that medium chain triglycerides (MCT) are released preferentially by gastric lipolysis over long chain fatty acids and are absorbed in the stomach of the newborn infant. In the light of these findings we recently filed a patent (26) covering the use of a regioselective immobilized lipase from *Rhizomucor miehei* for the manufacture of triglycerides in which the 1,3-positions are occupied by MCTs and the 2-position contains preferentially long chain fatty acid as DHA. This process allows the restructuring of DHA-containing oils (i.e., marine oils), producing a lipid material containing at least 50% of true structured triglycerides with a large proportion of MCT-DHA-MCT structures. Comparative bioavailability studies on animals are underway.

El Boustani et al. (27) showed recently that the kinetics of absorption of EPA in man depends on its chemical structure: their data confirm that 2-EPA in the form of 1,3 dioctanoyl-2 eicosapentaenoic is well absorbed, is not randomly distributed during the absorption process, and behaves better than other EPA-containing structures such as free fatty acids and ethyl esters. Chernenko (28) also found that the DHA in fish oil is primarily in the sn-2-position, whereas EPA is more randomly distributed, so that pancreatic lipase and probably carboxyl ester lipase will leave a DHA-enriched monoacylglycerol fraction (Table 4). It is interesting to note that triacylglycerols of marine mammal oils have an atypical fatty acid distribution pattern, where LCFA are enriched in the sn-1,3-position. Ackman (29) reported the different distributions in the oils of marine fish and marine mammals.

Conflicting results, however, are still reported on the stereospecificity of lipoprotein lipase, the enzyme bound to the endothelial surface through heparin sulfate and responsible for the breakdown of chylomicrons and very low density lipoprotein (VLDL) particles.

REACTIVITY OF LONG CHAIN POLYUNSATURATED FATTY ACIDS

Formulations of products containing increasing levels of double bound structures raises the problem of the interaction of oxygen with highly unsaturated lipids. Although the rate of peroxidation of pure lipids or unsaturated fatty acids is extremely slow, since oxidation requires an active form of oxygen, the spin restriction of molecular oxygen can be overcome by the so-called initiation mechanisms.

TABLE 4. *Fatty acid composition of products of pancreatic lipase digestion of fish oil*

Fatty acid	Monoacyl-glycerol fraction	Free fatty fraction	Substrate
14:0	13.8	4.9	5.6
14:1	1.1	0.5	N.D.
16:0	23.3	17.8	17.9
16:1	8.0	7.8	7.7
18:0	2.3	11.1	5.0
18:1	6.5	17.2	16.1
18:2	1.1	1.5	1.7
18:3	0.3	0.8	N.D.
18:4	2.6	1.9	2.4
20:0	0.2	0.3	0.6
20:1	1.9	2.8	3.6
20:2	N.D.	0.3	0.6
20:3	N.D.	0.1	N.D.
20:4	1.1	0.8	0.6
20:5	11.2	13.8	14.6 ←
22:1	1.1	2.1	3.2
22:4	0.4	0.5	0.6
22:5	3.0	1.7	2.0
22:6	14.3	5.8	11.1 ←
24:0	0.8	0.3	0.6
24:1	0.3	0.5	1.3
Unknowns	4.0	5.9	4.0

From Chernenko GA (28).

PUFA are the ideal target for the activated oxygen species due to their diene structure and the presence of the allylic hydrogen, which, via its abstraction, forms pentadienylradicals for the subsequent oxygen and/or enzymatic attack (30). The resulting fat oxidation products promote interaction with the other food components affecting the overall nutritional value of the product. We did some experiments (31) on a model system where methyl linoleate was emulsified in whey protein and the emulsion was subsequently dried and stored under well-defined conditions. This model allows us to check the protein-lipid oxidation interaction, to identify the various parameters affecting the kinetics of reaction, and to quantify the losses of essential fatty acids.

Figure 2 shows the losses of lysine and methionine during the storage of our dried emulsions under various experimental conditions. Sulphydric groups seem to be most sensitive to oxidative phenomena: methionine is readily oxidized to methionine sulphoxide during lipid oxidation and to a lesser extent to methionine sulphone.

It is known that an increase in the ratio of disulphides/sulphydric groups, as in glutathione and dimethylsulphides, represents a metabolic marker of an oxidative degradation affecting *in vivo* the activity of different enzymes. Peroxidation of n-6, n-3 fatty acids also produces high concentrations of cytotoxic aldehydic products, i.e., 4-hydroxynonenal and 4-hydroxyhexanal, as reported recently by Van Kuijk et al. (32).

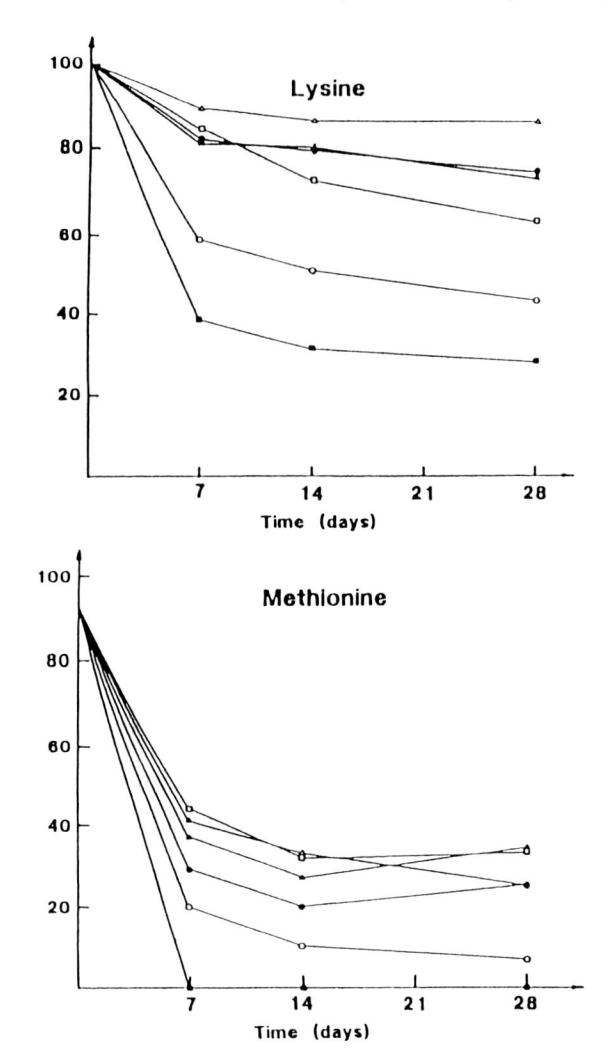

SYMBOL	TEMP. °C	A$_w$	MOISTURE CONTENT %	MOLE OXYGEN / MOLE LIPID
△	37	0.28-0.33	2	4
●	37	0.85-0.90	17	1
▲	37	0.67	7	4
□	20	0.90	17	4
○	37	0.85-0.90	17	4
■	55	0.85-0.90	17	4

FIG. 2. Losses of lysine and methionine (%) under various storage conditions.

TABLE 5. *Rat feeding studies: PER (weight gain/protein intake) and NPU (N-retained/N-intake) (4 weeks)*

	Storage conditions			PER	NPU
	Temp., °C	A_W	O_2/lipid		
Control protein	—	—	—	4.70 ± 0.15	5.82 ± 0.10
A	37	0.84	4	−0.97 ± 0.25	1.92 ± 0.10
B	37	0.33	4	4.62 ± 0.17	5.72 ± 0.20
C	37	0.84	1	1.77 ± 0.44	4.00 ± 0.27
D	55	0.84	4	−0.78 ± 0.25	1.70 ± 0.27

We measured *in vivo* the effect of the lipid oxidation on the overall protein quality and amino acid availability, by feeding rats the delipidized whey protein of our dried emulsion after incubation with methlylinoleate under the conditions already reported. Growth assays and nitrogen balance studies showed clearly how lipid peroxidation affects the overall nutritional value of the diet. Table 5 reports data on NPU (net protein utilization) and PER (protein efficiency ratio) of whey protein after storage with methyl-linoleate. High water activity in the product and high storage temperature result in the lowest biological value of proteins in the diet.

THE TECHNOLOGICAL APPROACH TO NEW LIPID INGREDIENTS FOR INFANT FORMULAS

The quality aspects concerning long chain fatty acids (LCFA) in infant formulas relate to 1) the composition of the oils (total n-6, n-3 content and structure, liposoluble vitamins); 2) purity of the oils (absence of nontriglyceride structures, heavy metals, pesticide levels); 3) stability of the oils.

Marine oils in particular are now postrefined by large-scale chromatography called displacement chromatography, based on the affinity of the various lipid classes for selected stationary phases. This process allows to separate and obtain specific lipid classes from complex natural oil mixtures and to select suitable ones for our formulations.

Figure 3 shows the cleaning up of refined fish and blackcurrant seed oil before and after the column absorbing process: The triglyceride species are separated and collected, guaranteeing the absence of interfering material (sterols, partial glycerides) and ensuring constant triglyceride purity. The adsorption process not only allows the lipid class separation but also improves the primary and secondary oxidation parameters of the oil.

A further improvement in the oxidative stability of LCFA concerns the use of appropriate antioxidant systems well adapted both to the oil blends and to the final formulation. We found, unexpectedly, and subsequently patented (33) the increasing antioxidant activity of ternary systems, in particular the synergy of vitamin C/vitamin

```
SAMPLE    Purified Blackcurrant Seed Oil, Nestec
DOCUMENT  Purity test
BATCH     K 90216
ORIGIN    M P 7/89, Nestec-Research
METHOD    HPLC      Injected: 20 ul (50 mg/ml)
                    Detector: ACS Mass Detector
                    Elution:  Isooctane/Isopropanol/Acetic acid
                              (gradient)
                    Column:   Diol phase 5 um; 250x4.0 mm
```

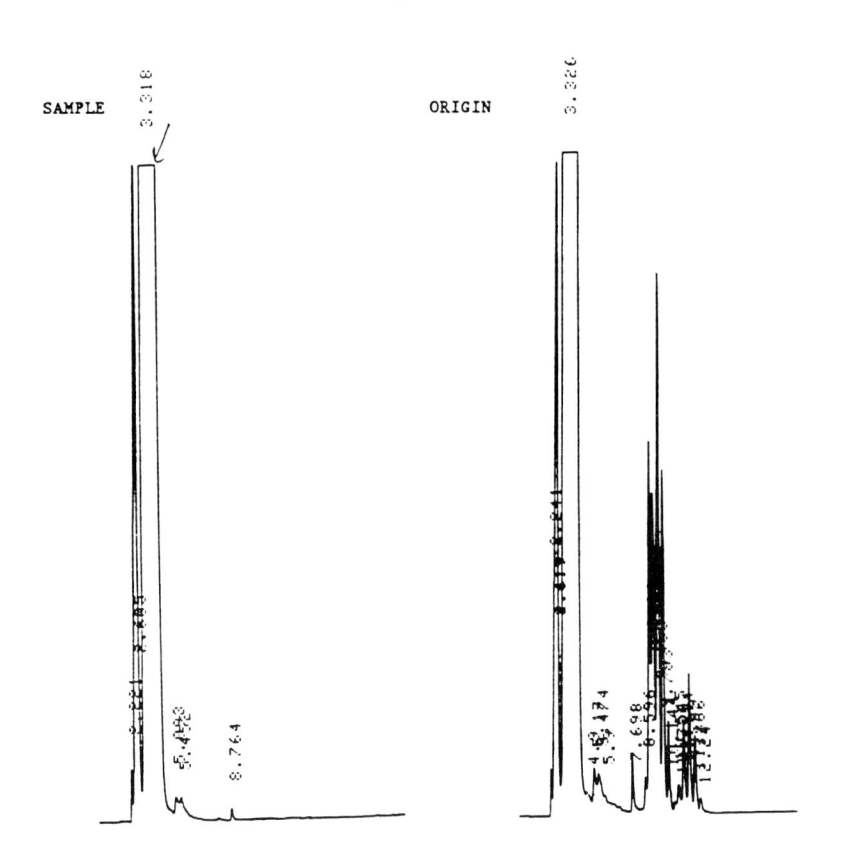

Peak identification:

2.605	Sterol esters	2.619	Sterol esters
3.318	Triglyceride species	3.326	Triglyceride species
		4.9 -	Fatty acids, diglyce-
8.764	Gammatocopherol	- 12.24	rides, unknowns

FIG. 3. Chromatographic cleaning of oils.

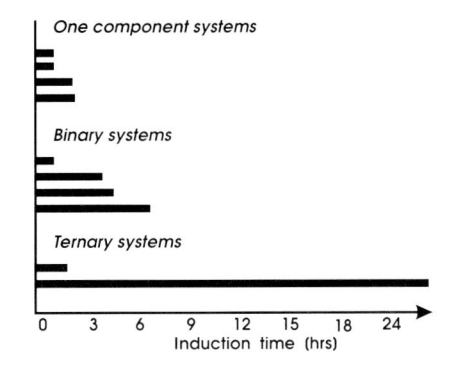

FIG. 4. Oxidative stability of fish oil added with different antioxidant systems.

E and natural phospholipids. As shown in Fig. 4, the oxidative induction time (resistance to peroxidation) in fish oil is practically unaffected by known single antioxidants such as vitamin E, vitamin C, and its esters, whereas moving to a more complex ternary system, we could identify very active blends. This is particularly important as, in the quest for ever better matching of human breast milk lipids, we are continuously increasing the number of diene structures. Thus, from the first cow's milk fat-based formulations, we have moved to linoleic-, α linolenic-, γ linolenic-, and finally to LCFA-rich oils.

Due to interchangeability of natural oils in food products, once the absolute and relative figures for each of the bioactive fatty acids have been established, we can set up formulations based on different oils and having suitable fatty acids compositions. Table 6 reports as an example the gross composition and the LCFA level of formulations based on LCFA-bearing oils. These formulations guarantee the presence of LCFA per dl of milk comparable to breast milk, together with a favorable ratio of fatty acids of both n-6 and n-3 families.

The effect of providing for the apparent DHA needs for growth and development of infants by feeding fish oil only should be evaluated in relation to the resulting arachidonic acid levels in red blood cells and plasma phospholipids (34). New lipid compositions should take into account the competition at the cell membrane level between long chain fatty acids of the n-6 and n-3 families: Our formulations contain

TABLE 6. *Infant formulae enriched in LCFA*

	Gross composition		LCFA-oils			mg in 100 g dry product		
	Weight %	Calories %	Egg lecithin %	Blackcurrant %	Fish %	AA	GLA	DHA
Protein	14–16	11–13	—					
Lipids	24–27	41–44	0.5–0.7	0.5–0.7	1.0–1.2	28–39	75–90	150–180
CHOs	58–61	44–48	—					

arachidonic-acid-bearing material (egg lecithin) and its precursor GLA (blackcurrant oil). Nevertheless, the ratio between these fatty acids is still not ideal when compared to breast milk.

CONCLUSION

The task of the food industries is to translate, in terms of suitable products, the biochemical and physiological evidence coming from *in vitro* animal and human studies on particular bioactive molecules. LCFA belong to this process as they govern the modification of the eicosanoid system and the functional changes in the cell.

Natural and biotechnology lipids, obtained, purified, and stabilized according to the latest knowledge in fat technology, allow us to prepare food products with specific activities and physiological responses. One field of growing importance in LCFA application is food for growth and development of infants, where the LCFA essentiality for brain structure and function is undisputed. The particular structure of LCFA-bearing oils and their reactivity require a rigorous monitoring of sources, technological processes, and storage stability in order to offer bioactive ingredients under the most controlled conditions.

REFERENCES

1. Clandinin MT, et al. Extrauterine fatty acid accretion in infant brain: implications for fatty acid requirements. *Early Hum Dev* 1980; 4: 131–8.
2. Kinsella J. *Seafoods and fish oils in human health and disease*. New York/Basel: Marcel Dekker; 1987.
3. Sidwell VA. *Chemical and nutritional composition of finfishes, whales, crustaceans, mollusks and their products*. NOAA Techn. Memo. NMFS F/SEC 11; 1981.
4. Traitler H, et al. Characterisation of gamma linolenic acid in ribes seed. *Lipids* 1984; 19: 923–8.
5. Nestlé SA. GLA extraction from ribes seeds. European patent 83110241.3—14.10.1983.
6. Hudson B. Evening primrose (Oenothera spp.) oil and seed. *J Am Oil Chem Soc* 1984; 61: 540–4.
7. Privett OS. Studies on the composition of egg lipid. *J Food Sci* 1962; 27: 463–8.
8. Inst. Merieux. Procédé de préparation de lipides riches en acides gras polyunsaturés à longue chaîne. French patent 2'596'988—14.4.1986.
9. Koletzko B. Fatty acid composition of mature human milk in Germany. *Am J Clin Nutr* 1988; 47: 954–9.
10. Grattan Roughan P. Spirulina: a source of dietary gamma linolenic acid. *J Sci Food Agric* 1989; 47: 85–93.
11. Kyle DJ. Microalgae as a source of EPA. IUFOST Symposium, Göteborg, Sept 17–20, 1989.
12. Suntory Ltd. Process for production of bis-homo GLA and EPA. European patent 0252716—13.1.1988.
13. Shimizu S, et al. Microbial conversion of an oil containing α-linolenic acid to an oil containing eicosapentaenoic acid. *J Am Oil Chem Soc* 1989; 66: 342–7.
14. Lyon Corp. Method for producing fat containing gamma-linolenic acid. European patent application 0269351—1.6.1988.
15. Nestlé SA. PUFAs by moss-cell culture. Patent application (Switzerland) 00146/90-2—17.1.1990.
16. Idemitsu Petroch Co. Method for the production of lipids containing bis-homo linolenic acid and/or arachidonic acid. European patent application 0304049—22.2.1989.
17. [Anonymous] Sturge plans biotech spend. Provess Eng 1986; 67: 11.
18. Lawson LD, et al. Triacylglycerol structure of plant and fungal oils containing γ-linolenic acid. *Lipids* 1988; 23: 313–7.

19. Perrin JL, et al. Analysis of triglycerides species of blackcurrant seed oil by HPLC via a laser light scattering detector. *Rev Fr Corps Gras* 1987; 34: 221–3.
20. Jensen RG. *The lipids of human milk*. Boca Raton, FL: CRC Press, 1989: 70.
21. Paltauf F, et al. Stereospecificity of lipases. *FEBS Lett* 1974; 40: 119–23.
22. Staggers JE. Studies on fat digestion and absorption in suckling rats. *J Lipid Res* 1981; 22: 675–9.
23. Bottino NR. Resistance of certain long chain polyunsaturated fatty acids of marine oils to pancreatic lipase hydrolysis. *Lipids* 1967; 2: 489–93.
24. Jandacek RJ, et al. The rapid hydrolysis and efficient absorption of triglycerides with octanoic acid in the 1 and 3 positions and long-chain fatty acid in the 2-position. *Am J Clin Nutr* 1987; 45: 940–5.
25. Hamosh M, et al. Gastric lipolysis and fat absorption in preterm infants: effect of medium chain triglycerides or long-chain triglyceride-containing formulas. *Pediatrics* 1989; 83: 86–92.
26. Nestlé-Novo. Triglycerides composition comprising such triglycerides and use of such composition. WO 90/04013—10.10.1989.
27. El Boustani S, et al. Enteral absorption in man of eicosapentanoic acid in different chemical forms. *Lipids* 1987; 22: 711–4.
28. Chernenko GA. Intestinal absorption and lymphatic transport of fish oil (Max EPA) in the rat. *Biochim Biophys Acta* 1989; 1004: 95–102.
29. Ackman RG. Some possible effects on lipid biochemistry of differences in the distribution on glycerol of long-chain n-3 fatty acids in the fats of marine fish and marine mammals. *Atherosclerosis* 1988; 70: 171–3.
30. Van Rollins M, et al. Autoxidation of docosahexaenoic acid: analysis of ten isomers of hydroxy docosahexanoate. *J Lipid Res* 1984; 25: 107–11.
31. Nielsen KH. Nutritional aspects of reactions between oxidizing lipid and protein with emphasis on tryptophan. Thesis No 865—Nestec, 1984.
32. Van Kuijk FG, et al. 4-Hydroxyhexenal: a lipid peroxidation product derived from oxidized docosahexaenoic acid. *Biochem Biophys Acta* 1990; 1043: 116–8.
33. Nestlé SA. European patent. Mélange Antioxydant Synergique, 0326829—13.1.1989.
34. Carlson SE, et al. Essentiality of omega-3 fatty acids in growth and development of infants. II. International Conference on health effects of omega-3 PUFA in Seafoods, Washington, DC, 1990.

DISCUSSION

Dr. Guesry: It seems to me that there is a consensus that we should try to provide at least arachidonic and docosahexaenoic acids in infant formulas and you showed an alternative source of these LCPUFA derived from algae. I may be wrong but I believe that Codex Alimentarius, FDA, and other regulatory institutions do not at present permit the use of this type of material. Could Dr. Glinsmann tell us whether he sees the possibility of our being able to use this type of raw material and what would be the possible timing?

Dr. Glinsmann: We always approve foods and additives for a given use. We do not approve items for general unrestricted use unless we have evidence that they are safe. The problem at the moment is that we have not been presented with data that document the nature of any standardized products containing the specific fatty acids mentioned, or information on exactly what type of use is intended for them. This is the basis of our inaction. Most of the uses of LCPUFA that we consider are therapeutic. Even in the case of premature infants, specialized formulas may be very different from standard infant formulas. Products for premature infants do not mimic human milk but some kind of placental nutriture that is delivered during the last trimester of fetal growth. We certainly agree with you on the importance of lipids for growth and development, but we do not want to simply add fish oil or long chain ω-3 polyunsaturates and interfere with arachidonic acid metabolism without being able to predict the outcome. This could result in other unanticipated effects on immune function and on long-term development that we need to evaluate. We need a very firm basis for establishing general safety. As you bring new products onto the market we want to facilitate the process as much as possible and will do so when safety can be clearly established. I also would not like to see claims for specific oils expand irrationally beyond the available scientific base.

Dr. Guesry: In your stabilizing system you show a difference between a system containing ascorbyl palmitate and a system containing vitamin C. Vitamin C is not fat soluble whereas ascorbyl palmitate is fat soluble. Why is there such a difference in your results?

Dr. Bracco: We found that the synergic activity of vitamin C with vitamin E is due to the tocopheryl anion, whereas ascorbyl palmitate shows less protective interaction on vitamin E due to reduced ionized forms. The reason for using lecithin is to enhance the liposolubility of vitamin C.

Dr. Crawford: At the start of your presentation you expressed great concern about putting long chain n-3 and n-6 fatty acids in milk. Can I put the question the other way around? What evidence have you got for leaving them out? Second, if you are thinking of incorporating these lipids, would it not be reasonable to think in terms of mimicking nature? The most unsaturated components in human milk are the phosphoglycerides and these are buried in the lipoproteins. This stabilizes the lipid. Also the bulk of the lipid supplied in human milk is in the form of droplets, so why not follow that approach and provide the lipid microencapsulated?

Dr. Bracco: In relation to your first point, there is at present no evidence for either risk or benefit of using these long chain fatty acids in infant formulas. As to your second point, yes, we can mimic nature in terms of fatty acid composition but probably not in terms of structural distribution. The docosahexaenoic acid we add is not really the same compound or in the same environment as in human milk. However, when this product is made it is indeed encapsulated in some way, depending on the formulation. It is not free-floating.

Dr. Cunnane: I wanted to address a question regarding the effectiveness of GLA in increasing arachidonic acid. Being fairly familiar with the literature I think the consensus is right now that you cannot raise arachidonic acid by feeding GLA to adult humans. I don't think it has been addressed in infants yet. So I am not so sure how effectively one can put in the intermediates between linoleic acid and arachidonic and raise arachidonic acid in adults.

Dr. Bracco: At least by using GLA you can increase without doubt the dihomo-γ-linolenic acid, which is the source of interesting precursors, of which all are found in human milk.

Dr. Clandinin: I should like to point out that we are rapidly approaching the point when a lot of our traditional sources of fats are going to become very untraditional. We are close to being able to move desaturases into various cells and probably to put some of these enzymes into our vegetable crops. We shall soon be buying things like corn oil with DHA, or corn oil with arachidonic acid, and so on. I suspect that within this decade as an industry you are going to have some fairly untraditional fats to change your mixtures with.

Polyunsaturated Fatty Acids in Human Nutrition,
edited by U. Bracco and R. J. Deckelbaum,
Nestlé Nutrition Workshop Series, Vol. 28,
Nestec Ltd., Vevey/Raven Press, Ltd., New York © 1992.

Long Chain Fatty Acid Metabolism and Essential Fatty Acid Deficiency with Special Emphasis on Cystic Fibrosis

Birgitta Strandvik

Department of Pediatrics, University of Göteborg, S-41685 Göteborg, Sweden

Cystic fibrosis (CF) is a recessive hereditary disease which for many years has been the most common serious disease of childhood in Caucasians (1). Although the cause of the disease is still unknown (as of November 1991), the identification of the gene locus at chromosome 7, and the determination of the protein it codes for, opens possibilities for both determination of the etiology and understanding of the pathophysiology and hopefully for therapy in the near future (2-4). The coded protein, named cystic fibrosis transmembrane conductance regulator (CFTR), has been found to be a complex transmembraneous large protein consisting of 1,480 amino acids and with two phosphorylation parts. One phenylalanine missing in the 508 position has been found to be the most common mutation, present in 55-70% of the probands (5,6). More than 125 different mutations have now been reported but the function of the CFTR is still unknown; it is therefore controversial whether or not it is the chloride channel (7). It is out of the question that it influences the chloride transport and it is the defective chloride conductance which up to now has been generally considered to be the basic cause of the disease (8).

CF PATIENTS HAVE ESSENTIAL FATTY ACID DEFICIENCY

In CF, the frequent occurrence of essential fatty acid deficiency (EFAD) has been known for many decades (9). It has, however, been neglected due to the fact that it has been considered as a consequence of pancreatic insufficiency, which is present in more than 90% of the patients (10). During later years several reports have also confirmed the presence of EFAD in patients without pancreatic insufficiency (11-16) and have indicated an increased turnover of essential fatty acids (17-19). The possibility that some of the clinical symptoms of CF may be influenced by correcting the EFAD has been presented (20), and the clinical benefit of supplying emulsions rich in essential fatty acids on a regular basis has been confirmed (21).

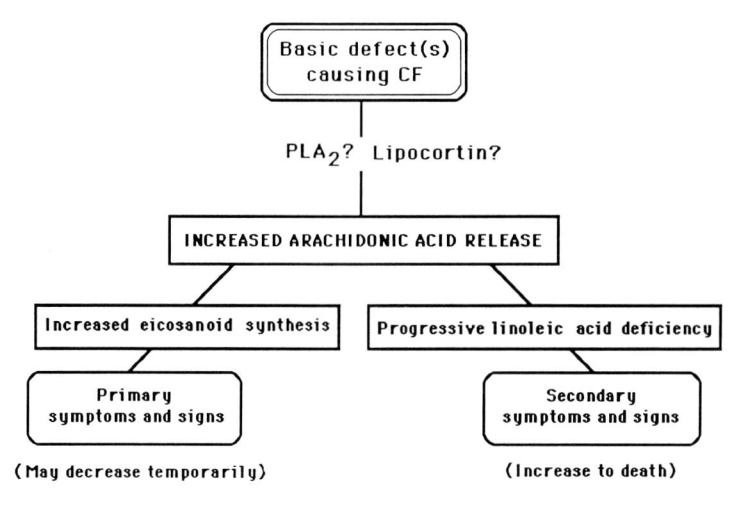

```
┌─────────────────┐
│  Basic defect(s)│
│   causing CF    │
└─────────────────┘
         │
   PLA₂? Lipocortin?
         │
┌─────────────────────────────┐
│ INCREASED ARACHIDONIC ACID RELEASE │
└─────────────────────────────┘
      ╱              ╲
┌──────────────────┐  ┌──────────────────────────────┐
│ Increased eicosanoid │  │ Progressive linoleic acid    │
│    synthesis         │  │       deficiency             │
└──────────────────┘  └──────────────────────────────┘
      │                            │
┌──────────────┐            ┌──────────────┐
│  Primary     │            │  Secondary   │
│ symptoms and │            │ symptoms and │
│   signs      │            │    signs     │
└──────────────┘            └──────────────┘
(May decrease temporarily)   (Increase to death)
```

FIG. 1. The major effects of arachidonic acid related to basic symptoms in CF.

A HYPOTHESIS OF THE PATHOPHYSIOLOGY IN CF

A hypothesis that the EFAD might influence some of the symptoms in CF and the progression of the disease has been proposed (22–25). Studies in animals with EFAD have further supported this view, since many organ systems frequently affected in CF are those which are early and seriously affected in the rats (26,27) and the chicken (28,29). All symptoms cannot of course be explained by EFAD. Some of the more specific symptoms, such as the disturbed chloride conductance (8), the increased mucus production (30), and the aberration in the response to β-adrenergic stimulus (31), are likely to be related to a defect which increases the turnover of the essential fatty acids, i.e., the defect should be sought in connection with an effect of these fatty acids or their products on different cells or tissues (Fig. 1).

In a previous study on lymphocytes from patients with CF, we found that the release of labeled arachidonic acid was not normally inhibited by dexamethasone (19). If this were due to a defective regulation of phospholipase A_2, which is also the rate-limiting enzyme in eicosanoid synthesis, the increased release of arachidonic acid would result in an increased production of these active products apart from arachidonic acid itself. This might be a possible model to explain the primary symptoms in CF.

PRIMARY SYMPTOMS ARE RELATED TO ARACHIDONIC ACID RELEASE

Interestingly, both arachidonic acid and its major products in the eicosanoid cascade have been shown to influence those mechanisms which are connected with the

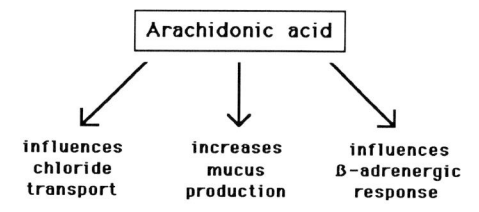

```
        ┌─────────────────┐
        │ Arachidonic acid │
        └─────────────────┘
         ↙       ↓       ↘
influences   increases   influences
 chloride      mucus     β-adrenergic
 transport   production    response
```

FIG. 2. The baselines of a hypothesis on the pathophysiology of CF.

basic symptoms in CF (Fig. 2). Arachidonic acid, as well as prostaglandins, thromboxanes, and leukotrienes, can regulate chloride transport in different cells (32–34), and it has also been reported to change sweat chlorides *in vivo* (35). Prostaglandins, leukotrienes, and hydroxyeicosatetraenoic acids (HETE) have been shown to increase mucus production in the gastrointestinal and respiratory tracts (36–38). Arachidonic acid has been shown to regulate the β-adrenergic response in a dose-dependent way, higher concentrations giving a lower release of ATP (39), which would be in congruence with the reported unresponsiveness of ATP to increase after β-adrenergic stimulation in CF (31). An increased arachidonic acid cascade would thus be a possible explanation to the primary symptoms in CF (Figs. 1, 2). The time of onset and the extension of clinical symptoms and the progression rate of the disease could well be explained by the rate of the release of the arachidonic acid cascade, which might be regulated by the type and/or extent of defective regulation of phospholipase A_2, other membrane-bound regulations, or other glucocorticosteroid-regulated mechanisms of the arachidonic acid release. Such a mechanism would explain the scatter of levels of arachidonic acid release which has been observed in different patients regardless of the congruent inability of dexamethasone to inhibit this release in CF (19). It may be speculated that the different mutations of CFTR would change the function or stereochemistry of this protein in a way giving directly or indirectly (via a transported product?) different degrees of influence on the release of arachidonic acid from the phospholipids in the membranes. Regardless of the mechanisms, the arachidonic acid cascade would be expected, theoretically, to be less pronounced in advanced disease with a high degree of EFAD. It has been observed that meconium ileus or its equivalent in older patients is rare in clinically advanced disease. Furthermore, the secretion richest in prostaglandins in the human, that of the seminal vesicles, seems completely lacking in prostaglandins in CF patients (40).

Support for an increased eicosanoid production *in vivo* has been obtained, since very high levels of some prostanoids have been found in urine of patients with CF (41). An increased production of leukotrienes in leukocytes from stable CF patients without clinical and biochemical signs of infection further supports the hypothesis (Lindgren and Strandvik, to be published). It has to be determined if the increased prostanoid production is a result of the arachidonic acid release or is the cause of an increased release of this fatty acid.

SECONDARY SYMPTOMS CAN BE EXPLAINED BY EFAD

In animal studies growth retardation is one of the initial symptoms of EFAD (26,27) and this is also a well-known phenomenon in CF, which might sometimes be overcome by generous nutritional supplementation (42). Pulmonary infection and fibrosis have been reported in chickens and rats, respectively (28,29,43), and the rabbit has been suggested as a clinical model to study lung involvement in CF (44). In rats, defective fatty acid composition has been reported in bronchial phosphatidylcholine (45), one of the major constituents of pulmonary surfactant. An increased minimal surface tension, a measure of the activity of pulmonary surfactant, has been found in these animals with EFAD (46), and interestingly, similar findings have been reported in bronchial secretions from CF patients (47,48). In rats with EFAD the basal amylase secretion in isolated pancreatic acini was significantly decreased, and, although it increased after carbachol stimulation, the levels remained at a much lower level than in controls (49). The insulin response after glucose stimulation was exaggerated in essential-fatty-acid-deficient rats (49), a pattern similar to that found in a subgroup of patients with CF (50). In the younger rat with EFAD the glomerular filtration rate was significantly increased, but it decreased gradually in parallel with a worsening of the EFAD (51). In the older animals with EFAD, renal calcification and hematuria were common findings. At autopsy renal calcification has been described as a characteristic finding in CF and hematuria is not uncommon in advanced disease (30). In CF patients an increased glomerular filtration rate can be normalized in parallel with a normalization of essential fatty acid status by regular administration of a fat emulsion (21). Increased reabsorption of sodium has been observed in the airways (52) and in the kidneys (53) of CF patients. After regular administration of essential fatty acids the renal excretion of sodium normalized (21). Before the use of amiloride as a therapeutic tool in these patients (54) becomes too widespread, it is important to study whether a similar result might be obtained in the airways by correcting the EFAD in CF patients. It is worth noting that lecithin membranes from rats with EFAD show an increased sodium flux (55).

The model of this hypothesis in regard to gastrointestinal symptoms in CF has been described previously (25). In Fig. 3 a corresponding overview of the pulmonary symptoms is given and from the data presented above it can easily be seen that similar drafts may also be constructed for other organ systems.

FUTURE RESEARCH

The data presented show convincing evidence that EFAD influences the symptomatology in CF and also that indications point to a role of arachidonic acid and/or its metabolites in CF. The function of CFTR will probably very soon be determined and this will give an opportunity to confirm or reject the hypothesis presented. The large size and complexity of CFTR opens many possibilities as to the ways in which a defective protein of this kind might interfere with fatty acid metabolism in the

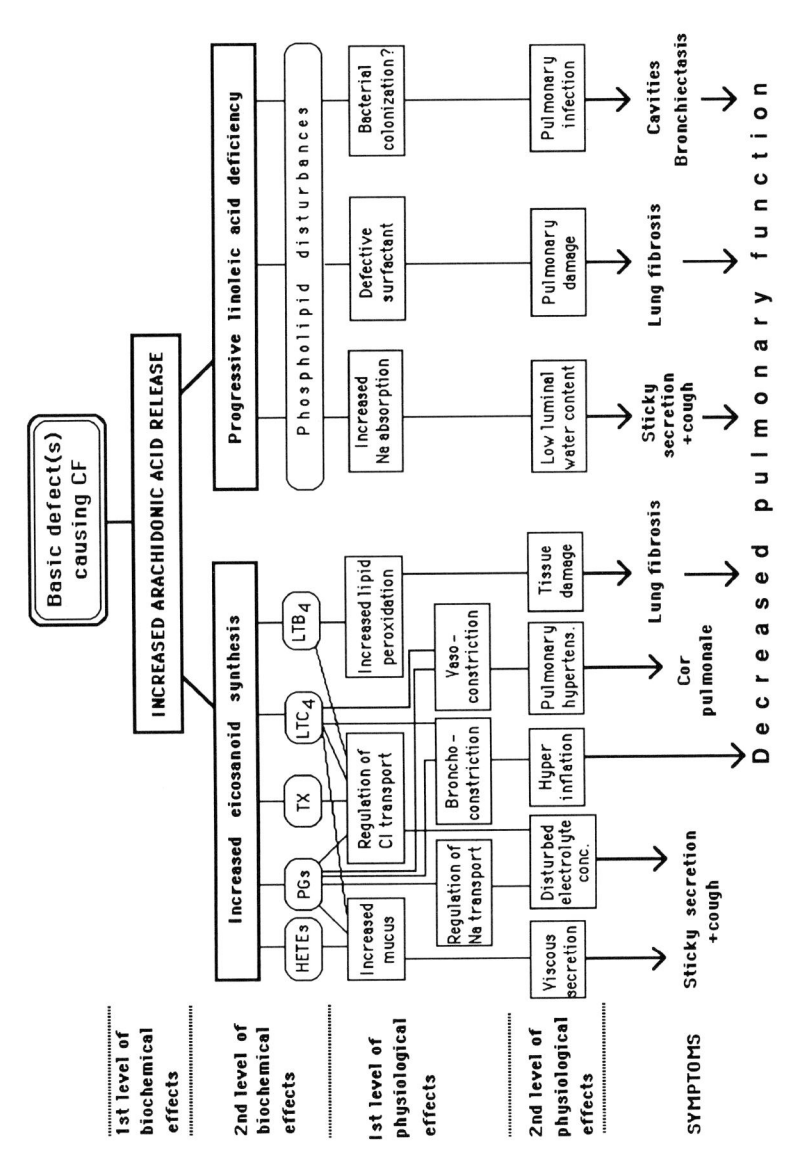

FIG. 3. Review of the existing knowledge and the arachidonic acid hypothesis related to pulmonary symptoms.

membranes, directly or indirectly. These facts may also enable explanation of the variability of disease severity and progression rate.

REFERENCES

1. Hodson ME, Norman AP, Batten JC, eds. *Cystic fibrosis*. London: Baillère Tindall; 1983.
2. Rommens JM, Iannuzzi MC, Kerem BS, *et al*. Identification of the cystic fibrosis gene: chromosome walking and jumping. *Science* 1989; 245: 1059–65.
3. Riordan JR, Rommens JM, Kerem B-S, *et al*. Identification of the cystic fibrosis gene: cloning and characterization of complementary DNA. *Science* 1989; 245: 1066–72.
4. Kerem B-S, Rommens JM, Buchanan JA, *et al*. Identification of the cystic fibrosis gene: genetic analysis. *Science* 1989; 245: 1073–80.
5. Dean M, White MB, Amos J, *et al*. Multiple mutations in highly conserved residual are found in mildly affected cystic fibrosis patients. *Cell* 1990; 61: 863–70.
6. Cutting GR, Kasch LM, Rosenstein BJ, *et al*. A cluster of cystic fibrosis mutations in the first nucleotide-binding fold of the cystic fibrosis conductance regulator protein. *Nature* 1990; 346: 366–8.
7. Boyd CAR. Function of cystic fibrosis gene product. *Lancet* 1990; ii: 938.
8. Quinton PM. Defective epithelial ion transport in cystic fibrosis. *Clin Chem* 1989; 35: 726–30.
9. Kuo PT, Huang NN, Bassett DR. The fatty acid composition of the serum chylomicrons and adipose tissue of children with cystic fibrosis of the pancreas. *J Pediatr* 1962; 60: 394–403.
10. Park RW, Grand RJ. Gastrointestinal manifestations of cystic fibrosis: a review. *Gastroenterology* 1981; 81: 1143–61.
11. Galabert C, Filliat M, Chazalette JP. Fatty acid composition of serum-lecithins in cystic fibrosis patients without steatorrhoea. *Lancet* 1978; i: 903.
12. Rogiers V, Dab I, Crokaert R, Vis HL. Long chain non-esterified fatty acid pattern in plasma of cystic fibrosis patients and their parents. *Pediatr Res* 1980; 14: 1088–91.
13. Rogiers V, Vercruysse A, Dab I, Baran D. Abnormal fatty acid pattern of the plasma cholesterol ester fraction in cystic fibrosis patients with and without pancreatic insufficiency. *Eur J Pediatr* 1983; 141: 39–42.
14. Henker J, Schimke E, Paul K-D, Leupold W. Fettsäuremuster bei Kindern mit Mukoviszidose in Beziehung zum Grad der exokrinen Pankreasinsuffizienz. *Helv Paediatr Acta* 1987; 42: 13–20.
15. Farrell PM, Mischler EH, Engle MJ, Brown DJ, Lau S-M. Fatty acid abnormalities in cystic fibrosis. *Pediatr Res* 1985; 19: 104–9.
16. Dimand RJ, Moonen CTW, Chu SC, Bradbury EM, Kurland G, Cox KL. Adipose tissue abnormalities in cystic fibrosis: noninvasive determination of mono- and polyunsaturated fatty acids by carbon-13 topical magnetic resonance spectroscopy. *Pediatr Res* 1988; 24: 243–6.
17. Roscher AA, Hadorn B. Regulation of beta-receptor-mediated biological signals on the cellular level. In: Kaiser D, ed. *Approaches to cystic fibrosis research*. Berlin: Maizena Diät; 1981: 61–7.
18. Rogiers V, Dab I, Michotte Y, Vercruysse A, Crokaert R, Vis HL. Abnormal fatty acid turnover in the phospholipids of the red blood membranes of cystic fibrosis patterns (in vitro study). *Pediatr Res* 1984; 18: 704–9.
19. Carlstedt-Duke J, Brönnegård M, Strandvik B. Pathological regulation of arachidonic acid release in cystic fibrosis: the putative basic defect. *Proc Natl Acad Sci USA* 1986; 83: 9202–06.
20. Elliott RB, Robinson PG. Unusual clinical course in a child with cystic fibrosis treated with fat emulsion. *Arch Dis Child* 1975; 50: 76–8.
21. Strandvik B, Berg U, Kallner A, Kusoffsky E. The effect on renal function of essential fatty acid supplementation in cystic fibrosis. *J Pediatr* 1989; 115: 242–8.
22. Strandvik B, Gilljam H, Kallner A, Wiman L-G. Fatty acid metabolism in cystic fibrosis. In: Warwick W, ed. *1000 years of cystic fibrosis*. Minneapolis: University of Minnesota; 1981: 304.
23. Strandvik B, Brönnegård M, Carlstedt-Duke J. Arachidonic acid release in CF. In: Mastella G, Quinton PM, eds. *Cellular and molecular basis of cystic fibrosis*. San Francisco: San Francisco Press, 1988: 445–50.
24. Strandvik B, Brönnegård M, Gilljam H, Carlstedt-Duke J. Relation between defective regulation of arachidonic acid release and symptoms in cystic fibrosis. *Scand J Gastroenterol* 1988; 23 [Suppl 143]: 1–4.

25. Strandvik B. Relation between essential fatty acid metabolism and gastrointestinal symptoms in cystic fibrosis. *Acta Paediatr Scand (Suppl)* 1989; 363: 58–65.
26. Burr GO, Burr MM. A new deficiency disease produced by the rigid exclusion of fat from the diet. *J Biol Chem* 1929; 82: 345–67.
27. Holman RT. Essential fatty acid deficiency. *Prog Med Chem* 1971; 9: 279–348.
28. Hopkins DT, Witter RL, Nesheim MC. A respiration disease syndrome in chickens fed essential fatty acid deficient diet. *Proc Soc Exp Biol Med* 1963; 114: 82–4.
29. Craig-Schmidt MC, Faircloth SA, Teer PA, Weete JD, Wu C-Y. The essential fatty acid deficient chicken as a model for cystic fibrosis. *Am J Clin Nutr* 1986; 44: 816–24.
30. Bodian M, ed. *Fibrocystic disease of the pancreas: a congenital disorder of mucus production-mucosis*. New York: Grune & Stratton; 1953.
31. Davis PB. Physiologic implications of the autonomic aberrations in cystic fibrosis. *Horm Metab Res* 1986; 18: 217–20.
32. Leikauf GD, Veki IF, Widdicombe JH, Nadel JA. Alteration of chloride secretion across canine tracheal epithelium by lipoxygenase products of arachidonic acid. *Am J Physiol* 1986; 250: 147–51.
33. Schaeffer BE, van Praag D, Greenwald L, Farber SJ, Zadunaisky JA. Effects of leukotrienes on chloride transport across frog cornea. In: Braquet P *et al.* eds. *Prostaglandins and membrane ion transport*. New York: Raven Press; 1984: 165–72.
34. Hwang T-C, Guggino SE, Guggino WB. Direct modulation of secretory chloride channels by arachidonic and other cis unsaturated fatty acids. *Proc Natl Acad Sci USA* 1990; 87: 5706–9.
35. Silverman BL, Lloyd-Still JD, Hazinski TA, Hunt CE. Increased sweat chloride levels associated with prostaglandin E_1 infusion. *J Pediatr* 1985; 106: 953–4.
36. Peatfield AC, Piper PJ, Richardson PS. The effect of leukotriene C4 on mucin release into the cat trachea in vivo and in vitro. *Br J Pharmacol* 1982; 77: 391–3.
37. Marom Z, Shelhamer JH, Sun F, Kaliner M. Effects of arachidonic acid monohydroxy eicosatetraenoic acid and prostaglandins on the release of mucous glycoproteins from human airways in vitro. *J Clin Invest* 1981; 67: 1695–702.
38. Lamorte WW, Lamont JT, Hale W, Booker ML, Scott TE, Turner B. Gallbladder prostaglandins and lysophospholipids as mediators of mucin secretion during cholelithiasis. *Am J Physiol* 1986; (*Gastrointest Liver Physiol* 14): G701–9.
39. Iizuka H, Kajita S, Mizumoto T, Kawaguchi H. Glucocorticoid-induced modulation of the beta-adrenergic adenylate cyclase response of epidermis: its relation to epidermal phospholipase A_2 activity. *J Invest Dermatol* 1986; 87: 577–82.
40. Bendvold E, Gottlieb C, Svanborg K, *et al.* Absence of prostaglandins in semen of men with cystic fibrosis is an indication of the contribution of the seminal vesicles. *J Reprod Fertil* 1986; 78: 311–4.
41. Strandvik B, Seyberth HJ. Prostanoid metabolites in urine of patients with cystic fibrosis. Taipei Conference on Prostaglandin and Leukotriene Research. Taipei, Taiwan; 1988: 166.
42. Shepard RW, Cooksley WGE, Cooke WDD. Improved growth and clinical nutritional and respiratory changes in response to nutritional therapy in cystic fibrosis. *J Pediatr* 1980; 97: 351–7.
43. Parnham MJ, Essed CE, Montfoort A, Spierings ELH. Inflammatory pleuropulmonary fibrosis in essential fatty acid deficient rats and the lack of response to methysergide. *Agents Actions* 1984; 14: 223–7.
44. Harper TB, Chase HP, Henson J, Henson PM. Essential fatty acid deficiency in the rabbit as a model of nutritional impairment in cystic fibrosis. *Am Rev Respir Dis* 1982; 78: 311–4.
45. Kyriakides EC, Beeler DA, Edmonds RH, Balint JA. Alterations in phosphatidylcholine species and their reversal in pulmonary surfactant during essential fatty acid deficiency. *Biochim Biophys Acta* 1976; 431: 399–407.
46. Burnell JM, Kyriakides EC, Edmonds RH, Balint JA. The relationship of fatty acid composition and surface activity of lung extracts. *Respir Physiol* 1978; 32: 195–206.
47. Gilljam H, Strandvik B, Ellin Å, Wiman L-G. Fatty acid pattern in bronchial secretion in patients with cystic fibrosis. In: Adam G, Valassi H, eds. Proceedings of the 12th Annual Meeting of the EWGCF, Athens, Greece; 1983: 207–13.
48. Gilljam H, Andersson O, Ellin Å, Robertson B, Strandvik B. Composition and surface properties of the bronchial lipids in adult patients with cystic fibrosis. *Clin Chim Acta* 1988; 176: 29–38.
49. Hjelte L, Ahrén B, Andrén-Sandberg Å, Böttcher G, Strandvik B. Pancreatic function in the essential fatty acid deficient rat. *Metabolism* 1990; 39: 871–5.
50. Strandvik B, Stanciulescu E, Hjelte L. Insulin response and oral glucose tolerance in cystic fibrosis. 16th Annual Meeting of ISGD, Oslo, Norway; September 6–9, 1990: 222.

51. Hjelte L, Larsson M, Alvestrand A, Malmborg AS, Strandvik B. Renal function in rats with essential fatty acid deficiency. *Clin Sci* 1990; 79: 299–305.
52. Boucher RC, Cotton CU, Gatzy JT, Knowles MR, Yankaskas JR. Evidence for reduced Cl^- and increased Na^+ permeability in cystic fibrosis human primary cell cultures. *J Physiol (Lond)* 1988; 405: 77–103.
53. Berg U, Kusoffsky E, Strandvik B. Renal function in cystic fibrosis with special reference to the renal sodium handling. *Acta Paediatr Scand* 1982; 71: 833–8.
54. App EM, King M, Helfesrieder R, Köhler D, Matthys H. Acute and long-term amiloride inhalation in cystic fibrosis lung disease. *Am Rev Respir Dis* 1990; 141: 605–12.
55. Moore JL, Richardson T, DeLuca HF. Essential fatty acids and ionic permeability of lecithin membranes. *Chem Phys Lipids* 1969; 3: 39–58.

DISCUSSION

Dr. Guesry: If you believe that cystic fibrosis symptoms are partly due to increased prostaglandin synthesis, did you check the levels of prostaglandins in the urine and did you try cyclo-oxygenase inhibitors such as aspirin or other anti-inflammatory agents?

Dr. Strandvik: When we first found these high levels we gave nonsteroidal anti-inflammatory agents to some patients, but they didn't work. The high level of excretion remained, which made me think our method was wrong. I have not repeated these studies but the amounts of prostaglandins we have now found using GLC-mass spectrometry are so great that I am not surprised that we did not influence them with the drugs we used. New drugs are becoming available, for leukotriene inhibition for instance, but it is too early yet to embark on trials.

Dr. Guesry: I am surprised because a long time ago we treated Bartter's syndrome which is also due to hypersecretion of prostaglandin, and it works very well.

Dr. Strandvik: Yes, but Bartter's syndrome is not the same as cystic fibrosis; it is different. I agree, we are using indometacin to treat patients with Bartter's syndrome and we can manage that, so this is the difference. However, this is a very relevant comment, because, interestingly, some of the patients with cystic fibrosis may debut with a very similar syndrome, but it is not Bartter's.

Dr. Cunnane: The effects of cystic fibrosis are in some respects very similar to those of zinc deficiency. I also think a proportion of CF patients are zinc deficient. I refer to the high free arachidonic acid and the more rapid phospholipase A_2 activity, increased prostaglandin excretion, and some of the clinical symptoms related to growth retardation, immune deficiency, and so on. Have you investigated zinc status in your patients?

Dr. Strandvik: It has been shown that zinc is not well absorbed in CF, but I have never found low levels in my patients. I have not treated with zinc under controlled conditions so I cannot say that it might not cause improvement in spite of normal serum concentrations.

Dr. Spielmann: Ashkenazy, from New York, recently investigated the effect of a lipid parenteral emulsion in CF and found that there were responders and nonresponders. Responders, who improved with the emulsion, had higher levels of 20:3 ω-6 after the parenteral nutrition. Since 20:3 ω-6 cannot be substrate for 5-lipoxygenase I would be interested in your comments.

Dr. Strandvik: Ashkenazy treated patients who were severely ill and needed parenteral nutrition. They are not at all comparable to our patients, who were clinically quite well and just had EFA deficiency. You are likely to see an improvement in lung function in any severely ill CF patient if you give sufficient calories. I have not found high levels of 20:3 ω-6 in any of my patients, but on the other hand I have not specifically looked for them.

Dr. Deckelbaum: Ashkenazy did not control for better nutritional status, which your study did. Yours suggest that the effect of the parenteral emulsion was not nutritional.

Dr. Strandvik: I do not think it was a nutritional effect because the control and treatment groups had similar weight gain and did not eat differently from ordinary people. They had a Z score of about zero and there was no change between the groups during the study.

Dr. Heim: Your patients were all steatorrhoic. Does this mean that treatment with pancreatic enzymes was insufficient and that therefore they were nutritionally deficient?

Dr. Strandvik: No. My patients have as much enzyme as they need to ensure one normal stool per day. You can never compensate completely for the absence of pancreatic enzymes in CF, so there will always be some degree of steatorrhoea.

Dr. Heim: What percentage of patients with cystic fibrosis develop EFA deficiency?

Dr. Strandvik: We don't know this. The interesting thing is that some patients without steatorrhoea develop EFA deficiency. Furthermore, not all patients who have steatorrhoea have EFA deficiency. The primary defect must be something that induces a high turnover, and this defect may differ in different patients, depending on the mutation. You can compensate if you have a diet containing adequate fat, since it is the percentage of fat that determines what is absorbed even if you have steatorrhoea.

Effects of Dietary Essential Fatty Acid Balance on Behavior and Chronic Diseases

Harumi Okuyama

Faculty of Pharmaceutical Sciences, Nagoya City University, 3-1 Tanabedori, Mizuhoku, Nagoya 467, Japan

Beneficial effects of supplementing fish oil have been studied extensively (1,2), and eicosapentaenoic acid (20:5n-3, EPA) ethylester was recently developed in Japan as a treatment for thrombotic disease. Supplementary EPA appears to competitively inhibit the metabolism of arachidonate and to change the overall eicosanoid balance in the body. This in turn constitutes the major basis for the beneficial effects of Ω-3 fatty acids in alleviating thrombotic diseases.

Despite extensive studies on the importance of arachidonate and EPA in animal physiology, relatively little attention has been paid to the effects of their 18-carbon precursors, linoleic (18:2n-6), and α linolenic (18:3n-3) acids in our diets. This is mainly because people have believed that the conversion of 18-carbon polyunsaturated fatty acids to 20-carbon highly unsaturated fatty acids (desaturation-elongation) is a relatively slow step in humans as compared with experimental animals. However, evidence has accumulated which indicates that the rate of desaturation-elongation activity is sufficient to supply 20-carbon highly unsaturated fatty acids in humans as well. The amounts of linoleic and α linolenic acids in human diets must then be considered more seriously in relation to eicosanoid balance and apart from the hypocholesterolemic activities of these polyunsaturates.

Our studies have indicated that the dietary α linolenate/linoleate balance has effects both on aspects of behavior and learning and on the development of chronic diseases such as cancer, allergy, thrombotic diseases, cerebral vascular disease, hypertension, and aging (3).

EVIDENCE THAT DESATURATION-ELONGATION ACTIVITY IN HUMANS IS ENOUGH TO PROVIDE 20-CARBON HIGHLY UNSATURATED FATTY ACIDS

Human cells in culture are known to have desaturation-elongation activity. Recently, the conversion of labeled α linolenic acid to EPA and docosahexaenoic acid (DHA) was estimated to be of the order of 5% of the ingested amount in 24 hours

(4). This rate of conversion is quite significant because most of the ingested polyunsaturated fatty acids are oxidatively catabolized. In this experiment, however, the conversion of linoleic acid to arachidonic acid was not detectable, probably due to the dilution of labeled linoleic acid with the large amount of nonlabeled acid ingested daily (ca. 15–20 g/day). In fact, the conversion of both linoleic and α linolenic acids to 20-carbon highly unsaturated fatty acids has been noted in a patient under total parenteral nutrition (Dr. K. Yamaguchi, Tokyo Kasei University, Tokyo; personal communication). Holman *et al.* (5) and Bjerve *et al.* (6) showed that ingestion of a vegetable oil containing α linolenic acid permitted patients to recover from n-3 fatty acid deficiency symptoms. Adam *et al.* (7) found that the amounts of arachidonate metabolites in urine varied depending on the amounts of linoleic acid ingested. Finally, it should be emphasized that strict vegetarians ingest only linoleate and α linolenate, and usually do not develop essential fatty acid deficiency (8).

All these data indicate that humans are no exceptions among mammals in the metabolism of linoleate and α linolenate, although the desaturation-elongation activities may be relatively lower in most humans probably due to the negative feedback control of the enzyme systems by large amounts of highly unsaturated fatty acids in their diets (9).

ESSENTIALITY OF α LINOLENIC ACID IN BRAIN AND NERVE FUNCTIONS

DHA derived from α linolenic acid is rich in brain, retina, and nerve tissues, and therefore has been assumed to be essential for their functions. Direct evidence came from observations in monkeys given safflower oil as a source of essential fatty acids (10). The animals showed mental disorders (self-mutilation), skin disorders, and hepatic lesions, which are not easily recognized in rats given safflower oil. Rats fed safflower oil showed lower learning ability in a simple Y-maze test (11), but this observation was not reproduced when an X-maze test was carried out under similar conditions, as reviewed by Bivins *et al.* (12). Furthermore, the learning ability of rats in a maze test was reported to be the lowest in the fish-oil-fed group as compared with the groups which were fed oils rich in saturated, oleic, or linoleic acids (13). These data did not appear to be consistent with one another.

We used a brightness discrimination learning test for the evaluation of learning abilities of rats fed linoleate-rich or α-linolenate-rich diets (see Table 1 for the fatty acid composition of the diets). There were no significant differences in the positive responses (the lever-pressing response under a bright light for which diet pellets were given), but the negative response (the lever-pressing response under a dark light) was significantly less in the perilla group than in the safflower group. Consequently, the correct response ratio was higher in the perilla group. So far, four strains of rats have been examined in the brightness-discrimination learning test and quite reproducible results have been obtained (14–16). In one set of experiments, the stimuli were reversed after 30 sessions (days) of the test, and the test was

TABLE 1. Fatty acid compositions of the diets[a]

Fatty acid	Safflower diet	Soybean diet	Perilla diet
14:0	0.5	0.5	0.6
16:0	8.6	15.5	8.1
16:1	nd	1.5	nd
18:0	2.2	2.5	1.9
18:1n-9	10.4	22.8	12.3
18:2n-6	78.0	48.8	12.8
18:3n-3	0.05	4.1	64.0
20:1	nd	0.9	nd
20:4n-6	0.2	0.4	0.2

[a] Semipurified diets containing 5% vegetable oils were used for the estimation of brain and nerve functions, and the fatty acid compositions of the diets are shown as wt %. For other experiments, a conventional diet (Nihon Clea Co., Tokyo) was treated with hexane, and then various oils (5% or 10%) and a vitamin mixture were added to the defatted diet.

continued for another 30 sessions to find even clearer differences between the safflower group and the perilla group (the former being inferior in the discrimination-learning ability; Table 1).

A series of behavior tests were carried out with mice fed the safflower diet or the perilla diet through two generations to distinguish significant differences in the behaviors of the two groups. It is now quite certain that the α linolenate/linoleate balance affects the behavior of animals.

Essential fatty acid (n-6 and n-3) deficiency during the gestational period is reported to induce irreversible damage to brain function; supplementation after this period does not allow rats to recover from decreased learning ability (17). Deficiency of n-3 in the presence of n-6 fatty acids appears to differ from the n-6 plus n-3 deficiency induced with fat-free diets. The decreased learning ability caused by n-3 deficiency was completely reversed by supplementing with n-3 fatty acids after weaning.

Wheeler et al. (18) have shown in rats that a fat-free diet induced a significant decrease in the amplitudes of electroretinogram, which was restored by both linoleate and α linolenate, the latter being more effective. We observed similar differences in rats fed a high linoleate (safflower oil) diet as compared with a high α linolenate (perilla oil) diet (19). Although we could not describe what the decreased amplitude means in terms of the function of the eye, Neuringer et al. (20) have found that n-3 fatty acid deficiency induces a decrease in visual acuity in monkey.

All these data have served to establish that α linolenic acid is essential for the maintenance of brain and nerve functions at higher levels.

THE MINIMUM AMOUNT OF n-3 FATTY ACID REQUIRED FOR THE MAINTENANCE OF BRAIN AND NERVE FUNCTIONS

Both in the brightness discrimination learning tests and the electroretinographic measurements, responses were better in the perilla oil group than in the soybean oil group, which, in turn, was better than in the safflower oil group (see Table 1 for the fatty acid compositions of the diets). Although the fatty acid compositions of brain and retina were quite similar between the soybean group and the perilla group, the physiological responses (learning ability and electroretinographic response) were not the same. These results indicate that a concentration of α linolenic acid of 0.55% of energy (soybean oil diet) is insufficient to induce the maximum physiological response seen in the group fed the perilla diet (α linolenic acid 8% of energy). Consistent with these observations, Wheeler *et al.* (18) showed that the amplitude in the electroretinogram was still higher in the group fed 2 wt % α linolenic acid than in the group fed 1 wt % linoleic acid and 1 wt % α linolenic acid (estimated to be 2.6% of energy intake). Thus, the minimum amount of α linolenic acid needed to induce a full response must be above 2.6% of energy which is higher than the values (0.3–0.5%) proposed by others, as reviewed (21). It is quite possible that there is no minimum amount of n-3 fatty acids required for the maintenance of brain and nerve functions, but that the physiological responses of these organs may change continuously, depending on the amounts and the ratios of linoleic and α linolenic acids in diets within a range broader than that suggested.

ALLERGIC HYPERREACTIVITY AS INFLUENCED BY DIETARY ESSENTIAL FATTY ACID BALANCE

In Japan, the number of allergic patients has increased severalfold in the past several decades, and now one-third of infants born in Japan are diagnosed as atopic. More or less similar situations appear to be seen in industrialized countries. Environmental antigens such as house dust mite, fungi, pollen, and food allergens have been identified, and much effort has been made to keep patients away from these antigens. However, the increases in these antigens do not appear to account for the severalfold increase in the numbers of allergic patients in the past 30 years in Japan. Now, we have evidence that the excess intake of linoleic acid and the changes in the essential fatty acid balance of diets have made our bodies hyperreactive to various allergens.

Leukotrienes, prostaglandins, and platelet-activating factor (PAF) are mediators of allergy and inflammation. Eicosanoids derived from the n-6 series fatty acids are known to have physiological activities severalfold to several hundredfold higher than those of eicosanoids derived from n-3 fatty acids. Furthermore, the release of PAF from neutrophils was found to be significantly less in the n-3-rich diet group as compared with n-6-rich diet group. Therefore, raising the n-3/n-6 ratios of cells responsible for allergy and inflammation would help to decrease the allergic reactivity of the body, as shown in animal models (22). It is understood that the increase in the intake of linoleic acid in the past several decades in the industrialized countries has made our bodies hyperreactive to various allergens.

SUCCESS AND FAILURE OF NUTRITIONAL RECOMMENDATIONS FOR THE PREVENTION OF CHRONIC DISEASES

The nutritional guidelines for the prevention of diseases of the elderly have called for decreases in the intakes of animal fats and cholesterol but increases in the intakes of vegetable oils and vegetable oil products rich in linoleic acid. In the Untied States, nutritionists have succeeded in persuading people to follow these guidelines; the intake of animal fats (except those included in meats and poultry products) has decreased by one-half and the intake of vegetable oil has increased three-fold in the past 50 years. However, the incidence of coronary heart disease is still high and has tended to increase, although mortality related to heart disease has decreased, mostly due to the improvement in medical care in the United States.

In Japan, the incidence of stroke (cerebral bleeding) has decreased but the incidences of thrombotic diseases such as cardiac infarction and cerebral infarction have increased significantly along with the westernization of the food environment. Studies with stroke-prone SHR rats have revealed that the major risk factors for this model are high salt and low protein, which had been characteristic features of foods in certain areas of Japan. The westernization of foods (high protein) and the recommendation to decrease salt intake appear to have been successful in decreasing the incidence of cerebral bleeding. On the other hand, the incidence of thrombotic diseases is increasing rapidly, despite great efforts to increase the P/S ratio of diets.

Starting from epidemiological studies on Eskimos and Danes, scientists have clarified that the n-3/n-6 ratio of diets is a major factor in the pathogenesis of thrombotic diseases (1,2). The n-3/n-6 ratios of Western diets are very low and the ratios are decreasing in Japan, mainly because of the increase in the intake of linoleic acid. Evidence was obtained from studies in our laboratories on the effects of vegetable oils on animal models of chronic diseases that the intake of excess linoleic acid is the major factor increasing the incidence of many chronic diseases including cancer (22–27). The results of such studies are summarized in Table 2.

TABLE 2. Effects of vegetable oils on behavior and chronic diseases

Perilla oil was better than soybean oil and safflower oil in
 Brightness discrimination learning ability, water maze learning ability, retinal response, suppression of carcinogenesis, spontaneous tumorigenesis, metastasis of tumor cells, thrombotic diseases, stroke (cerebral bleeding), hypertension, allergic reactivity and aging

Safflower oil was better than perilla oil in
 Suppression of anti-GBM antibody-induced nephritis and LPS-GalN-induced hepatitis

No significant difference was found between perilla & safflower oils in
 Growth, appearance, teratogenicity, reproductive physiology (gestational period, litter size), radiation damage, lipofuscin content, membrane lipid peroxidizability, erythrocyte deformability, LPS-induced hepatitis and nephritis in autoimmune mice (MRL)

EFFECT OF DIETARY ESSENTIAL FATTY ACID BALANCE ON CARCINOGENESIS

Most of the available data support the conclusion that dietary linoleic acid promotes but that n-3 fatty acids suppress carcinogenesis (28). Metastasis of tumor cells is also stimulated by linoleic acid but suppressed by n-3 fatty acids (23). Prostaglandin E_2 promotes the transcription of certain oncogenes and stimulates growth. This may be the mechanism for the stimulatory effects of linoleic acid. Prostaglandin E_2 also suppresses the immunological system of the host, allowing the tumor cells to grow faster. On the other hand, platelet aggregability is stimulated with dietary linoleic acid, and this, in turn, is positively correlated with the metastatic potential of tumor cells (29). These appear to form at least a part of the basis for the modification of carcinogenesis and metastasis by dietary essential fatty acid balance. The cancers so far reported to be enhanced by dietary linoleic acid are lung (adenocarcinoma type), mammary, colon, kidney, pancreatic, skin, esophageal, and prostate.

AN n-3/n-6 RATIO THAT IS OPTIMAL FOR ALL HUMANS DOES NOT EXIST

We compared the effects of safflower oil (n-3/n-6 ratio < 0.01), soybean oil (n-3/n-6 = 0.1–0.2), and perilla oil (n-3/n-6 ratio = 4–5) on several aspects of animal physiology. Learning ability and retinal function were higher in the perilla group than in the other groups. The dietary essential fatty acid balance also affected other types of behavior. However, it is difficult to conclude which type of general behavior is better. For most chronic diseases, perilla oil was better than soybean oil and safflower oil. However, there are pathological conditions under which prostaglandins derived from n-6 fatty acids play protective roles, and the safflower oil diet is better than the perilla oil diet for suppressing the symptoms (e.g., endotoxin shock and anti-GBM antibody-induced nephritis) (30). Therefore, the optimum n-3/n-6 ratio must be different among individuals under different physiological conditions. For the prevention of most of the chronic diseases listed in Table 2, perilla oil with an n-3/n-6 ratio of 4–5 was better than soybean oil with a ratio of 0.1–0.2. Therefore, to avoid these chronic diseases one should decrease the intake of n-6 fatty acids and increase the intake of n-3 fatty acids. It should be noted that n-3/n-6 ratios of diets now ingested in industrialized countries (Fig. 1) are lower than the ratios in the Danish diet (0.28) and in the Eskimo diet (3.0) (39).

A NEW NUTRITIONAL RECOMMENDATION FOR THE PREVENTION OF CANCER AND CHRONIC DISEASES

Based on the results from animal experiments and epidemiological studies, I recommend the following nutritional guidelines for the prevention of the chronic diseases listed in Table 2.

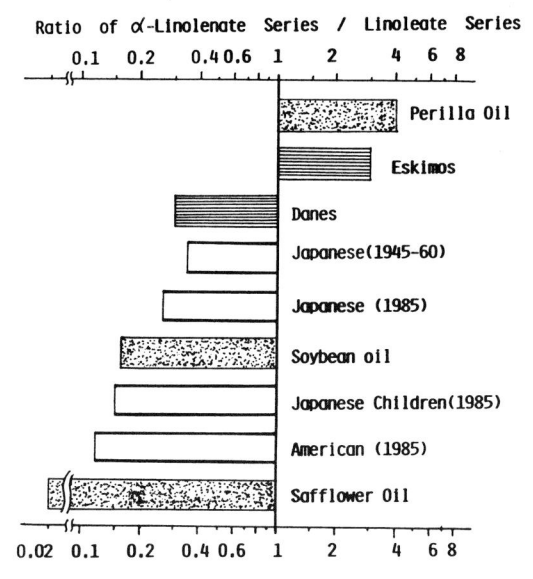

FIG. 1. The n-3/n-6 ratios of diets ingested. The n-3/n-6 ratios of Danes and Eskimos were calculated from data reported by Dyerberg (31) while those of Japanese and American diets were taken from Lands et al. (32).

1. The intake of linoleic acid should be greatly decreased. An intake of linoleic acid of 1% of dietary energy is known to satisfy the requirements. This is 1–2 g/day even for a growing person with a 60 kg body weight. More than twice the amounts required would be supplied through regular meals that include bread, rice, meat, and eggs. These days, average people are ingesting ~10 times the required amount of linoleic acid.

2. The intake of saturated and monoenoic fatty acids (animal fats) should be decreased. Total fat intake of less than 20% of energy is preferable. The average Japanese is now consuming 25% of energy as fats, and the incidences of fat-related chronic diseases and cancers have begun to increase rapidly since ~1965 when the fat intake was 15% of energy.

3. The intake of n-3 fatty acids should be increased. The amount of α linolenic acid as high as 8.4% of energy (perilla diet) was still the best in animal models examined for the prevention of cancer and chronic diseases.

PERSPECTIVES FOR FUTURE RESEARCH

Two major aspects of progress have been noted in Japanese food industry in 1990; some infant formulas were supplemented with α linolenic acid (perilla oil) and DHA (fish oil), and a part of premium oils was changed to high oleate type from high linoleate type. To extend further the changes in this direction in our food environment, clinical (long-term perspective) studies should be started, based on the results obtained with experimental animals.

REFERENCES

1. Lands WEM. *Fish and human health.* Orlando, FL: Academic Press; 1986.
2. Lees RS, Karel M, eds. *Omega-3 fatty acids in health and disease.* New York: Marcel Dekker; 1990.
3. Okuyama H. *Abura, kono oisikute huan na mono* (in Japanese, "Oils, very delicious but in anxiety"). Tokyo: Nobunkyo Pub. Co.; 1989.
4. Emken EA, Adlof RO, Rakoff H, Rohwedder WK. Synthesis and application of isotopically labeled compounds. In 1988 Proceedings of the Third International Symposium, Innsbruck, Austria; 1988: 713–6.
5. Holman RT, Johnson SB, Hatch TF. A case of human linolenic acid deficiency involving neurological abnormalities. *Am J Clin Nutr* 1982; 35: 617–23.
6. Bjerve KS, Mostad IL, Thoresen L. Alpha-linolenic acid deficiency in patients on long-term gastric-tube feeding: estimation of linolenic acid and long-chain unsaturated n-3 fatty acid requirement in man. *Am J Clin Nutr* 1987; 45:66–77.
7. Adam O, Wolfram G, Zollner N. Effect of α-linolenic acid in the human diet on linoleic acid metabolism and prostaglandin biosynthesis. *J Lipid Res* 1986; 27: 421–6.
8. Sanders TAB, Ellis FR, Dickerson JWT. Studies in vegans: the fatty acid composition of plasma choline phosphoglycerides, erythrocytes, adipose tissue and breast milk, and some indicators of susceptibility to ischemic heart disease in vegans and normal controls. *Am J Clin Nutr* 1978; 31:805–13.
9. DeGomez Dumm INT, DeAlaniz NJT, Brenner RR. Effect of dietary fatty acids on Δ5 desaturase activity and biosynthesis of arachidonic acid in rat liver microsomes. *Lipids* 1983; 18: 781–8.
10. Fiennes RNTW, Sinclair AJ, Crawford MA. Essential fatty acid studies in primates, linolenic acid requirements of capuchins. *J Med Primatol* 1973; 2: 155–69.
11. Lamptey MS, Walker BL. A possible essential role for dietary linoleic acid in the development of the young rat. *J Nutr* 1976; 106: 86–93.
12. Bivins BA, Bell RM, Rapp RP, Griffin WO, Jr. Linoleic acid versus linolenic acid: What is essential? *J Parenter Enter Nutr* 1983; 7: 473–8.
13. Harman D, Hendricks S, Eddy DE, Seibold J. Free radical theory of aging: effect of dietary fat on central nervous system function. *J Am Geriatr Soc* 1976; 24: 301–7.
14. Yamamoto N, Saitoh M, Moriuchi A, Nomura M, Okuyama H. Effect of dietary α-linolenate/linoleate balance on brain lipid compositions and learning ability of rats. *J Lipid Res* 1987; 28: 144–51.
15. Yamamoto N, Hashimoto A, Takemoto Y, *et al.* Effect of dietary α-linolenate/linoleate balance on lipid compositions and learning ability of rats. II. Discrimination process, extinction process, and glycolipid compositions. *J Lipid Res* 1988; 29: 1013–21.
16. Yamamoto N, Okaniwa Y, Mori S, Nomura M, Okuyama H. Effects of a high-linoleate and a high-α-linolenate diet on the learning ability of aged rats. Evidence against an autoxidation-related lipid peroxide theory of aging. *J Gerontol* 1991; 46: B17–22.
17. Morgan BLG, Oppenheimer J, Winick M. Effects of essential fatty acid deficiency during late gestation on brain N-acetylneuraminic acid metabolism and behavior in progeny. *Br J Nutr* 1981; 46: 223–30.
18. Wheeler TG, Benolken RM, Anderson RE. Visual membranes: specificity of fatty acid precursors for the electrical response to illumination. *Science* 1975; 188: 1312–4.
19. Watanabe I, Kato M, Aonuma H, *et al.* Effect of dietary alpha-linolenate/linoleate balance on the lipid composition and electroretinographic responses in rats. *Adv Biosci* 1987; 62: 563–70.
20. Neuringer M, Connor WE, Oetten CV, Barstad L. Dietary omega-3 fatty acid deficiency and visual loss in infant rhesus monkeys. *J Clin Invest* 1984; 73: 272–6.
21. Anonymous, Omega-3 event focuses on functional changes. *INFORM* 1990; 1: 520–4.
22. Hashimoto A, Katagiri M, Torii S, Dainaka J, Ichikawa A, Okuyama H. Effect of the dietary α-linolenate/linoleate balance on leukotriene production and histamine release in rats. *Prostaglandins* 1988; 36: 3–16.
23. Hori T, Moriuchi A, Okuyama H, Sobajima T, Tamiya-Koizumi K, Kojima K. Effect of dietary essential fatty acids on pulmonary metastasis of ascites tumor cells in rats. *Chem Pharm Bull* 1987; 35: 3925–7.
24. Watanabe S, Suzuki E, Kojima N, Kojima R, Suzuki Y, Okuyama H. Effect of dietary α-linolenate/

linoleate balance on collagen-induced platelet aggregation and serotonin release in rats. *Chem Pharm Bull* 1989; 37: 1572–1575.
25. Shimokawa T, Moriuchi A, Hori T, *et al.* Effect of dietary alpha-linolenate/linoleate balance on mean survival time, incidence of stroke and blood pressure of hypertensive rats. *Life Sci.* 1988; 43: 2067–75.
26. Kamano K, Okuyama H, Konishi R, Nagasawa H. Effects of a high-linoleate and a high-α-linolenate diet on spontaneous mammary tumourigenesis in mice. *Anticancer Res* 1989; 9: 1903–8.
27. Hirose M, Masuda A, Ito N, Kamano K, Okuyama H. Effects of dietary perilla oil, soybean oil and safflower oil on 7,12-dimethylbenz(a)anthracene (DMBA) and 1,2-dimethylhydrazine (DMH)-induced mammary gland and colon carcinogenesis in female SD rats. *Carcinogenesis* 1990; 11: 731–5.
28. Ip C, Birt DF, Rogers AE, Mettlin C, eds. *Dietary fat and cancer,* New York: Alan R. Liss; 1986.
29. Sugimoto Y, Oh-hara T, Watanabe M, Saito H, Yamori T, Tsuruo T. Acquisition of metastatic ability in hybridomas between two low metastatic clones of murine colon adenocarcinoma 26 defective in either platelet-aggregating activity or in vivo growth potential. *Cancer Res* 1987; 47: 4396–401.
30. Watanabe S, Suzuki E, Kojima R, Suzuki Y, Okuyama H. Effect of dietary α-linolenate/linoleate balance on crescent type anti-glomerular basement membrane nephritis in rats. *Lipids* 1990; 25: 267–72.
31. Dyerberg J. Linolenate-derived polyunsturated fatty acids and prevention of atherosclerosis. *Nutr Rev* 1986; 44: 125–34.
32. Lands WEM, Hamazaki T, Yamazaki K, Okuyama H, Sakai K, Goto Y, Hubbard VS. A story of changing dietary patterns. *Am J Clin Nutr* 1990; 51: 991–3.

DISCUSSION

Dr. Juhlin: What type of plant is perilla?

Dr. Okuyama: It grows naturally in the northern parts of China and Japan and probably also grows in Canada and northern United States. It grows to 1.5 m in height and comes from the family that includes lavender.

Dr. Jeremy: I find your epidemiologic data interesting, since breast and endometrial cancer are both etiologically related to estrogens. Thus the disparity in incidence between the two cancers may be indicative of a diet-related etiology, independent of estrogens.

Dr. Merrill: Numerous studies over the years, conducted with different models of carcinogens, different fatty acids, different regimes, multiple nutrient combinations, and so on, have indicated that drawing conclusions about fat and carcinogenesis is very risky because the results tend to be specific to the organ examined as well as to the type of carcinogen. Do you think you can extrapolate the data from your models to other kinds of cancer?

Dr. Okuyama: I don't think I can make such an extrapolation on the basis of our limited data. However for most cancers which have high incidences in Western countries and rapidly increasing incidences in Japan there is enough evidence to conclude that linoleic acid (n-6) promotes and n-3 fatty acids suppress carcinogenesis.

Dr. Glinsmann: Rats get certain types of tumors spontaneously. Was there any difference between the groups in these tumors?

Dr. Okuyama: We examined the effects on spontaneous mammary carcinogenesis and found a significant reduction in the perilla oil group.

Dr. Jeremy: It is important to establish reversibility of a learning defect. Most studies so far have come to the conclusion that many of these defects are irreversible. At the same time one feels instinctively that there has to be a degree of plasticity during brain development. Presumably if reversibility is induced at 3 weeks of age it cannot be associated with any change in cell number because it is too late for this. It could be a neurotransmitter effect, or due to changing numbers of synaptic junctions.

Dr. Okuyama: In our system the decrease in learning ability induced by ω-3 deficiency was reversed by supplementing with ω-3 after weaning. So far we have not investigated neurotransmitters or synaptic junctions.

Dr. Galli: We found the effects of EFA deficiency induced in the rat during brain development to be irreversible. We studied the effects on neurotransmitters and found no changes.

Dr. Widhalm: Your final recommendations that total fat intake should not exceed 20% of dietary energy are in contrast with the present dietary habits in Japan. Is there any subpopulation in Japan in which you have shown that these recommendations are practical?

Dr. Okuyama: At present in Japan the average fat intake is about 25% of energy intake, but the incidence of fat-related diseases began to increase dramatically following the westernization of our food in the early 1960s, when fat intake was about 15% of energy intake. It should not be impracticable to return to an intake of 20% or less.

Polyunsaturated Fatty Acids in Human Nutrition,
edited by U. Bracco and R. J. Deckelbaum,
Nestlé Nutrition Workshop Series, Vol. 28,
Nestec Ltd., Vevey/Raven Press, Ltd., New York © 1992.

Long Chain Fatty Acids in Obstetrics, Gynecology, and Fertility: A Focus on Non-Eicosanoid-Mediated Mechanisms

Jamie Y. Jeremy

Department of Chemical Pathology and Human Metabolism, Royal Free Hospital School of Medicine, University of London, London, NW3 2QG England

It has long been recognized that certain fatty acids (for example, linoleic and arachidonic) are essential for all aspects of mammalian reproductive function, at least in the laboratory animal (1–4). In women, the picture is not so clear, since no systematic studies on prolonged depletion of dietary essential fatty acids (EFA) on reproductive function have been carried out. However, an understanding of the relative significance of EFAs in mediating normal and abnormal reproductive function in women is potentially of extreme value in obstetric and gynecological practice. In other areas of medicine, manipulation of dietary fatty acid intake with foods and oils containing high levels of certain polyunsaturated fatty acids (PUFA) has proved successful in treating or ameliorating other diseases [e.g., cardiovascular disease, psoriasis, rheumatoid arthritis, and atherosclerosis (5–11)]. It is generally accepted that the effects of dietary oils are mediated by the high contents of three PUFA, eicosapentaenoic acid (EPA), docosahexaenoic acid (DHA), and dihomo-γ-linolenic acid (DGLA). In turn, since arachidonic acid, DGLA, and EPA are precursors of eicosanoids (prostaglandins, leukotrienes, and lipoxins; see ref. 12) the effects of EFA deficiency and the success of treating disease with dietary fatty acid supplementation have largely been interpreted as being mediated by alterations in eicosanoid synthesis. However, fatty acids possess other important non-eicosanoid-related properties that may determine their biological actions.

The aim of this paper, therefore, is to review how fatty acids may play a role in normal and abnormal reproductive function in women. The first part of this review will discuss effects of fatty acids and fatty acid-containing lipids on hormone dynamics, plasma membrane functions, signal transduction mechanisms, and eicosanoid synthesis as well as hormone effects on lipid metabolism and eicosanoid synthesis. The second part will discuss how these aspects may come into play in some selected areas, i.e., infertility, gynecological cancers, premature labor, hypertension, and premenstrual syndrome.

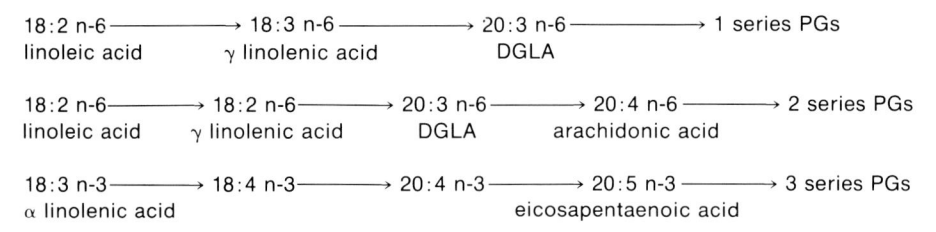

```
18:2 n-6 ─────────→ 18:3 n-6 ─────────→ 20:3 n-6 ─────────→ 1 series PGs
linoleic acid      γ linolenic acid     DGLA

18:2 n-6 ────→ 18:2 n-6 ────→ 20:3 n-6 ────→ 20:4 n-6 ────→ 2 series PGs
linoleic acid  γ linolenic acid  DGLA        arachidonic acid

18:3 n-3 ────→ 18:4 n-3 ────→ 20:4 n-3 ────→ 20:5 n-3 ────→ 3 series PGs
α linolenic acid                              eicosapentaenoic acid
```

FIG. 1. Formation of 1, 2, and 3 series eicosanoids.

FATTY ACIDS AS PRECURSORS OF EICOSANOIDS

Monoenoic ("1" series) and dienoic prostaglandins and thromboxanes ("2" series) are derived biosynthetically from DGLA and arachidonate, respectively. Eicosapentaenoic acid (EPA) is the precursor of the "3" series prostaglandins and thromboxanes (Fig. 1). On cell activation, precursor fatty acids are released from phospholipid stores by the action of phospholipases (12). The fatty acids are then metabolized to eicosanoids (depending on cell type). Since the prostaglandins and thromboxanes of the 1, 2, and 3 series possess markedly different properties, the mode of action of dietary fatty acids is thought to be mediated largely via changes in eicosanoid type (13). How this modulation of eicosanoid synthesis by fatty acids relates to selected areas of obstetrics, gynecology, and fertility will be discussed in the second part of this review.

STEROID HORMONE-FATTY ACID INTERACTIONS

Reproductive cycles and related functions in women are governed by a complex interaction of hormones of pituitary, ovarian, adrenal or placental origin. Hence, estrogens, progestogens, and gonadotrophins are used therapeutically in all areas of obstetrics and gynecology. Hormones are transported in the blood by specific carrier proteins prior to binding with specific receptors on plasma membranes or in the cytosol of target cells. There is considerable evidence that fatty acids, altered lipid metabolism, and nutritional status can profoundly influence hormone production, distribution, and metabolism.

In vitro experiments have shown that PUFA strongly inhibit the binding of steroid hormones to carrier and other blood-borne proteins such as human sex hormone-binding globulin (SHBG) (14), murine α fetoprotein (15), and human sex steroid-binding protein, whereas saturated fatty acids potentiate binding (15–18). Thus the fatty acid content of binding proteins may influence the increased free hormone levels (the hormone fraction known to be bioactive). The binding of estradiol to human uterine breast and melanoma tissue has also been reported to be potentiated by unsaturated fatty acids, an effect apparently elicited by irreversible binding (19). Vallette *et al.* have shown that, depending on the estradiol/nonesterified fatty acid

(NEFA) ratio, there may be a decrease in the reversible binding of estradiol and/or a dramatic increase in irreversible binding to uterine protein (20). Similar results have been observed with brain glucocorticoid and progestin receptors (21,22). Apart from steroid hormones, fatty acids also inhibit thyroxine binding to serum proteins (23) and angiotensin and opioid binding to tissue receptors, the extent of inhibition relating directly to the degree of unsaturation of the fatty acid (24,25). Little is known of the effects of fatty acids on gonadotrophin binding, but this may also follow the pattern of other hormones.

In the clinical context, hormone binding data in relation to fatty acids are sparse. However, it has been demonstrated that sex hormone binding to SHBG as well as to albumin is diminished in obese patients (26). Bruning and Bonfrer (27) found that the non-protein-bound fraction of estradiol in plasma correlated with the total NEFA in healthy nonfasting premenopausal women. In a more recent study on fasted nonpregnant women where free fatty acid concentrations were doubled, the percentage of bound estradiol was significantly lower in the fasted as compared to fed subjects (28).

SEX HORMONES AND LIPID METABOLISM

Not only can fatty acids influence hormone dynamics but, conversely, estrogens and progestogens (and as such, gonadotrophins) may markedly influence lipid metabolism in the nonpregnant and pregnant state. In oral contraceptive users, fasting levels of NEFA appear to be unaltered, whereas plasma triglycerides, lipoproteins, and phospholipids are markedly elevated (29). Generally, contraceptive progestogens have no effect on blood lipids (30–32), whereas when estrogen alone is administered there is a significant elevation of blood triglyceride and phospholipid levels (33). The mechanism of this action of estrogens appears to be via a reduction in the activity of tissue lipoprotein lipase (LPL), an enzyme present in the endothelium of blood vessels that degrades triglycerides to glycerol and free fatty acids. Progesterone alone tends to lower triglyceride levels in hypertriglyceridemic patients (34), apparently due to an activation of LPL (35). Similarly, pregnancy is characterized by a marked increase in concentrations of circulating estrogens and triglycerides. Again this has been ascribed to a generalized estrogen-elicited decrease in tissue lipoprotein lipase activity (36). Two notable exceptions to this are the abrupt increase in mammary gland and placental LPL activity in the later stages of pregnancy (37,38), indicating the existence of subtle differential mechanisms governing LPL activity in tissue function. These may involve prolactin and/or fetal hormones.

It is clear that fatty acids may potentially elicit effects on reproductive functions via modulation/disruption of normal hormonal action. These aspects are discussed where relevant in ensuing sections.

CONTROL OF PROSTAGLANDIN SYNTHESIS BY HORMONES

The above effects of fatty acids on hormones may also influence prostaglandin synthesis indirectly, since hormone action is thought to be mediated, at least in part, through eicosanoids (39–41). In general, estrogens stimulate and progesterone inhibits prostaglandin synthesis, though the precise mechanisms remain obscure. The effects of these steroid hormones on the various prostaglandin synthesizing enzymes (i.e., cyclo-oxygenase, synthetases, and phospholipase A_2 [PLA_2]) have been reported (42–44). It is also generally accepted that progesterone priming is a prerequisite for estrogen stimulation of prostaglandin synthesis. More recently, estrogens have been shown to enhance calcium uptake into the myometrium, whereas progesterone was a potent inhibitor of calcium mobilization in the same tissue (45). Estrogens are also known to increase excitability of the uterus, whereas progesterone renders the myometrium refractory to excitation (46). It has also become apparent that calcium mobilization is an obligatory step in receptor-linked prostaglandin synthesis through activation of PLA_2 [liberating prostaglandin precursors from phospholipid stores in the plasma membrane (47)]. It follows, therefore, that inhibition of calcium mobilization by progesterone would result in diminished prostaglandin production, whereas the converse would be true for estrogens. In turn, fatty acids may influence steroid-eicosanoid interactions indirectly. Such possibilities warrant further investigation.

SIGNAL TRANSDUCTION MECHANISMS AND MEMBRANE PROPERTIES OF FATTY ACIDS

Although this topic is covered in more depth by Dr. Merrill elsewhere in this volume (also see refs. 48–52 for reviews), a few brief comments on how these mechanisms may relate to reproductive processes is warranted. Briefly, the binding of various hormones and neurotransmitters to cell surface receptors triggers the activation of phospholipase C (PLC), a process mediated by receptor-associated G proteins, which catalyzes the breakdown of phosphatidyl 4,5-bisphosphate to inositol 1,4,5-trisphosphate (IP_3) and diacylglycerol (DAG) (see refs. 49–52). DAG activates phospholipid/Ca^{2+}-dependent protein (protein kinase C [PKC]) by increasing the apparent affinity of the enzyme for Ca^{2+} (49–51). DAG is therefore considered to be the physiological activator for PKC. In turn, phosphoinositol degradation is accompanied by PLA_2-mediated release of arachidonic acid from phospholipids (51). It has also been suggested that activated PKC may elicit prostaglandin synthesis via activation of calcium channels, which results in the activation of PLA_2 and the generation of prostaglandin substrate (47). In turn, there is increasing evidence that arachidonic acid and its cyclo-oxygenase and lipoxygenase metabolites play an important role in hormone signal transduction (52), possibly via modulation of cyclic nucleotides (53). PKC and IP_3 act ultimately on cellular processes by phosphorylating proteins and stimulating the release of intracellular calcium, respectively (49–52).

These basic signal transduction mechanisms have been demonstrated in all reproductive processes, since phorbol esters (DAG mimetics) stimulate steroidogenesis, prostaglandin synthesis, gonadotrophin release, uterine contractility and endometrial proliferation (54–59).

Fatty acids alone, depending on the degree of saturation and spatial conformation, are capable of activating PKC (60–64). For example, cis-unsaturated fatty acids, but not trans-unsaturated elaidic acid or saturated fatty acids, induce neuronal and platelet activation and phosphorylation of specific proteins (62). In elegant studies, Seifert et al. demonstrated that both cis- and trans-unsaturated fatty acids activate PKC purified from rat brain as well as in platelets (63,64). Furthermore, these actions were potentiated by DAG. The authors demonstrated that trans-unsaturated fatty acids with 16- and 18-carbon atoms, with the exception of elaidic acid, activated PKC to a similar extent as their cis-isomers. Notwithstanding the biological significance of these findings, trans-unsaturated fatty acids may prove useful experimental tools to study the regulation of PKC since they are not metabolized by cyclo-oxygenase or lipoxygenase and they do not increase membrane fluidity (63,64). Cis-unsaturated fatty acids, but not trans-unsaturated fatty acids, stimulate other cellular signaling systems such as adenylate and guanylate cyclase (65,66).

Other key membrane functions are altered by fatty acids. For example, the activity of the Ca^+-Mg^+-ATPase reconstituted into bilayers of phosphatidyl cholines depends on the fatty acyl length of the phospholipids (67). Fatty acids, as cholesteryl esters or alone, modify calcium-dependent potassium channel activity in smooth muscle cells from human aorta (68–70), possibly via changes in membrane fluidity (71,72).

Thus, there are several ways whereby fatty acids can influence cellular functions associated with reproductive processes:

1. Substrate for (or competitive inhibitors of) eicosanoid synthesis
2. Inhibition or potentiation of hormone action/availability
3. As determinants of the physicochemical properties of membranes
4. As components of intracellular second messengers (DAG, sphingosine, platelet-activity factor [PAF])
5. Activators/inhibitors of PKC in their own right
6. Modulators of ion (for example Ca^{2+}) mobilization and of cyclic nucleotides.

Possible ways in which these properties, in concert with prostaglandins and hormones, affect the female reproductive cycle are now explored in some selected but diverse areas in obstetrics and gynecology.

INFLUENCE OF FATTY ACIDS ON CELLULAR FUNCTION IN REPRODUCTIVE PROCESSES

Infertility

In the normal cycle, following menses, follicle-stimulating hormone (FSH) brings about maturation of a selected Graafian follicle, while a midcycle surge of leuteinizing hormone (LH) leads to follicle rupture and expulsion of the mature oocyte (73). During the preovulatory phase estrogens secreted by the developing follicle stimulate proliferation and thickening of the endometrium, and progesterone secreted by the follicle and corpus luteum induces the secretory phase, which prepares for implantation of the fertilized ovum. Defects in any of these steps leads to ovulatory failure and infertility. Infertility of endocrine etiology can be treated with administration of the antiestrogen, clomiphene, and human chorionic gonadotrophin. The mechanisms leading to ovulation remain unknown. However, it has been established that there is a marked increase in the concentration of prostaglandins (principally $PGF_{2\alpha}$ and PGE_2) in the follicular fluid of the maturing follicle (74) and prostaglandins have been ascribed roles in follicular and oocyte maturation and ovulation (75).

Although little is known of the effects of dietary fatty acid manipulation on fertility, it is well known that women with anorexia nervosa are liable to develop amenorrhea and failure to ovulate when their weight falls to 35 kg or less. In contrast, obesity and infertility also seem to be associated, since fat women ovulate and menstruate with reduced frequency (76). Plasma levels of fatty acids are raised in patients with anorexia nervosa and bulimia nervosa following episodes of severe fasting (76). In general, LH and FSH levels are low in anorectics, and such individuals do not possess normal circadian LH patterns (76). Data obtained from responses to clomiphene citrate (an antiestrogen that acts by blocking the negative feedback of estrogen on hypothalamic releasing factors) suggest that dysfunction occurs at the level of the hypothalamus. Interestingly, binding of hormones to their binding globulins is also altered, suggesting a possible involvement of circulating fatty acids (76).

It is also of interest that autonomic function in anorectics and obese women is markedly disturbed. There appears to be an overall increase in α adrenoceptor activity accompanied by a reduction of β-adrenoceptor activity (76). Similar changes are found in the central nervous system of starved or fasted rats (77). We have also recently demonstrated that calcium mobilization in platelets from anorectic patients is increased in response to α-adrenoceptor activation but markedly diminished in response to β-adrenoceptor activation (78). As was mentioned earlier, fatty acids have been shown to modulate adrenoceptors in other cells (65,66). The possibility that not only hormone receptors but also receptors to other transmitters (e.g., serotonin, histamine, and acetylcholine) are influenced differentially by fatty acids of different chain length, degree of saturation, or configuration warrants further investigation.

It is also pertinent to mention some aspects of male infertility. Seminal fluid contains large amounts of prostaglandins, principally of the E type (as much as a microgram per ejaculate [79]). Their precise role remains unknown, but they have been shown to exert direct effects on the motility of spermatozoa, are of importance in the fertilizing ability of sperm, may be of relevance to the ejaculation mechanisms, and may act on the female genital tract by enhancing sperm migration (79). Few studies have been carried out to investigate the relationship between sperm dysfunction and seminal fluid prostaglandins. However, in a recent study of insulin-dependent diabetic men, sperm function was found to be significantly abnormal and the prostaglandin content of seminal fluid markedly increased (80). Furthermore, it has been established that Leydig cell function is mediated, in part, by prostaglandins

(81). It is also of interest that prostaglandins may be involved in erection of the penis (82,83). Clearly, impotence is an indirect cause of infertility. In this context, experimental diabetes results in markedly diminished PGI_2 synthesis by the penis (84). In turn, since diabetes is associated with an increased incidence of impotence, it was suggested that impaired prostaglandin synthesis by the penis and associated vasculature may play an etiological role in impotence (84). Thus, the possibility that dietary manipulation of fatty acid intake may ameliorate testicular and sperm dysfunction and improve impotence warrants consideration.

Gynecological Cancers

Although an area of some controversy, there is considerable epidemiological evidence of a relationship between high fat diets and the incidence of breast and endometrial cancers (85,86). Results with animal experiments confirm that dietary fat may be involved in tumorigenesis (87–90). Other studies suggest that NEFA may influence cell growth and multiplication by modifying membrane fluidity, with accompanying changes in enzymatic and receptor activity (91). It has also been reported that high fat diets composed of comparatively high levels of linoleic acid increased spontaneous metastasis in comparison to high fat diets containing lower levels of this fatty acid (92). However, deposition in the lungs of radiolabeled mammary tumor cells did not alter, nor did metastasis of a mammary tumor in rat fed high concentrations of linoleic acid (93).

Malignant tumors of the breast also synthesize more prostaglandins than do benign tumors (94). Certainly prostaglandins have been shown to modulate cell proliferation in various cell types (95), and nonsteroidal anti-inflammatory drugs (NSAID) have been shown to inhibit malignant cell proliferation *in vitro* (96). However, data on NSAID should be treated with caution since it has recently been shown that these drugs inhibit the mobilization of calcium, probably at the level of the plasma membrane, at lower concentrations than are required to inhibit cyclo-oxygenase (97–99). In this context, NSAID have been shown to inhibit cell proliferation at the G1 phase through a non-prostaglandin-mediated mechanism (100). It has been proposed that NSAID may act by disrupting a "trigger pool" of calcium associated with signal transduction mechanisms (G proteins, PLC, and PKC) (101). Furthermore, PKC and IP_3 are becoming increasingly prominent as mediators of malignant cell proliferation (102). Thus, although this area (fatty acids and malignancy) is in its infancy, the investigation of the role of fatty acids in cell proliferation is an area of much promise.

Pregnancy-Induced Hypertension

Pregnancy-induced hypertension (PIH; formally pre-eclampsia) is characterized by an increasing sensitivity to the pressor effect of infused angiotensin II prior to clinical manifestation of the disease (103). This vascular pressor response is dependent on the reactivity of the vascular smooth muscle rather than on the level of circulating pressor substance (104,105). Prostaglandins not only markedly influence vascular refractoriness to pressor substances but pressor substances themselves elicit the synthesis of endogenous vascular prostaglandins (47). Inhibitors of prostaglandin synthesis (indomethacin, aspirin) can abolish the decrease in vascular refractoriness of healthy pregnant women after the 28th week of pregnancy (106). Furthermore, low dose aspirin has been shown to prevent PIH in angiotensin-sensitive primigravidae (107). This led to the concept that dietary deficiency of fatty acids (and hence decreased vascular prostaglandin synthesis) may contribute to vascular hyperreactivity (108,109). In pregnant rabbits dietary deficiency of EFA resulted in increased vascular reactivity (110). However, in a double blind trial of dietary supplementation with linoleic acid, there was no significant difference in the incidence of PIH between placebo and treatment groups (111), although O'Brien *et al.* (112) found increased vascular refractoriness to angiotensin infusion in pregnant patients whose diets were supplemented with linoleic and γ linolenic acids.

Thus, from a mechanistic point of view, effects of dietary supplementation with fatty acids, such as EPA, DGLA, or linoleic acid, on vascular reactivity have been largely interpreted as being mediated by alterations in endogenous prostaglandin synthesis. However, vascular reactivity also involves PKC and calcium mobilization (113). Since fatty acids, particularly PUFA, possess the capacity to alter such processes, studies on these alternative systems may shed further light not only on PIH but also on the etiology of hypertension *per se.*

Premenstrual Syndrome

Premenstrual syndrome (PMS) is a widespread and distressing condition of menstruating women. Ovariectomy abolishes PMS, indicating an etiological role for the ovarian steroid hormones, estrogens and progesterone (114). However, no consistent abnormalities of hormone concentrations have been found in women with PMS (115). In a study on fatty acid concentrations in women with PMS, α linoleic acid and linoleic acid levels were found to be normal, but the levels of the 6-destaturated metabolites of linoleic acid were significantly reduced in plasma (116). It was therefore proposed that PMS may be related to a failure of PGE_1 formation. In subsequent studies, six double blind placebo-controlled trials conducted at eight university hospitals have all shown evening primrose oil to be significantly better than placebo at relieving symptoms of PMS (for review, see ref. 115). Although the mechanisms mediating this beneficial effect of dietary fatty acid manipulation are unknown, effects on hormone dynamics, as expressed earlier in this review, have been postulated (115).

Parturition

Although the trigger for the onset of parturition remains an enigma, it is clear that prostaglandins play a pivotal role in uterine contractility at term (117,118). It is known that the myometrium, endometrium, amnion, and chorion all synthesize prostaglandins (117,118) and that these eicosanoids influence contractility of the myometrium (119). That the endocrine milieu of the pregnant woman influences endogenous prostaglandin synthesis was largely expounded by Csapo, who postulated that progesterone and uterine prostaglandins are inversely related at term (46). Other endocrine factors known to influence prostaglandin synthesis are estrogens, corticosteroids, and gonadotrophins (117,118). For example, oxytocin, released by the pituitary at term, has also been shown to stimulate the synthesis of uterine prostaglandins (120). PGE_2 and PGI_2, principally under the control of estrogens, are also key modulators of cervical ripening and dilatation (121,122).

Few epidemiological studies on the timing of parturition and dietary fatty acid intake have been carried out. However, in a comparison between Faroese and Danish women, Olsen et al. (123) found that gestation was prolonged in Faroese women when compared to Danish women. They concluded that the high dietary intake of (n-3) PUFAs by Faroese women increases birthweight through prolongation of gestation, possibly by inhibiting the production of dienoic prostaglandins, these prostanoids being involved with uterine contractility and cervical ripening and dilatation.

In horses, sheep, and monkeys, food withdrawal has been shown to be followed not only by an increase in prostaglandin metabolites detectable in fetal or maternal plasma, but also by an earlier onset of parturition (124). Furthermore, there was an increase in electromyographic (uterine) activity in the monkey (125). Although no equivalent data exist for women, increased frequency of births has been reported for Jewish women following the 24 hour fast of Yom Kippur (126). Since fasting elicits an increase in circulating NEFA due to increased lipolysis, it is tempting to speculate that the increased levels of prostaglandins are due to increased prostaglandin precursors (e.g., arachidonate). Certainly fasting or semistarvation in the rat is associated with an increase of both vascular and platelet prostaglandin synthesis (127). The converse occurs in experimental diabetes mellitus, a state in which circulating arachidonic acid is diminished (128). It is tempting, therefore, to speculate that fasting-induced increases in fatty acids may result in increased prostaglandin synthesis ubiquitously. Clearly such an effect could be a precipitating factor for the onset of parturition.

Given the key role of prostaglandins in the onset of labor and the other events in the onset of parturition (uterine contractility, calcium mobilization, hypothalmic-pituitary activity) it is possible that changes in fatty acids, both in their free and esterified forms, may precede the onset of labor. Certainly maternal hypertriglyceridemia is one of the most striking and consistent changes occurring at late gestation in both humans and experimental animals but its physiological relevance is not yet understood.

In the elegant study of Friedman et al. (129) the fatty acid composition of blood from mother and fetus was analyzed over the third trimester of pregnancy. There appeared to be no marked increase in phospholipids, cholesterol esters, triacylglycerols, or free fatty acids in maternal blood immediately preceding labor. In contrast, although the proportion of linoleic acid in fetal blood lipids was far less (40%) than in maternal lipids, arachidonate was significantly higher at term than in maternal lipids. Since arachidonate is a precursor for the dienoic prostaglandins (i.e., PGF_2, PGI_2 and PGE_2), it may contribute to the enhanced synthesis of these prostaglandins when delivered to the uterus from the fetal side. In human placental tissue culture experiments it was demonstrated that arachidonate was released to its nonesterified state much more quickly than it could be metabolized by the placenta to prostaglandins (130). Others have found that the placenta possesses a weak capacity to generate prostaglandins from arachidonate (131). This may lead to a locally high concentration of arachidonic acid in the fetal blood present in the placental villous space juxtapositioned to the uterus prior to parturition, which in turn would enhance dienoic prostaglandin formation and therefore the contractility of the myometrium. Indeed, in a recent study, Delmis found significantly raised arachidonate levels in placentas from preterm deliveries as well as in chorioamnionitis (132). Furthermore, Filshie and Anstey demonstrated that the arachidonic acid content in uterine tissues from women undergoing cesarean section in labor was significantly raised in comparison with women undergoing elective cesarean section (133). The possibility of such a mechanism, as well as any direct effects of fatty acids (alone or as components of other bioactive lipids) on uterine activity, warrants further investigation.

AREAS FOR FUTURE RESEARCH

It is conceded by the author that much of this paper has been speculative. This is largely due to the sparse data available on the topics discussed. Nevertheless, it is clear that the ever-emerging diverse properties of fatty acids constitute an exciting avenue for future research. These include the following:

1. The relationship between circulating fatty acid status and hormone binding to carrier proteins and tissue receptors. Areas where these interactions may yield innovative results include the onset of parturition, the etiology and treatment of gynecological cancers, and infertility.

2. Effects of fatty acids, alone or as components of other bioactive lipids, on reproductive processes. It is becoming clear that fatty acids do not only influence signal transduction mechanisms on their own (e.g., PKC activation) but also as components of other bioactive lipids (diacyl glycerol, PAF). Since these signal transduction mechanisms are universal, *in vitro* experimentation coupled with effects of dietary fatty acid manipulation on these mechanisms as they relate to specific reproductive processes will undoubtedly furnish novel insights.

3. Effects of fatty acids on cell membrane function, for example, the mobilization of ions (calcium, potassium, sodium, chloride, protons, etc.). Ion mobilization is universal to all cell activity, including reproductive cells. Given the fundamental role of fatty acids on the physicochemical nature of membranes, studies on the mobilization of ions in contractile and secretory cells hold considerable promise.

4. Effects of fatty acids on eicosanoid synthesis in reproductive tissues. Apart from effects on eicosanoid substrates, fatty acids may influence eicosanoid synthesis

by indirect mechanisms, including PKC activation, IP_3 generation, and calcium mobilization. Apart from prostaglandins, leukotrienes, lipoxins, and PAF also play key roles in reproductive processes. Clearly, further research into the effects of fatty acids on these processes and substances is warranted.

REFERENCES

1. Burr GO, Burr MM. On the nature and role of the fatty acids essential in nutrition. *J Biol Chem* 1929; 86: 587–621.
2. McKenzie CG, McKenzie JB, McCollum EV. Growth and reproduction on a low fat diet. *Biochem J* 1939; 33: 935–9.
3. Quackenbush FW, Kummerow FA, Steenbock HJ. The effectiveness of linoleic, arachidonic and linolenic acids in reproduction and lactation. *J Nutr* 1942; 24: 213–4.
4. Deuel JH, Martin CR, Alfin-Slater RB. The effect of fat level of the diet on general nutrition. XII. The requirement of essential fatty acids for pregnancy and lactation. *J Nutr* 1954; 54: 193–8.
5. Horrobin DF. The role of essential fatty acids in the development of diabetic neuropathy and other complications of diabetes mellitus. *Prostaglandins Leukotrienes Essential Fatty Acids Rev* 1988; 31: 181–97.
6. Leaf A, Weber PC. Cardiovascular effects on n-3 fatty acids. *N Engl J Med* 1988; 318: 549–57.
7. von Schacky C. Prophylaxis of atherosclerosis with marine omega-3 fatty acids. *Ann Intern Med* 1987; 107: 890–9.
8. Darlington LG. Do diets rich in polyunsaturated fatty acids affect disease in rheumatoid arthritis? *Ann Rheum Dis* 1988; 47: 169–72.
9. Wright S. Essential fatty acids and the skin. *Prostaglandins Leukotrienes Essential Fatty Acids Rev* 1989; 38: 229–36.
10. Hollander D. Dietary essential fatty acids in the prevention of gastric mucosal injury. *Drug Invest* 1990; 2: 7–9.
11. Horrobin DF. Low prevalences of coronary heart disease, psoriasis, asthma and rheumatoid arthritis in eskimos: Are they caused by high dietary intake of eicosapentaenoic acid, a genetic variation of essential fatty acid metabolism or a combination of both? *Med Hypotheses* 1987; 22: 421–35.
12. Waite M. The phospholipases. In: Hanahan DJ, ed. *Handbook of lipid research*, Vol 5. New York: Plenum Press; 1988; 111–33.
13. Crawford MA. Background to essential fatty acids and their prostanoid derivatives. *Br Med Bull* 1983; 39: 210–5.
14. Martin M-E, Vranckx R, Benassayag C, Nunez EA. Modifications of the properties of human sex steroid binding protein by non-esterified fatty acids. *J Biol Chem* 1986; 261: 2954–9.
15. Benassayag C, Savu L, Vallette G, Delorme J, Nunez EA. Relationship between fatty acids and oestrogen binding properties of pure alpha -1-fetoprotein. *Biochem Biophys Acta* 1979; 587: 227–37.
16. Martin M-E, Vranckx R, Benassayag C, Nunez EA. In: Forest MG, Pugeat M, eds. *Binding proteins of steroid hormones*. Colloque INSERM, Vol 149; 1986: 637.
17. Apter D, Bulton NJ, Hammond GL, Vihko R. Serum sex hormone binding globulin during puberty in girls and in different types of adolescent menstrual cycle. *Acta Endocrinol* 1984; 107: 413–9.
18. Siiteri PK, Murai JT, Hammond GL, Nisker JA, Raymoure WJ, Kuhn RW. The transport of steroid hormones. *Recent Prog Horm Res* 1982; 38: 474–8.
19. Bennassayag C, Vallette G, Hassid J, Raymond JP, Nunez EA. Potentiation of estradiol binding to human steroid transport proteins by unsaturated nonesterified fatty acids. *Endocrinology* 1986; 118: 1–7.
20. Vallette G, Christeff N, Bogard C, Benassayag C, Nunez E. Dynamic pattern of estradiol binding to uterine receptors of the rat. Inhibition and stimulation by unsaturated fatty acids. *J Biol Chem* 1988; 263: 3639–45.
21. Kato J, Takano A, Mitsuhashi N, *et al*. Modulation of brain progestin and glucorticoid receptors by unsaturated fatty acids and phospholipid. *J Steroid Biochem* 1987; 27: 641–8.
22. Mitsuhashi N, Takano A, Kato J. Inhibition of the binding of R-5020 and rat uterine progesterone receptors by long chain fatty acids. *Endocrinol Jpn* 1986; 33: 251–6.
23. Chopra IJ, Huang T-S, Hurd RE, Beredo A, Solomon DH. A competitive ligand binding assay for measurement of thyroid hormone binding inhibitor in serum and tissues. *J Clin Endocrinol Metab* 1984; 58: 619–28.

24. Goodfriend TL, Ball DL. Fatty acid effects on angiotensin receptors. *J Cardiovasc Pharmacol* 1986; 8: 1276-83.
25. Ho WKK, Cox BM. Reduction of opioid binding in neuroblastoma X glioma cells grown in medium containing unsaturated fatty acids. *Biochim Biophys Acta* 1982; 688: 211-7.
26. Lee IR, Greed LC, Hahnel R. Comparative measurements of plasma binding capacity and concentration of human sex hormone binding globulin. *Clin Chim Acta* 1984; 137: 131-9.
27. Bruning PF, Bonfrer JM. Free fatty acid concentrations correlated with the available fraction of estradiol in human plasma. *Cancer Res* 1986; 46: 2606-9.
28. Key TJ, Pike MC, Moore JW, Wang DY, Morgan B. The relationship of free fatty acids with the binding of oestradiol to SHBG and to albumin in women. *J Steroid Biochem* 1990; 35: 35-8.
29. Seng P, Hasche HH, Rebensburg W, Voight KD. Systematic investigations on the influence of a contraceptive on some biochemical parameters of fat and carbohydrate metabolism. *Acta Endocrinol* 1969; 623: 181-6.
30. Zorilla E, Hulse M, Hernandez A, Gershberg H. Severe endogenous hypertriglyceridaemia during treatment with estrogen and oral contraceptives. *J Clin Endocriol* 1968; 28: 1793-5.
31. Barton GMG, Freeman PR, Lawson JP. Oral contraceptives and serum lipids. *J Obstet Gynaecol Br Cwlth* 1970; 77: 551-5.
32. Larsson-Cohn U, Berlin R, Vikrot O. Effects of combined and low gestagen oral contraceptives on plasma lipids, including individual phospholipids. *Acta Endocrinol* 1970; 63: 717-21.
33. Bazzanno G, Welch RG. The effect of intermittent fasting and estrogen treatment on serum lipids of an obese patient. *Clin Res* 1969; 17: 378-84.
34. Glueck HI, Glueck CJ. Clotting mechanisms in patients with hypertriglyceridemia during therapy with anabolic or progestational drugs. *Clin Res* 1970; 18: 611-6.
35. Glueck CJ. Progestins, anabolic androgens estrogens: effects on triglycerides and lipases. *Clin Res* 1971; 29: 475-82.
36. Herrera E, Lasuncion MA, Gomez-Coronado D, Aranda P, Lopez-Luna P, Maier I. Role of lipoprotein lipase activity on lipoprotein metabolism and the fate of circulating triglycerides in pregnancy. *Am J Obstet Gynecol* 1988; 6: 1575-83.
37. DeSoye G, Schweditsch MO, Pfeiffer KP, et al. Correlation of hormones with lipid and lipoprotein levels during normal pregnancy and postpartum. *J Clin Endocrinol Metab* 1987; 64: 704-12.
38. Rotherwell JE, Elphick MC. Lipoprotein lipase activity in human and guinea pig placenta. *J Dev Physiol* 1982; 4: 153-9.
39. Jeremy JY, Mikhailidis DP, Dandona P. Eicosanoids in obstetrics, gynaecology and fertility. *Prostaglandins Leukotrienes Essential Fatty Acids Rev* 1988; 34: 193-5.
40. Peplow P, Jeremy JY. Antiestrogens: structure, mode of action and relationship to eicosanoids. *Prostaglandins Leukotrienes Essential Fatty Acids Rev* 1989; 37: 241-54.
41. Jeremy JY, Dandona P. RU486 antagonises the inhibitory action of progesterone on prostacylin and thromboxane A_2 synthesis in cultured rat myometrial explants. *Endocrinology* 1986; 19: 661-5.
42. Castracane VD, Jordan VC. The effect of estrogens and progestins on uterine PG biosynthesis on ovariectomised rat. *Biol Reprod* 1975; 13: 587-92.
43. Dey SK, Hoversland RC, Johnson DC. Phospholipase A_2 activity in the rat uterus: modulation by steroid hormones. *Prostaglandins* 1982; 23: 619-25.
44. Jeremy JY, Dandona P. Mifepristone reverses corticosteroid and progesterone inhibited prostanoid synthesis in cultured myometrial vascular and gut tissue explants. In: Agrawal MA, ed. *Receptor-mediated antisteroid action*. Berlin: Walter de Gruyter; 1987: 99-119.
45. Batra S. Effect of estrogen and progesterone treatment on calcium uptake by the myometrium and smooth muscle of the lower urinary tract. *Eur J Pharmacol* 1986; 127: 37-42.
46. Csapo AI. The see saw theory of parturition. In: *The fetus and birth*. Ciba Foundation Symposium 47. Amsterdam: Elsevier, 1977: 159-79.
47. Jeremy JY, Mikhailidis DP, Dandona P. Excitatory receptor-prostanoid synthesis coupling in mammalian smooth muscle: mediation by calcium, protein kinase C and G proteins. *Prostaglandins Leukotrienes Essential Fatty Acids Rev* 1988; 34: 215-35.
48. Berridge MJ. Inositol trisphosphate and diacyl glycerol as second messengers. *Biochem J* 1984; 220: 345-55.
49. Abdel-Latif AA. Calcium-mobilising receptors, polyphosphoinositides and the generation of 2nd messengers. *Pharmacol Rev* 1986; 38: 227-72.
50. Nishizuka Y. The role of protein kinase C in cell surface signal transduction. *Nature* 1984; 308: 693-8.

51. Burch RM, Luini A, Axelrod J. Phospholipase A_2 and phospholipase C are activated by distinct GTP-binding proteins in response to alpha 1 adrenergic stimulation in FRTL 5 thyroid cells. *Proc Natl Acad Sci USA* 1986; 83: 7201–5.
52. Needleman P, Turk J, Jackshcik BA, Morrison AR, Lefkowith JB. Arachidonic acid metabolism. *Annu Rev Biochem* 1986; 55: 69–102.
53. Lagarde M. Cyclic nucleotides and prostaglandins. In Curtis-Prior PB, ed. *Biology and chemistry of prostaglandin and related eicosanoids.* Edinburgh: Churchill Livingstone; 1988: 147–55.
54. Kawai Y, Clark MR. Phorbol ester regulation of rat granulosa cell prostaglandin and progesterone accumulation. *Endocrinology* 1985; 116: 2320–5.
55. Wang J, Lee V, Leung PCK. Differential role of protein kinase C in the action of leutinizing hormone-releasing hormone on hormone production in rat ovarian cells. *Am J Obstet Gynecol* 1989; 160: 984–9.
56. Noland TA, Dimino MJ. Characterisation and distribution of protein kinase C in ovarian tissue. *Biol Reprod* 1986; 35: 863–9.
57. Cowell A-M, Buckingham JC. Eicosanoids and the hypothalamic-pituitary axis. *Prostaglandins Leukotrienes Essential Fatty Acids Rev* 1989; 36: 235–50.
58. Harman I, Zeitler P, Ganong B, Bell RM, Handwerger S. Sn-1,2 diacylglcerols and phorbol esters stimulate the synthesis and release of human placental lactogen from placental cells: a role for protein kinase C. *Endocrinology* 1986; 119: 1239–44.
59. Stachura ME, Tyler JM, Kent PG. Effect of growth hormone releasing factor-44 upon release of concurrently synthesised hormone by perifused rat pituitary tissue. *Endocrinology* 1986; 119: 1245–52.
60. McPhail LC, Clayton CC, Snyderman R. A protein second messenger role for unsaturated fatty acid activation of Ca^{2+} dependent protein kinase C. *Science* 1984; 224: 622–5.
61. Murakami K, Routtenberg A. Direct activation of purified protein kinase C by unsaturated fatty acids (oleate and arachidonic acid) in the absence of phospholipids and calcium. *FEBS Lett* 1985; 192: 189–93.
62. Lindsen DJ, Murakami K, Rottenberg A. A newly discovered protein kinase C activator (oleic acid) enhances long-term potentiation in the intact hippocampus. *Brain Res* 1986; 379: 358–63.
63. Seifert R, Schachtele C, Schultz G. Activation of protein kinase C by cis- and trans-octadecaedienoic acids in intact human platelets and its potentiation by diacylglycerol. *Biochem Biophys Res Commun* 1988; 149: 762–8.
64. Seifert R, Schachtele C, Rosenthal W, Schultz G. Activation of protein kinase C by cis- and trans-fatty acids and its potentiation by diacylglycerol. *Biochem Biophys Res Comm* 1988; 154: 358–65.
65. Orly J, Schramm M. Fatty acids as modulators of membrane function: catecholamine activated adenyl cyclase of the turkey erythrocyte. *Proc Natl Acad Sci USA* 1975; 72: 3433–7.
66. Glass DB, Frey W, Carr DW, Goldberg ND. Stimulation of human platelet guanylate cyclase by fatty acids. *J Biol Chem* 1977; 252: 1279–85.
67. Froud RJ, East JM, Jones OT, Lee AG. Effects of lipids and long chain alkyl derivatives on the activity of $(Ca^{2+}-Mg^{2+})$-ATPase. *Biochemistry* 1986; 25: 7544–52.
68. Bregetovski PD, Boltina VM, Serebryakov VN. Fatty acids modifies Ca^{2+}-dependent K^+ channel activity in smooth muscle cells. *Proc R Soc Long [Biol]* 1989; 237: 259–66.
69. Bolotina V, Omelyanenko V, Heyes B, Ryan U, Bregestovski P. Variations of membrane cholesterol alter the kinetics of calcium dependent K^+ channel and membrane fluidity in vascular smooth muscle cells. *Pflugers Arch* 1989; 415: 262–8.
70. Bregetowski PD, Prinseva O Yu, Serebryakov V, Stinnakre J, Turmin A, Zamoyski V. Comparison of Ca^{2+} dependent K^+ channels in the membrane of smooth muscle cells isolated from adult and fetal human aorta. *Pflugers Arch* 1988; 413: 8–13.
71. Karnovsky MJ, Kleinfeld AM, Hoover RL, Klausner RD. The concept of lipid domains in membranes. *J Cell Biol* 1982; 94: 1–6.
72. Takenaka T, Hori H, Hori H, Kawasaki Y. The correlation between the lateral motion of membrane lipids and nerve membrane excitability. *Biomed Res* 1986; 7: 49–51.
73. Ross GT, Vande Wiele RL. The ovaries. In: Williams RH, ed. *Textbook of endocrinology.* Philadelphia: WB Saunders; 1974: 368–74.
74. Jeremy JY, Okonofua F, Thomas M, Smith A, Craft I, Dandona P. Oocyte maturity and human follicular fluid prostanoids, gonadotrophins and prolactin after administration of clomiphene and pergonal. *J Clin Endocrinol Metab* 1987; 65: 402–7.
75. Darling MRN, Jogee M, Elder MG. Prostaglandin F levels in the human ovarian follicle. *Prostaglandins* 1982; 23: 551–60.

76. Ploog DW, Pirke KM. Psychobiology of anorexia nervosa. *Psychol Med* 1987; 17: 843–60.
77. Spyra B, Pirke KM. Binding of clonidine and WB 4101 to pre- and post synaptic alpha adrenoceptor of the basal hypothalamus of the starved male rat. *Brain Res* 1982; 245: 179–85.
78. Gill J, De Souza V, Dandona P, Wakeling A, Jeremy JY. Profound changes in alpha- and beta adrenoceptor-linked calcium uptake by platelets from patients with anorexia nervosa. *J Clin Endocrinol Metab* 1992; 74: 441–6.
79. Gottlieb C, Bygdeman M. Prostanoids in sperm function. *Prostaglandins Leukotrienes Essential Fatty Acids Rev* 1988; 34: 205–15.
80. Shrivastav P, Swann J, Jeremy JY, Craft I, Dandona P. Sperm function and seminal plasma prostanoid concentrations in type I (insulin dependent) diabetic men. *Diabetes Care* 1989; 12: 223–5.
81. Abayasakara DRE, Kurlak LO, Cooke MA, Jeremy JY, Dandona P, Sharpe RM. Role of arachidonic acid metabolites in mediating the HcG-induced increases in interstitial fluid volume in rats. *Int J Androl* 1990; 13: 408–8.
82. Jeremy JY, Mikhailidis DP. Prostaglandins and the penis. *Sexual Marital Ther* 1990; 5: 155–65.
83. Jeremy JY, Morgan RJ, Mikhailidis DP, Dandona P. Prostacylin synthesis by the corpus cavernosa of the human penis: evidence for muscarinic control. *Prostaglandins Leukotrienes Essential Fatty Acids* 1985; 23: 211–6.
84. Jeremy JY, Mikhailidis DP, Thompson CS, Dandona P. Experimental diabetes mellitus inhibits prostacylin synthesi by the rat penis: pathological implications. *Diabetologia* 1985; 28: 365–8.
85. Dunn JE Jr. Cancer epidemiology in populations of the United States with emphasis on Hawaii and California and Japan. *Cancer Res* 1975; 35: 3240–5.
86. Enig MG, Munn RJ, Keeney M. Dietary fat and cancer trends—a critique. *Fed Proc* 1978; 37: 2215–20.
87. Carroll KK, Khor HT. Dietary fat in relation to tumorigenesis. *Prog Biochem Pharmacol* 1969; 10: 2215–20.
88. Carroll KK, Khor HT. Effect of dietary fatty acids and dose level of 7,12-dimethyl benz anthracene on mammary tumor incidence in rats. *Cancer Res* 1970; 30: 2260–4.
89. Carroll KK, Khor HT. Effect of level and type of dietary fat on incidence of mammary tumours induced in female Sprague-Dawley rats by 7,12-dimethyl benz anthracene. *Lipids* 1971; 6: 415–20.
90. Erickson KL, Schlanger DS, Adams DA, Fregau DR, Stern JS. Influence of dietary fatty acid concentration and geometric configuration on murine mammary tumorigenesis and experimental metastasis. *J Nutr* 1984; 114: 1834–42.
91. Burns CP. Effect of modification of plasma membrane fatty acid composition on fluidity and methotrexate transport in L 1210 murine leukaemia cells. *J Steroid Biochem* 1987; 27: 641–8.
92. Hubbard NE, Erickson KL. Enhancement of metastasis from a transplantable mouse mammary tumour by dietary linoleic acid. *Cancer Res* 1987; 47: 6171–8.
93. Kort WJ, Wiejma IM, Stehmann TEM, Vergroesen AJ, Westbroek DL. Diets rich in fish oil cannot control tumor cell metastases. *Ann Nutr Metab* 1987; 31: 342–9.
94. Karim SMM. Prostaglandins and tumours. In: Karim SMM, ed. *Advances in prostaglandin research*, Vol 2, Oxford, England: MTP Press; 1976.
95. Wickremasinghe RG. The role of prostaglandins in the reguation of cell proliferation. *Prostaglandins Leukotrienes Essential Fatty Acids Rev* 1988; 31: 171–6.
96. Fulton AM. The role of eicosanoids in tumor metastasis. *Prostaglandins Leukotrienes Essential Fatty Acids Rev* 1988; 34: 229–38.
97. Jeremy JY, Mikhailidis DP, Dandona P. Differential inhibitory potencies of NSAIDs on smooth muscle prostanoid synthesis. *Eur J Pharmacol* 1990; 182: 83–9.
98. Jeremy JY, Mikhailidis DP. NSAID-induced side effects. Are they wholly prostaglandin mediated? *J Drug Devel* 1990; 3: 3–4.
99. Gill J, Dandona P, Jeremy JY. Indomethacin and ibuprofen inhibit calcium uptake in washed human platelets by a thromboxane A_2 independent mechanism. *Eur J Pharmacol* 1990; 187: 135–8.
100. De Mello MCF, Bayer BB, Beaven MA. Evidence that prostaglandins do not have a role in the cytostatic action of antiinflammatory drugs. *Biochem Pharmacol* 1980; 29: 311–5.
101. Abramson SB, Weissman G. The mechanism of action of non steroidal antiinflammatory drugs. *Arthritis Rheum* 1989; 32: 1–8.
102. Wickremasinghe RG, Jeremy JY. Phospholipase C and A_2 in malignant cell proliferation. *Prostaglandins Leukotrienes Essential Fatty Acids Rev* 1989; 36: 199–201.
103. Gant NF, Daley GL, Chand S, Whalley PJ, MacDonald PC. A study of angiotensin II pressor response throughout primigravid pregnancy. *J Clin Invest* 1973; 52: 2682–7.

104. Weir RJ, Brown JJ, Fraser R. Plasma renin, renin substrate, angiotensin II and aldosterone in hypertensive disease of pregnancy. *Lancet* 1973; 1: 291–3.
105. Whalley PJ, Everett RB, Gant NG. Pressor responsiveness to angiotensin II in hospitalised primigravidae with pregnancy induced hypertension. *Am J Obstet Gynecol* 1983; 145: 481–6.
106. Everett RB, Worley RJ, MacDonald PC, Gant NF. Effect of prostaglandin synthetase inhibitors on pressor response to angiotensin II in human pregnancy. *J Clin Endocrinol Metab* 1978; 46: 1007–11.
107. Wallenberg HCG, Dekker GA, Makowitz JW, Rotmans P. Low dose aspirin prevents pregnancy induced hypertension and preeclapmsia in angiotensin sensitive primigravidae. *Lancet* 1986; i: 1–4.
108. Pedersen EB, Christensen NJ, Christensen P. Preeclampsia—a state of prostaglandin deficiency. *Hypertension* 1983; 5: 105–10.
109. England MJ, Atkinson PM, Sonnerdecker EWW. Pregnancy induced hypertension: will treatment with dietary eicosapentaenoic acid be effective? *Med Hypotheses* 1987; 24: 179–86.
110. O'Brien PMS, Broughton-Pipkin F. The effects of deprivation of prostaglandin precursors on vascular sensitivity to angiotensin II and on the kidney in the pregnant rabbit. *Br J Pharmacol* 1979; 65: 29–34.
111. Gant NF, Worley RJ. In: Gant NF, ed. *Hypertension in pregnancy: concepts and management*. New York: Appleton; 1980: 16–30.
112. O'Brien PMS, Morrison R, Broughton-Pipkin F. The effect of dietary supplementation of linolenic acid and gammalinolenic acids on the pressor response to angiotensin II—a possible role in pregnancy-induced hypertension. *Br J Clin Pharmacol* 1985; 19: 335–8.
113. Colucci WS, Gimbrone MA, Alexander RW. Phorbol diester modulates alpha adrenergic receptor coupled calcium efflux and alpha adrenergic receptor number in cultured vascular smooth muscle cells. *Circ Res* 1986; 58: 393–9.
114. Muse KN, Cetel NS, Futterman LA, Yen SCC. The premenstrual syndrome. Effects of 'medical ovariectomy.' *N Engl J Med* 1984; 311: 1345–9.
115. Horrobin DF, Manku S. Premenstrual syndrome and premenstrual breast pain (cyclical mastalgia): disorders of essential fatty acid (EFA) metabolism. *Prostaglandins Leukotrienes Essential Fatty Acids Rev* 1988; 37: 255–62.
116. Brush MG, Watson SJ, Horrobin DF, Manku MS. Abnormal essential fatty acid levels in plasma of women with premenstrual syndrome. *Am J Obstet Gynecol* 1984; 10: 363–6.
117. Keirse MJNC. Prostaglandins and the onset of labour. In: Anderson ABM, Bennebroek A, Gravenhorst J, eds. *Human parturition*. Leiden: University Press; 1979: 101–10.
118. Lundin-Schiller S, Mitchell MD. The role of prostaglandins in human parturition. *Prostaglandins Leukotrienes Essential Fatty Acids Rev* 1990; 39: 1–10.
119. Bremme K, Bygdeman M. Induction of labor by oxytocin and prostagldnin E_2. *Acta Obstet Gynecol Scand Suppl* 1980; 92: 11–16.
120. Mitchell MD, Flint AP, Turnbull AC. Stimulation by oxytocin of prostagldnin F levels in uterine venous effluent in pregnant and puerperal sheep. *Prostaglandins* 1975; 9: 47–55.
121. Mackenzie IZ, Emburey MP. A comparison of PGE2 and PGF2 vaginal gel for ripening the cervix before induction of labour. *Br J Obstet Gynaecol* 1979; 86: 167–72.
122. Ellwood DA, Mitchell MD, Turnbull AC. Oestrogens, prostaglandins and cervical ripening. *Lancet* 1980; i: 376–7.
123. Olsen SF, Hansen HS, Sorensen TIA, et al. Intake of marine fat rich in (n-3) polyunsaturated fatty acids may increase birthweight by prologation of gestation. *Lancet* 1986; ii: 367–9.
124. Fowden AL, Silver M. The effects of food withdrawal on uterine contractile activity and on plasma cortisol concentrations in ewe and their fetuses during late gestation. In: Jones CT, Nathanielz PW, eds. *The physiological development of the fetus and newborn*. Orlando, Florida: Academic Press; 1985: 157–70.
125. Binienda Z, Massman A, Mitchell MD, Gleed RD, Figueroa JP, Nathanielsz PW. The effect of food withdrawal on blood glucose and arterial plasma 13, 14 dihydro-15-keto prostaglandin F2alpha (PGFM) concentrations and electromyographic activity in the pregnant rhesus monkey in the last third of gestation. A model for preterm labor? *Am J Obstet Gynecol* 1988; 160: 746–50.
126. Kaplan M, Eidelman AI, Aboulafia Y. Fasting and the precipitation of labor: the Yom Kippur Effect. *JAMA* 1983; 250: 1317–8.
127. Jeremy JY, Thompson CS, Dandona P. Differential regional changes in the synthesis of prostacylin and thromboxane A_2 in the small intestine and mesenteric vasculature of the fasted and semi starved rat. *Pflugers Arch* 1987; 408: 68–72.
128. Jeremy JY, Mikhailidis DP, Thompson CS, Barradas MA, Dandona P. Platelet TXA_2 synthesising

capacity is enhanced by fasting but diminished by diabetes mellitus in the rat. *Diabetes Res* 1988; 8: 177–81.
129. Friedman Z, Danon A, Lamberth EL, Mann WJ. Cord blood fatty acid composition in infants and in their mothers during the third trimester. *J Pediatr* 1978; 92: 461–6.
130. Ogburn PL, Rejeshwari M, Turner SI, Hoegsberg B, Haning RV. Lipid and glucose metabolism in human placental culture. *Am J Obstet Gynecol* 1988; 159: 629–35.
131. Jeremy JY, Barradas MA, Mikhailidis DP, Craft I, Dandona P. Does the human placenta produce prostacylin? *Placenta* 1985; 6: 45–52.
132. Delmis J. Placental lipid contents in preterm labor complicated by chorioamnionitis. *J Perinat Med* 1989; 17: 417–22.
133. Filshie GM, Anstey MD. The distribution of arachidonic acid in plasma and tissue of patients near term undergoing elective or emergency caesarean section. *Br J Obstet Gynaecol* 1978; 85: 119–23.

DISCUSSION

Dr. Galli: It is not surprising that the placenta has little capacity for making prostaglandins from exogenous arachidonic acid. There are other examples of this situation. The limiting factor in a given cell is the K_m of the oxygenases for converting arachidonic acid to its metabolites. In platelets for instance, the formation of cyclo- and lipoxygenase products occurs immediately after incubation with 1 μM arachidonic acid, but you have to incubate polymorphonuclear leukocytes with high concentrations of substrate in order to see formation of products.

Dr. Jeremy: In our experience the placenta has a very low capacity to synthesize prostacyclin, either when studied by conversion of radiolabeled arachidonic acid to prostanoid or by measurement of release of PGI_2. This may constitute a mechanism by which arachidonic acid is presented to the myometrium from the fetal compartment for synthesis of contractile prostaglandins at term.

Dr. Crawford: Could you comment on the thrombosis that is so frequently found in the placenta, especially in small-for-dates and diabetic pregnancies?

Dr. Jeremy: The etiology of this is unknown. However we found that the placenta synthesizes large amounts of ADPase, a potent inhibitor of platelet aggregation. Fatty acids markedly inhibit this enzyme. Thus it is possible that thrombosis associated with diabetes is mediated by local effects of fatty acids on ADPase activity.

Dr. Guesry: Could the relative efficacy of the placenta in transforming arachidonic acid to prostaglandin be age dependent? Is there a difference in the 4–5 month placenta compared with the 9 month placenta?

Dr. Jeremy: That is a very good question. We have only studied term placentas. It could well be that as term approaches the conversion of arachidonic acid to prostaglandins is turned off, whereas it may be more active in early pregnancy. This warrants further investigation.

Dr. Clandinin: One of the things you always find in diabetes is low levels of arachidonic acid. It is also peculiar that the testes Leydig cells are the only ones I know of that have extremely high 22:5 n-6. This is somehow involved in testosterone production by these cells.

Dr. Jeremy: We found that prostaglandins are important mediators of function in these cells. We have also found profound sperm dysfunction in type 1 diabetics as well as altered prostaglandin profiles in their seminal fluid. There is also marked impairment of testosterone production by the testes of diabetic rats. Given the high concentrations of DHA in testicular tissue, the possible role of this fatty acid in testicular and sperm function is certainly worth investigation.

Thymus Eicosanoids Are Involved in Tolerance to Self

Norbert Gualde

Université de Bordeaux II and Fondation Bergonié, URA CNRS 1456, 33076, Bordeaux Cedex, France

The thymus is the major site for generating mature thymocytes with a broad repertoire of T cell receptors for the recognition of foreign epitopes (1). During development in the thymus, T cells are rendered tolerant to self antigens (2). It is now accepted that thymocytes bearing antiself T cell receptors are either eliminated (clonal deletion) or functionally inactivated (clonal anergy) (3). Nevertheless since autologous sensitive cells exist (4-11) we speculate that suppressor cells may be involved in tolerance to self by suppressing autologous sensitive cells. In other words we propose a third mechanism for attaining self-tolerance. This phenomenon may operate outside the thymus but we discuss here the mechanism that generates antiself suppressor thymocytes within the thymus and that is linked to a local production of eicosanoids. It is accepted that thymus accessory cells which express self major histocompatibility complex products participate in the education of immature thymocytes, "teaching" them how to distinguish self from non-self (12,13). Since it was observed that cells from the thymic microenvironment synthesize eicosanoids from the cyclo-oxygenase or the lipoxygenase pathway (14,15), the question remains whether eicosanoids have a major role in thymocyte differentiation and education. Considering the fact that an eicosanoid such as leukotriene B4 (LTB4) is involved in the generation of suppressor cells we were then interested in studying its effect on the function of prothymocytes, trying to determine if LTB4 participates in the generation of self antigen-specific suppressor cells. LTB4 is produced by a large variety of cells involved in immune and/or inflammatory responses (16) and it has been demonstrated that LTB4 acts as an immunomodulator (17). There is a good deal of evidence that some thymic accessory cells produce eicosanoids (14,15) and that LTB4 influences the function of immature cells (18,19). For instance we previously studied the effects of LTB4 on the proliferative response of lectin-stimulated PNA positive thymocytes (PNA+) in the presence of interleukin-2 (IL-2). We observed that the lectin-driven proliferative response of immature thymocytes increased with LTB4 (20). It is also well known that within the thymus, immature thymocytes differentiate (21) and that these intrathymic T cell precursors are double negative lymphocytes for both CD4 and CD8 differentiation molecules (22). In the thymus approximately 50% of the double negative thymocytes proliferate and give rise to progeny cells expressing either CD4 or CD8 markers or both (23). The thymic microenvironment plays an important role for immature thymocyte proliferation and differentiation; such is the case for accessory cells which influence immature T cells by both direct cell-to-cell contact and by releasing soluble mediators such as IL-1 and prostaglandin E_2 (24,25). To assess the role of eicosanoids in the education of immature thymocytes we studied 1) the expression of lipoxygenase and 2) the production of LTB4 by thymus accessory cells. We also investigated the behaviour of LTB4-treated double negative thymocytes. For that purpose autologous erythrocytes which stimulate *in vitro* T lymphocyte proliferative response (10,11) as do cells of the thymic stroma were used as self antigen expressing cells (26,27) and exogenous LTB4 was added to the cultures.

MATERIAL AND METHODS

Isolation of Thymus Accessory Cells

Macrophages were separated by using a slight modification of the method described by Papiernik *et al.* (24). Thymic fragments were cultivated in plastic flasks in RPMI 1640 complemented with 10% fetal calf serum, glutamine, and antibiotics. Cultures were continued for 12 days (medium was changed twice a week). By day 12, nonadherent round cells were recovered from the culture medium, washed, resuspended at 5×10^5 cells/ml, and replaced in flat-bottomed culture plates. Thereafter, cells became adherent and were available 24 h later either for assessment of eicosanoid production or hybridization with P388-D1 cells.

Hybridization

An azaguanine-resistant mutant cell line of the mouse macrophage-like cell line P388-D1 was established. P388-D1 cells and thymus macrophages were mixed in a plastic tube at a ratio of 1:1 and fused in RPMI 1640 medium containing 20% polyethylene glycol 1000. The cells were distributed (1×10^6/well) in a flat-bottomed 24 well microplate and selected in HAT medium (1×10^{-4} M hypoxanthine, 4×10^{-7} M aminopterine, 1.5×10^{-5} M thymidine). Cell growth was apparent 21 to 30 days after the fusion. Each colony was grown to a mass culture and cloned by limiting dilution in a flat-bottomed 96 well microplate.

Assessment of Eicosanoids

LTB4, LTC4, and LTD4 produced were assessed by high-pressure liquid chromatography or radioimmunoassay. For that purpose, thymic-macrophage hybridomas were pulsed for 15 min by 10 µg of arachidonic acid.

5-Lipoxygenase mRNA Analysis

Total RNA was isolated by the method of Chomczynski and Sacchi (28). Briefly cells from 150 mg of thymus were lysed in guanidine thiocyanate. Samples were extracted with phenol/chloroform/isoamyl alcohol and precipitated in ethanol. Purified RNA was separated on a 1.2% agarose gel containing formaldehyde. The electrophoresis was performed for 2 h at 100 mV. Gel was rinsed with water and transferred onto hybond messenger affinity paper. The prehybridization was performed during 2 h at 46°C under stringent conditions, hybridization was performed at 46°C during 48 h. 5-Lipoxygenase specific oligonucleotides probes (2) were labeled with ^{32}P-deoxycytidine triphosphate. After hybridization the blots were washed twice, dried, and exposed to X-ray film.

In Situ Hybridization

5-Lipoxygenase mRNA expression was analyzed by *in situ* hybridization technique. Thymus slices were deposited on a gelatin-coated glass slide and then treated by the prehybridization buffer. Oligonucleotides were then applied to the tissues. Hybridization was allowed to occur overnight at 40°C.

Slides were prepared for autoradiography using K5 emulsion, developed after 1 month's exposure and then stained with toluidine blue and analyzed under a light microscope.

Mice

C57B1/6 (B6-H2^b) DBA/2 (D2-H2^b) and C3H (C3-H2^k) 6 week old female mice were purchased and maintained on a standard pellet diet and water *ad libitum*.

Cells

Thymocytes and splenocytes were obtained from mice that had been killed with ether. Cell suspensions were prepared by mincing spleen and thymi in RPMI 1640 medium supplemented with either inactivated 10% fetal calf serum or inactivated 5% mouse serum (MS). Mononuclear cells were then separated from red blood cells by centrifugation over a lympholyte gradient. The cells were then washed twice in RPMI 1640 medium and resuspended in RPMI 1640 medium completed as described above.

LTB4 was kindly supplied by Dr. J. Rokach, stored in ethanol at −80°C, and diluted in RPMI 1640 medium before use.

Mouse Serum

MS was obtained by cardiac puncture from C57B1/6 mice anesthetized with ether, using 1 ml syringes. Between 0.2 and 0.7 ml of blood was obtained per mouse. After clotting, all sera containing hemoglobin were discarded; the remaining normal sera were then pooled and inactivated (56°C, 30 mn). The nontoxicity of diluted mouse serum was controlled as described below.

Monoclonal Antibodies and Immunofluorescence Analysis of the Cells

Antimouse Ly-2 (CD8) monoclonal antibody and MAS 110, a rat monoclonal antibody against mouse L3T4 marker (CD4), were purchased. A cell pellet containing 10^6 double negative thymocytes was incubated with 100 μl of an appropriate dilution of monoclonal antibodies for 1 h at 4°C. The cells were washed twice in a refrigerated centrifuge with RPMI 1640. The cells were then separated from debris by centrifugation over a lympholyte gradient and incubated with fluorescein-conjugated sheep F (ab')2 antimouse immunoglobulins (*NEN*) for the antimouse Ly-2; for the MAS 110 monoclonal antibody, a fluorescein-conjugated mouse antirat immunoglobulin was used. Cells were incubated with the second antibody for 30 min at 4°C. The cell pellet was washed twice and cells were separated from debris by centrifugation over a lympholyte gradient. The cells were then resuspended in 1 ml phosphate-buffered saline (PBS). Fluorescence of individual cells was measured using a cell sorter equipped with helium neon and Argon 90-4 lasers. The stored data were analyzed with a computer interfaced to the cytofluorimeter. Green fluorescence of labeled cells was collected between 500 and 540 nm. Cell size was determined by measuring the pulse width of the axial light signal according to Cambier *et al.* (29).

Assessment of Mouse Serum Cytotoxicity

We used a specific chromium release as described before (30). About 1×10^7 thymocytes or erythrocytes were labeled with 100 mCi of $(Na)_2\ ^{51}CrO4$ for 2 h. Cells were washed twice in Hanks' balanced salt solution and adjusted in RPMI 1640 medium to 1×10^6 cells/ml. One milliliter of cell suspension (in a disposable plastic tube) was preincubated for 6 h in the presence of 10% FCS and 10% and 5% MS, respectively. Cells preincubated without serum were used as background release cpm. After preincubation, tubes were centrifuged at $250g$ for 10 mn. Then 0.5 ml of supernatant of each tube was removed, placed in a glass tube, and counted in a gamma counter. Labeled cells were freeze-thawed three times in order to measure the total release of ^{51}Cr. Each experimental point was run in duplicate. The percentage of serum-induced mortality was calculated as

$$\frac{\text{Experimental cpm } - \text{ background cpm}}{\text{Total release cpm } - \text{ background cpm}}$$

Assessment of Mouse Serum Validity for Lymphocyte Stimulation

Splenocytes (2×10^6/ml) were suspended in RPMI 1640 medium prepared as described but supplemented with either fetal calf serum (FCS) (10%) or MS (either

10% or 5%). The cells were cultured for 72 h in 200 ml flat-bottomed wells. Each test was set up in triplicate. Cells were stimulated by concanavalin A, phytohemagglutinin, or pokeweed mitogen. After 72 h the cultures were pushed with 5 µCi ^{3}H-thymidine per well and were continued for 6 h. The cells were then washed and absorbed onto glass fiber filters in an automatic cell harvester, dried at 60°C, transferred to glass vials containing scintillation fluid, and the radioactivity determined in a β scintillation counter.

The proliferative response of B6 splenocytes was not significantly affected by the presence of 5% inactivated MS compared to the 10% FCS generally used for experiments dealing with lymphocyte proliferation assessment. On the other hand MS used at 10% final concentration always diminished thymidine uptake; it is likely that this phenomenon is linked to an inhibitory process rather than an actual cytotoxicity since the specific chromium release by mouse lymphocytes or erythrocytes (B6 or D2 or C3) was not increased when final concentration of MS was 20% (data not shown). Since it was demonstrated that the proliferative response of B6 lymphocyte was not affected by 5% MNS, we used this concentration of serum in the further experiments assessing the proliferative response of B6 lymphocytes in the presence of autologous antigens either with or without LTB4.

Separation of C57B1/6 CD4$^-$ Splenocytes

CD4$^-$ splenocytes were obtained by negative selection. Briefly 1×10^6 spleen cells were treated with a 1/500 final dilution of the anti-L3T4 monoclonal antibody for 1 h at room temperature. The cells were washed twice and then preincubated for 1 h at 37°C in the presence of 1/20 final dilution of rabbit complement. The remaining cells were separated from the debris on a lympholyte gradient; they contained less than 1% of CD4$^+$ lymphocytes.

Separation of Double Negative Thymocytes

Double negative thymocytes were obtained by negative selection using a protocol similar to the one we already reported (30). Thymic lymphocytes were first separated from other thymic cells by centrifugation on a lympholyte gradient. Lymphocytes (2×10^8 per tube) were then suspended in RPMI 1640 supplemented by 20% FCS and incubated for 1 h at 4°C with the appropriate final dilution (1/1,000) of both anti-L3T4 and anti-Ly-2 monoclonal antibodies. The tubes were centrifuged, the supernatant discarded, and the treated cells were resuspended in 1/20 final dilution (in RPMI 1640) of low toxicity rabbit complement for 30 min at 37°C. This treatment was made twice. Then the living cells were separated on a lympholyte gradient. The final recovery of living cells was $5 \pm 3\%$ from the total thymic lymphocytes; 0.5–1% of the remaining cells were either CD4$^+$ or CD8$^+$.

C57B1/6 Lymphocyte Cultures in the Presence of C57B1/6 Red Blood Cells

B6 mouse lymphocyte cultures were performed in flat-bottomed Falcon microtest II plates; 200 µl of cell suspension (whole splenocytes or CD4$^-$ splenocytes, whole thymocytes or double negative thymocytes) were combined with 20 µl of B6 red blood cells (RBC, 1×10^7/ml) and cultured in RPMI 1640 supplemented with 5% inactivated MNS, 1% hepes, 2-mercapthoethanol (5×10^{-5} M), 1% glutamine, and antibiotics. Some cultures were supplemented with 10 units per ml of interleukin 2 and LTB4. After 4 days, cultures were pulsed by 5 µCi of ^{3}H-thymidine per well and the cultures were continued for 12 h. Thereafter the cells were harvested as after stimulation by lectins.

Preincubation of C57B1/6 Double Negative Thymocytes

Prior to performing the cultures, double negative thymocytes (1×10^6/ml) were suspended in 2 ml of RPMI 1640 supplemented with 5% inactivated MS, and then incubated for 24 h in the presence of 10 units per ml of IL-2 2×10^6/ml red blood cells (B6 or D2 or C3) either with or without LTB4. Thus, beside the presence of IL-2, preincubations of double negative thymocytes were performed under six different conditions: 1) plus B6RBC, 2) plus B6RBC and LTB4, 3) plus D2RBC, 4) plus D2RBC and LTB4, 5) plus C3RBC, 6) plus C3RBC and LTB4.

After preincubation double negative thymocytes were separated from erythrocytes by centrifugation on lympholyte gradient. Living cells were counted by a trypan blue exclusion test.

Coculture of C57B1/6 Splenocytes and Preincubated Double Negative Thymocytes in the Presence of Red Blood Cells

Cultures were performed in flat-bottomed Falcon microtest II plates: 2×10^5 B6 splenocytes were combined with 2×10^5 preincubated double negative thymocytes and 1×10^6 RBC (B6 or D2 or C3) and cultured in RPMI 1640 supplemented with 5% inactivated MNS, 1% hepes, 2-mercaptoethanol (5×10^{-5} M), 1% glutamine, and antibiotics. After 4 days, cultures were pulsed by 5 mCi of ^{3}H-thymidine per well and continued for a further 18 h. Thereafter the cells were harvested as for B6 lymphocyte cultures.

RESULTS

Nothern blots and *in situ* hybridization to thymus macrophage RNA demonstrated the presence of 5-lipoxygenase transcripts within the thymus (data not shown). Weak nonspecific hybridization was also seen to the ribosomal RNAs. The specificity of the observed hybridization was confirmed by an absence of hybridization after

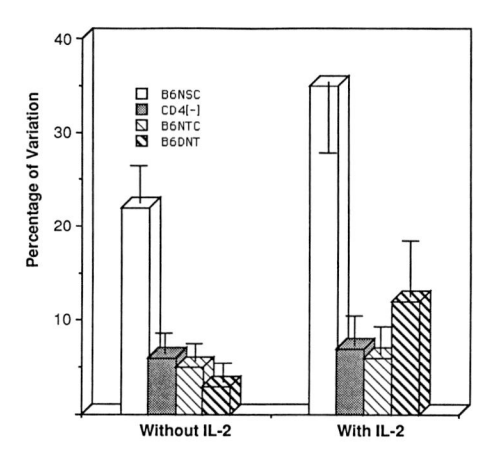

FIG. 1. Proliferative response of C57 B1/6 normal spleen cells (B6 NSC), CD4$^-$ splenocytes (CD4$^-$), C57 B1/6 normal thymocytes (B6 NTC), and double negative thymocytes (B6 DNT) cultured in the presence of autologous erythrocytes. IL-2 was used at 10 units/ml final concentration (mean ± SEM of five experiments).

reprobing duplicates of the blots used with various oligonucleotides for neuropeptides. The activity of the 5-lipoxygenase enzyme was demonstrated by assessment of leukotrienes. It was observed that the average production of LTB4 was 257 ± 40 pg per 1×10^7 cells (mean of 11 experiments). Figure 1 shows that B6 spleen cells proliferate in the presence of autologous erythrocytes. This proliferative response was increased by exogenous IL-2 (+45%) but strongly diminished when CD4$^+$ cells were eliminated before the culture. On the other hand when B6 thymocytes were cultured in the presence of B6 RBC they expressed a low thymidine uptake which was almost unchanged by addition of IL-2. Double negative thymocytes had very low proliferation on culture with autologous erythrocytes. However, IL-2 caused a substantial increase in the double negative thymocyte cell proliferation (225 ± 40%, $p < 0.05$, Student's paired t test) in the presence of autologous red blood cells but not when double negative thymocytes were cultured without autologous erythrocytes (data not shown).

We were then interested in determining the effects of LTB4 on these models of *in vitro* autologous stimulation. Similar experiments were set up, and LTB4 was added to the cultures, which were supplemented by exogenous IL-2 (Fig. 2). LTB4 inhibited the proliferation of whole splenocytes and had little effect on CD4$^-$ splenocytes. With thymocytes and double negative thymocytes, however, LTB4, used at 10^{-11} M final concentration, stimulated the proliferation of these cells when cultured with autologous RBC. We were then interested in determining the functions of double negative thymocytes treated with both LTB4 and IL-2. For this purpose we first assessed whether double negative thymocytes expressed CD4 or CD8 markers after preincubation in the presence of both IL-2 and LTB4. Table 1 shows no change in CD4 expression in the presence of IL-2, LTB4, or both; no change in CD8 expression with either IL-2 or LTB4; but a clear increase of CD8$^+$ cells with LTB4 in combination with IL-2.

Since, within the thymus, thymocytes differentiate in the context of self antigens plus IL-2 and eventually LTB4, the aim of the subsequent experiments was to assess

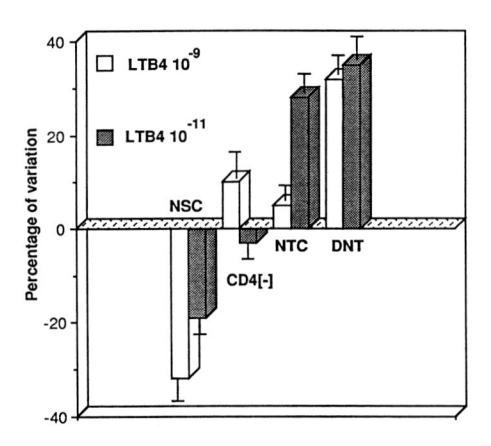

FIG. 2. Proliferative response of C57 B1/6 normal spleen cells (B6NSC), CD4⁻ splenocytes (CD4⁻), C57 B1/6 normal thymocytes (B6 NTC), and double negative thymocytes (B6 DNT) cultured in the presence of autologous erythrocytes and of both LTB4 (10^{-9} M) and IL-2 (10 units/ml final concentration). Results were expressed as percentage of variation compared to the controls (similar cultures but without LTB4) (mean ± SEM of five experiments).

the functional activity of LTB4-generated $CD8^+$ thymocytes on the proliferation of autologous mature T cells. For these experiments B6 double negative thymocytes were preincubated with IL-2 and erythrocytes (either auto or allo), with or without LTB4, and then combined with fresh B6 splenocytes stimulated by either autologous or allogeneic RBC. Allogeneic red cells were used in parallel with autologous for two reasons. First, allogeneic cells were used as "controls" for experiments in the presence of autologous red cells; the second purpose was to check whether immature thymocytes were, at least in our type of experiment, able to become tolerant to foreign antigens. Results are expressed in Fig. 3. Briefly, double negative thymocytes were preincubated with or without LTB4; the response of B6 splenocytes to B6 red blood cells was diminished when cocultured with B6 double negative thymocytes that had been preincubated in the presence of B6 RBC plus IL-2 and LTB4 (column 2) compared to B6 double negative thymocytes preincubated in similar conditions but without LTB4 (column 1). In the same figures columns 3 and 4 show the results when double negative thymocytes were treated with D2 RBC and then combined with D2 RBC-stimulated B6 splenocytes; columns 5 and 6 concern double negative

TABLE 1. *Expression of CD4 or CD8 markers by preincubated double negative thymocytes*[a]

Added products	$CD4^+$ thymocytes[b]	$CD8^+$ thymocytes
—	8 ± 4	16 ± 4
IL-2	8 ± 5	6 ± 4**
LTB4	10 ± 5	12 ± 6**
IL-2 + LTB4	10 ± 6	33 ± 11**

[a] Double negative thymocytes, 1×10^6/ml, were suspended in 2 ml of RPMI 1640 supplemented with 5% inactivated mouse normal serum. The cells were preincubated for 16 hr either alone or with IL-2 (10 units/ml) or LTB4 (10^{-9} M final concentration) or both of them.
[b] Percentage of positive cells.
* p nonsignificant (Student's paired t test).
** $p < 0.01$ (Student's paired t test).

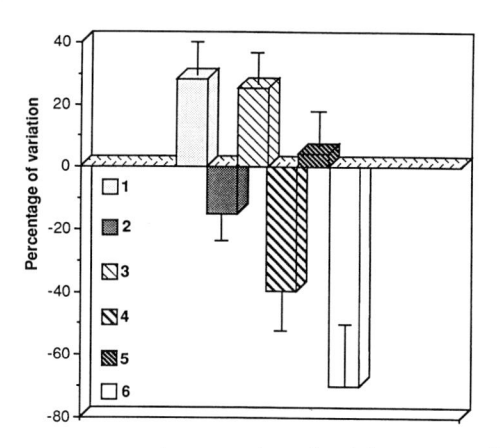

FIG. 3. Effects of C57 B1/6 preincubated double negative thymocytes on the C57 B1/6 fresh splenocytes stimulated by autologous red blood cells. Double negative thymocytes (1×10^6/ml) suspended in mouse normal serum supplemented RPMI were incubated overnight in the presence of IL-2 (10 units/ml) and B6, D2, or C3 red blood cells. Then B6 erythrocyte-treated thymocytes (2×10^5) were combined with fresh B6 splenocytes (2×10^5) stimulated by B6 erythrocytes (column 1). Under similar conditions D2 erythrocyte-treated thymocytes were combined with fresh B6 splenocytes stimulated by D2 erythrocytes (column 3) and C3 red blood cell-treated thymocytes were combined with C3 erythrocyte-stimulated B6 spleen cells (column 5). Results were expressed as percentage of variation compared to the controls (similar culture but with double negative thymocytes preincubated in the presence of IL-2 but without erythrocytes). B6 double negative thymocytes were LTB4 plus IL-2 treated in the presence of C3 red cells. Then they were combined with B6 spleen cells stimulated by either B6 (column 3) or C3 red cells (column 4). Similarly B6 thymocytes were preincubated in the presence of B6 erythrocytes and then mixed with B6 splenocytes activated by either C3 (column 1) or B6 red cells (column 2) (mean ± SEM of three experiments).

thymocytes preincubated in the presence of C3 RBC and cocultured with B6 splenocytes stimulated by C3 RBC. The results show that when B6 double negative thymocytes were preincubated with LTB4 they inhibited the proliferative response of fresh B6 splenocytes whatever the nature of mouse RBC used, either during the preincubation of double negative thymocytes or for the stimulation of splenocytes.

On the other hand, if the preincubation did not contain LTB4 the thymidine uptake was enhanced. Therefore it is likely that *in vitro* treatment of B6 double negative thymocytes by LTB4 plus IL-2 induces them to suppress the proliferative response of B6 spleen cells to allogenic or autologous RBC. The suppression was more effective when RBC used for the stimulation were the same as the RBC used to stimulate double negative thymocytes during the preincubation in the presence of LTB4 and IL-2. For instance (Fig. 4), when double negative thymocytes were first preincubated in the presence of C3 RBC, they strongly inhibited the proliferative response of C3 RBC-stimulated B6 splenocytes (column 4) compared to autologous RBC-stimulated B6 spleen cells (column 3). Similarly, when B6 double negative thymocytes were first preincubated with B6 RBC they were then more efficient at suppressing response to B6 RBC (column 2) compared to the same response induced by C3 erythrocytes (column 1).

CONCLUSION

The data reported in the present paper deal with some important immunological phenomena, i.e., 1) reactivity of mature lymphocytes to autologous antigens, 2)

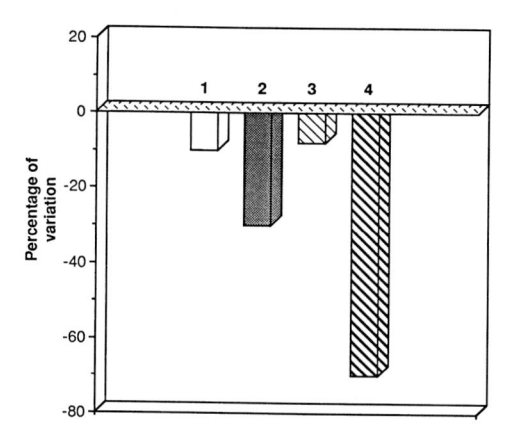

FIG. 4. Effects of C57 B1/6 preincubated double negative thymocytes on the C57 B1/6 fresh splenocytes stimulated by autologous red blood cells. Double negative thymocytes (1×10^6/ml) suspended in mouse normal serum supplemented RPMI were incubated overnight in the presence of IL-2 (10 units/ml)plus LTB4 (10^{-9} M) and B6, D2, or C3 red blood cells. Then B6 erythrocyte-treated thymocytes (2×10^5) were combined with fresh B6 splenocytes (2×10^5) stimulated by B6 erythrocytes (column 2). Under similar conditions D2 erythrocyte-treated thymocytes were combined with fresh B6 splenocytes stimulated by D2 erythrocytes (column 4), and C3 red blood cell-treated thymocytes were combined with C3 erythrocyte-stimulated B6 spleen cells (column 6). Results were expressed as percentage of variation compared to the controls (similar culture but with double negative thymocytes preincubated in the presence of both IL-2 and LTB4 but without erythrocytes) (mean ± SEM of three experiments).

immunomodulatory functions of LTB4, and 3) involvement of the thymus in tolerance to self. First we demonstrated that cells from the thymic microenvironment contain lipoxygenase and synthesize leukotrienes. These data support the fact that immature thymocytes differentiate in the context of lipoxygenase metabolites. Since our protocol needed to assess the autologous RBC-driven proliferative response of mature lymphocytes we performed these experiments in the presence of mouse syngeneic serum, hence avoiding any splenocyte or thymocyte stimulation by fetal calf serum xenoproteins. We observed that MS supports the proliferative response of lectin-stimulated splenocytes, depending on the concentration of added MS. MS concentrations higher than 5% had an inhibitory effect on thymidine uptake without any clear effect on cell viability.

Under such conditions we have observed that B6 splenocytes but not B6 thymocytes proliferate in the presence of autologous RBC and that elimination of $CD4^+$ splenocytes strongly inhibits (-70%) this RBC-induced proliferative response, suggesting that most autologous erythrocyte-sensitive cells carry the helper T cell phenotype. This phenomenon was reported by Hooper who suggests that helper T cells specific for autologous erythrocytes exist in the immunological repertoire of normal animals and that tolerance to erythrocytes is produced by immune regulation (10,11). Therefore it is likely that suppressor T cells play an important role in self tolerance (31–33) and this is probably the case for avoiding any antierythrocyte autoimmunization (10,11,34,35).

When recombinant IL-2 was added to cultures it did not significantly enhance the proliferative response of $CD4^-$ splenocytes stimulated with autologous RBC, but the thymidine uptake of double negative thymocytes was enhanced with IL-2, suggesting that among B6 double negative thymocytes there were some that were able to recognize B6 erythrocytes but needed IL-2 to proliferate.

In fact the experiments reported in Fig. 2 showed that in the presence of both IL-2 and LTB4, autologous erythrocyte-stimulated double negative thymocytes experienced an enhancement of their proliferative response. The same cells suppressed thymidine uptake of normal spleen cells stimulated under similar conditions.

Hence these results were similar to some already reported, i.e., LTB4 inhibits proliferative response of mature peripheral T cells (36) but stimulates the immature thymocyte response (37). It should be emphasized that even if IL-2 has already increased thymidine uptake by double negative thymocytes (Fig. 1) this increase is then augmented by LTB4 (Fig. 2). The data reported in Table 1 show that LTB4 plus IL-2 treatment of double negative thymocytes induces them to express the CD8 marker. We have observed that very few of $CD8^+$ cells expressed CD4 (less than 5%, data not shown) and it is likely that even if some LTB4-treated double negative thymocytes expressed the CD4 marker most of them show the suppressor-cytotoxic differentiation antigen. This is in agreement with data already reported showing that LTB4 induces suppressor T cells (38–40), that $CD8^+$ cells are highly sensitive to LTB4 (39), and that "IL-2 was found to play a major role in promoting the growth of $CD8^+$ cells *in vitro*" (41). The further experiments (Fig. 3) sustained the fact that LTB4-sensitive double negative thymocytes act as suppressor cells when combined with fresh splenocytes. Therefore it is likely that IL-2 and LTB4 induce double negative thymocyte differentiation into mainly $CD8^+$ suppressor lymphocytes. We have observed that the suppressive efficiency depended upon the origin of erythrocytes. For instance, double negative thymocytes preincubated in the presence of allo erythrocytes had a more suppressive effect on fresh splenocytes proliferative response to red blood cells from the same origin than to red blood cells from a different lineage. This discrepancy may be explained by the fact that thymocytes used to set up our experiments were already educated to suppress the response to autologous RBC, and that the *in vitro* procedure failed to have any potent effect on this preexisting suppression. It was also obvious that even if the suppressive effect was linked to H-2 markers (Fig. 3) it was also partly nonspecific (Fig. 4). This may be explained either by the fact that mouse erythrocytes from different strains may share common markers (27) and/or because the suppression induced in our experimental procedure is not totally specific. Nevertheless the data support the evidence that LTB4 plus IL-2 generates $CD8^+$ suppressor thymocytes among a population of double negative immature T cells, and that some of them are self-antigen-specific suppressor T cells.

Since it was observed that IL-2 is produced within the thymus (42), that cells from the thymic microenvironment express self-determinants and synthesize eicosanoids from the cyclo-oxygenase or the lipoxygenase pathway (43–45), and that IL-2 plus LTB4 plays a role in thymocyte differentiation (46), we speculate that LTB4 plus

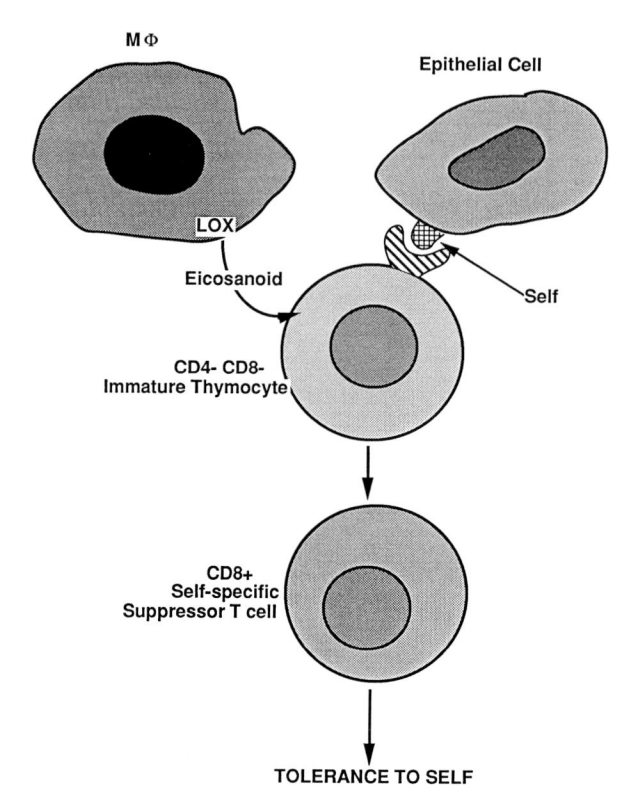

FIG. 5. A predicted pathway for differentiation of immature thymocytes in the context of presenting-self epithelial cell and eicosanoid-producing macrophage.

IL-2 generates $CD8^+$ suppressor thymocytes involved in tolerance to self. More precisely, immature double negative thymocytes, in the context of self-environment and leukotrienes, are induced to differentiate into CD8+ self-specific suppressor T cells involved in tolerance to self (Fig. 5).

REFERENCES

1. Von Boehmer H, Kisielow P. Self-non self discrimination by T cells. *Science* 1990; 248: 1369–73.
2. Blackman M, Kappler J, Marrack P. The role of the T cell receptor in positive and negative selection of developing T cells. *Science* 1990; 248: 1335–41.
3. Schwartz RH. A cell culture model for T lymphocyte clonal anergy. *Science* 1990; 248: 1349–56.
4. Cohen IR, Globerson A, Feldman M. Autosensitization in vitro. *J Exp Med* 1971; 133: 834–45.
5. Cohen IR, Wekerle H. Regulation of autosensitization. The immune activation and specific inhibition of self-recognizing thymus-derived lymphocytes. *J Exp Med* 1973; 137: 224–38.
6. Guilbert B, Dighiero D, Avrameas S. Naturally occurring antibodies against nine common antigens in human sera. I. Detection, isolation and characterization. *J Immunol* 1982; 128: 2779–92.
7. Dighiero G, Limbery P, Mazié JC, *et al*. Murine hybridomas secreting natural monoclonal antibodies reacting with self antigens. *J Immunol* 1983; 131: 2267–74.

8. Champion BR, Varey AM, Katz D, Cooke A, Roitt IM. Autoreactive T-cell lines specific for mouse thyroglobulin. *Immunology* 1985; 54: 513–9.
9. Karray S, Lymberi P, Avrameas S, Coutinho A. Quantitative evidence against inactivation of self-reactive B-cell clones. *Scand J Immunol* 1986; 23: 475–80.
10. Hooper DC. Self-tolerance for erythrocytes is not maintained by clonal depletion of T helper cells. *Immunol Today* 1987; 8: 327–30.
11. Hooper DC, Taylor RB. Specific helper T cell reactivity against autologous erythrocytes implies that self tolerance need not depend on clonal deletion. *Eur J Immunol* 1987; 17: 797–802.
12. Rock KL, Benacerraf B. Thymic T cells are driven to expand upon interaction with self-class II major histocompatibility complex gene products on accessory cells. *Proc Natl Acad Sci USA* 1984; 81: 1221–4.
13. Tutschka PJ. The role of the thymus in regulating tolerance to self and non self. *Transplant Proc* 1987; 19: 486–8.
14. Milicevic NM, Milicevic Z, Mujovic S. Histochemical characterization of the lipid content in the macrophages of the cortico-medullary zone of the rat thymus. *Anat Histol Embryol* 1986; 15: 355–8.
15. Duval D. Effect of dexamethasone on arachidonate metabolism in isolated mouse thymocytes. *Prostaglandins Leukotrienes Essential Fatty Acids* 1989; 37: 149–56.
16. Bonney RJ, Humes JL. Physiological and pharmacological regulation of prostaglandin and leukotriene production by macrophages. *J Leukocyte Biol* 1984; 35: 1–10.
17. Rola-Pleszczynski M. Immunoregulation by leukotrienes and other lipoxygenase metabolites. *Immunol Today* 1985; 6: 302–7.
18. Claesson HE, Dahlberg N, Gahrton G. Stimulation in human myelopoiesis by leukotriene B4. *Biochim Biophys Res Commun* 1985; 131: 579–85.
19. Snyder DS, Desforges JF. Lipoxygenase metabolites of arachidonic acid modulate hematopoiesis. *Blood* 1986; 67: 1675–9.
20. Delebassée S, Cogny Van Weydevelt F, Gualde N. Effects of eicosanoids on thymocyte physiology. *Immunobiol* 1987; 3: 227–8.
21. Penit C, Vasseur F. Cell proliferation and differentiation in the fetal and early postnatal mouse thymus. *J Immunol* 1989; 141: 3369–77.
22. Scollay R, Bartlett P, Shortman K. T-cell development in the adult murine thymus: changes in the expression of the surface antigens Ly2, L3T4 and B2A2 during development from early precursor cells to emigrant. *Immunol Rev* 1984; 80: 103–27.
23. Crispe IN, Moore MW, Husman LA, Smith L, Bevan MJ, Shimonkevitz RP. Differentiation potential of subsets of $CD4^-$ 8^- thymocytes. *Nature* 1987; 329: 336–8.
24. Papiernik M, Penit C, Elrouby S. Control of prothymocyte proliferation by thymic accessory cells. *Eur J Immunol* 1987; 17: 1303–10.
25. Dennings SM, Kurtzberg J, Le PT, Tuck D, Singer KH, Haynes BF. Human thymic epithelial cells directly induce activation of autologous immature thymocytes. *Proc Natl Acad Sci USA* 1988; 85: 3125–9.
26. Brent L, Medawar PB, Ruszkiewicz M. Studies on transplantation antigens. In: Wolstenholme GEW, Cameron MP, eds. *Ciba Foundation Symposium on Transplantation*. London: Churchill; 1962: 6–24.
27. Lejeune-Ledant G. Transplantation antigens, production of haemagglutinins and inhibition of the haemagglutination reaction. In: Wolstenholme GEW, Cameron MP, eds. *Ciba Foundation Symposium on Transplantation*. London: Churchill; 1962: 25–44.
28. Chomczynski P, Sacchi N. Single step method of RNA isolation by acid guanidium thiocyanate-phenol-chloroform extraction. *Ann Biochem* 1987; 162: 156–9.
29. Cambier JC, Havran WL, Fernandez de Albornoz T, Corley RB. Identification of a brain theta positive secretory cell from hematopoietic tissues. *J Immunol* 1981; 127: 1685–91.
30. Gualde N, Weinberger O, Ratnofsky S, Benacerraf B, Burakoff SJ. In vitro generation of helper T cells and suppressor T cells that regulate the cytolytic T lymphocyte response to trinitrophenyl-modified syngeneic cells. *Transplantation* 1982; 33: 422–6.
31. Lo D, Ron Y, Sprent J. Induction of MHC-restricted specificity and tolerance in the thymus. *Immunol Res* 1986; 5: 221–32.
32. Sprent J, Lo D, Gao EK, Ron Y. T cell selection in the thymus. *Immunol Rev* 1988; 101: 173–90.
33. Nossal GJU. Cellular mechanisms of immunological tolerance. In: Paul EW, Fathman CG, Metzger H, eds. *Annu Rev Immunol* 1983; 33–62.

34. Gibson J, Basten A, Walker KZ, Loblay RH. A role for suppressor T cells in induction of self-tolerance. *Proc Natl Acad Sci USA* 1985; 82: 5150–4.
35. Miller RD, Calkins CE. Suppressor T cells and self-tolerance active suppression required for normal regulation of anti-erythrocyte autoantibody responses in spleen cells from non autoimmune mice. *J Immunol* 1988; 140: 3779–85.
36. Rola-Pleszczynski M. Differential effects of leukotriene B4 on T4$^+$ and T8$^+$ lymphocyte phenotype and immunoregulatory functions. *J Immunol* 1985; 135: 1357–60.
37. Delebassée S, Gualde N. Effect of arachidonic acid metabolites on thymocyte proliferation. *Ann Inst Pasteur Immunol* 1988; 139: 383–99.
38. Atluru D, Goodwin JS. Control of polyclonal immunoglobulin production from human lymphocytes by leukotrienes; leukotriene B4 induces an OKT8(+) radiosensitive suppressor cell from resting human OKT8(-) T cells. *J Clin Invest* 1984; 74: 1444–50.
39. Gualde N, Alturu D, Goodwin JS. Effect of lipoxygenase metabolites of arachidonic acid on proliferation of human T cells and T cell subsets. *J Immunol* 1985; 134: 1125–9.
40. Rola-Pleszczynski M, Borgeat P, Sirois P. Leukotriene B4 induces human suppressor lymphocytes. *Biochim Biophys Res Commun* 1982; 4: 1531–7.
41. Sprent J. T lymphocytes and the thymus. In: Paul WE, ed. *Fundamental immunology*, 2nd ed. New York: Raven Press; 1989: 69–93.
42. Ceredig R, Glasebrook AL, Macdonald HR. Phenotypic and functional properties of murine thymocytes. I. Precursors of cytolytic T lymphocytes and interleukin 2-producing cells are all contained within a subpopulation of "mature" thymocytes as analyzed by monoclonal antibodies and flow microfluorometry. *J Exp Med* 1982; 155: 358–62.
43. Papiernik M, Homo-Delarche F. Thymic reticulum in culture secrete both prostaglandin E2 and interleukin 1 which regulate thymocyte proliferation. *Eur J Immunol* 1983; 13: 689–92.
44. Homo-Delarche F, Duval D, Papiernik P. Prostaglandin production by phagocytic cells of the mouse thymic reticulum in culture and its modulation by indomethacin and corticosteroids. *J Immunol* 1985; 135: 506–12.
45. Duval D, Huneau JF, Homo-Delarche F. Effect of serum on the metabolism of exogenous arachidonic acid by phagocytic cells of the mouse thymic reticulum. *Prostaglandins Leukotrienes Med* 1986; 23: 67–72.
46. Delebassée SF, Cogny Van Weydevelt F, Gualde N. Effect of arachidonic acid metabolites on thymus tolerance. *Ann NY Acad Sci* 1988; 524: 227–39.

DISCUSSION

Dr. Bazan: Is it possible that one of the missing links might be platelet-activating factor retention inside the cell? Have you investigated the effect of a platelet-activating factor antagonist?

Dr. Gualde: Yes, we have. We found no difference, so I don't think platelet-activating factor is involved in this model. We have to be very careful in that what we observe *in vitro* with eicosanoids might not be true *in vivo*. The immune system is a huge black box. When you combine it with the great number of metabolites issuing from arachidonic acid it is hard to understand exactly what happens *in vivo*. I proposed a model but I can't guarantee it is true.

Dr. Spielmann: Do you think that a deficiency of a fatty acid in very early life could have a bearing on the development of autoimmune disease?

Dr. Gualde: This is a possibility. The genetic background of autoimmune diseases partly explains their occurrence but there are other factors too. It may be relevant that neonatal mice with arachidonic acid depletion are eaten by the mother within a few days of birth.

Dr. Merrill: In your scheme where you show a macrophage releasing a factor that alters the CD4-/CD8- cell leading to your tolerance to self-cascade, the macrophage is itself interacting with self cells. Is it possible that there is direct communication between the cell acquiring tolerance to self and the macrophage releasing factors, which are then translated to the T cells, resulting in self-tolerance? In this way there would be a very local effect of the macrophage interacting with the cell and initiating the signal.

Dr. Gualde: I think this is very likely. We observed that few macrophages in the thymus express 5-lipoxygenase. This phenomenon is probably relevant to the role played by the thymus during life; and it is somewhere in the thymus that certain macrophages are involved in the generation of suppressive cells. It is not the whole organ that is involved, but only a part of it. These suppressor T cells are even able to suppress the response of B cells, so you can imagine an autoimmune disease with autoantibodies against erythrocytes. Probably everyone has helper T cells directed against their own erythrocytes but most people do not produce autoantibodies because the suppressor T cells are present to switch off the production of antibodies.

Long Chain Fatty Acids and Atopic Dermatitis

Lennart Juhlin

Department of Dermatology, University Hospital, S-751 85 Uppsala, Sweden

Atopic dermatitis (atopic eczema) is a common skin disorder which typically begins in the 3rd to 6th month of life and affects at least 3% of infants. The onset is often delayed until childhood but is rare in adult life. The disease tends to wax and wane. The course is unpredictable but in over 90% of the children the disease has cleared by 15 years of age. The few patients in whom the disease persists into later adult life often have pronounced epidermal changes.

In infancy the lesions tend to be erythematous, vesicular, and weeping on the face, trunk, and limbs. The child scratches whenever given the opportunity. In childhood the dermatitis becomes increasingly flexural on the limbs, leathery, dry, and excoriated. Coccal infections are common. In adults the distribution is the same as in childhood, with a marked tendency toward dryness and thickening of the flexural skin but a low-grade involvement of the trunk, face, and hands. The cardinal sign is itching and the scratching may account for most of the clinical pictures. Bacterial and viral infections such as herpes simplex often complicate the dermatitis.

Atopic dermatitis may later be associated with bronchial asthma, allergic rhinitis, conjunctivitis (hay fever), or urticaria. Other associated conditions include various types of dry scaly skin such as ichthyosis and keratosis pilaris. Keratoconus, cataract, and alopecia areata (patchy hair loss) are rarer associated features. The predisposition to these disorders is at least partly genetic and is called atopic diathesis or atopy, which is present in about 10–15% of the population.

The exact pathogenesis of atopic eczema is obscure. The presence of high levels of circulating IgE represents reaginic antibodies directed mainly against pollen, cat and dog dander, house dust mite, and certain foods. There is some evidence that infants with eczema have a low level of IgA secretion into the intestines together with a deficiency of suppressor T cells which could suggest abnormal entry of potentially antigenic ingested material causing abnormal IgE response. Dietary antigens, particularly cow's milk and eggs, may play a part in provoking dermatitis in some infants. It is advised that babies from atopic families should be breast-fed for at least 3–6 months as this may decrease the risk of eczema. Food allergens tend to be less important in older age groups and rarely provoke eczema in adults, in whom external factors such as airborne antigens, heat, and woolen clothing cause itching and scratching. Besides the removal of causative factors and irritants, the main treatments for atopic dermatitis have focused on measures to avoid scratching. Topical corticosteroids are the mainstay of suppressive treatment followed by regular use of bland emollients. Oral antihistamines also have their place at certain times, as does UV irradiation. In recent years ingestion of long chain fatty acids has been advocated. In this review I shall discuss the rationale for such a treatment and the results obtained, as well as the difficulties in judging the results.

There are two families of essential fatty acids (see Hernell, Fig. 1., this volume). First we have the n-3 or Ω-3 family, which is so called because one double bond is three carbon atoms distant from the methyl end. α-Linolenic acid, eicosapentaenoic acid, and docosahexaenoic acid are the fatty acids in fish oil belonging to this group. The other is the n-6 or Ω-6 family where the first double bond six carbon distant from the methyl end. The fatty acids in this series are linoleic, γ-linolenic, dihomo-γ-linolenic, and arachidonic acid. Arachidonic acid is the precursor for active inflammatory regulators such as most prostaglandins, leukotrienes, hydroxyeicosatetraenoic acid (HETE), and thromboxanes. Arachidonic acid is unstable and its content is low in most foods except cream.

Terestrial plants contain both series. The same desaturase enzymes metabolize both families in man. Diets rich in fish oil decrease the ratio of arachidonic acid to eicosapentaenoic acid in mononuclear cells and inhibit production of interleukin-1 and tumor necrosis factor (1). The two types of fatty acids can interact by competitive inhibition and thus have vastly different metabolic effects (see ref. 2 for review).

Burr and Burr discovered in 1929 that rats placed on a completely fat-free diet soon developed a syndrome including scaliness of the skin and cessation of growth (3). They became normal when fats were added to the diet. The studies disclosed the essential nature of the highly unsaturated fatty acids, particularly linoleic and arachidonic acid (4). In 1933 Hansen found that patients with atopic dermatitis had low concentrations of essential fatty acids in the blood (5). By feeding the infants fat rich in unsaturated fatty acid, such as lard, raw linseed oil, or corn oil, Hansen and coworkers reported a number of clinical cures (6). In atopic patients fed large amounts of linoleic acid, blood linoleic levels were normal whereas those of arachidonic acid were reduced (7). Cornbleet showed good results from treatment with corn oil in 87 adult patients with atopic dermatitis (8). Thereafter others reported a favorable effect in about half of the subjects (9–11), while some found fair or negative results in a small number of patients (12,13). When a controlled trial showed that linolenic and linoleic acid (130 mg and 270 mg, respectively, daily) produced no effect in children with atopic dermatitis research into this mode of treatment was for a time interrupted (14).

Interest was renewed in 1981 when Lovell *et al.* reported that oral treatment of atopic dermatitis with evening primrose seed oil for 3 weeks produced a small but significant improvement (15). The following year Wright and Burton (16) published the results of a 12 week double blind, controlled, crossover study of various doses of evening primrose oil in patients with atopic dermatitis. Each capsule contained

360 mg of linoleic acid and 45 mg of γ-linolenic acid. The placebo capsules contained 500 mg of liquid paraffin. Sixty adults received either two, four, or six capsules twice daily, while 39 children (8 months to 14 years of age) received one or two capsules twice a day. In the two low dose groups in children and adults no objective improvements were noticed but patients did feel that pruritus was improved compared to placebo ($p < 0.05$). In the higher dose groups evening primrose oil was better than placebo with regard to itch, scaling, and general severity ($p < 0.01$). These responses were noted most prominently in the adult groups and less so among children. Adult patients in the high dose group noted an overall improvement in severity of about 43%. No side effects were found.

In a similar Finnish study, 25 young adult patients with atopic dermatitis randomly received either evening primrose oil or placebo for 12 weeks (17). The patients receiving evening primrose oil noted a statistically significant reduction in the severity and grade of inflammation as well as the percentage of body surface area involved. In addition they felt less dryness and itch. Patients in the placebo group also showed a significant reduction in inflammation and clinical improvement but it was less than in the group receiving evening primrose oil therapy. Evening primrose oil caused a significant rise in the amount of dihomo-γ-linolenic acid but plasma levels of thromboxane and prostaglandins were not changed. Evening primrose oil (6×0.5 g capsules) was compared to olive oil in 24 Italian children with atopic dermatitis (18). After 4 weeks the skin lesions had improved in eight of the primrose-oil-treated patients compared to one in the placebo group. Meigel *et al.* found an improvement after primrose oil in 14 of 17 patients as compared to 11 of 17 patients after olive oil or fish liver oil (19). Bamford *et al.* (20) were unable to show any favorable effect in a double blind study of 123 children and adult patients with atopic dermatitis. The doses were similar to those of Wright and Burton but the patients were less severe (11% had >50% skin involvement *vs.* 50% in the earlier study). In a smaller uncontrolled series of eight respectively 50 patients no convincing effects of evening primrose oil were reported (21,22). The controlled trials have recently been included in a meta-analysis by a Research Institute claiming significant benefits for evening primrose oil in atopic dermatitis (23). The findings of Bamford *et al.* were rejected in this study because the serum levels of dihomo-γ-linolenic acid also increased in their placebo-treated patients, indicating that placebo and active drugs could have been mixed. This has caused further discussion as to whether treatment with evening primrose oil is justified or not (24,25).

An intriguing rationale for treatment with evening primrose oil is the finding of raised levels of linoleic and α-linolenic acid in patients with atopic dermatitis but with reduced levels of their metabolites, suggesting that the patients have a functional defect of the desaturating enzymes, especially δ-6-desaturase (26). These findings were confirmed by Strannegård *et al.* (27) who also found that linoleic acid in umbilical cord serum was higher in babies with high serum IgE levels, who are known to be prone to the development of atopic disease. A therapeutic effect of evening primrose oil could thus be due to the fact that it bypasses the 6-desaturation step, since γ-linolenic acid provides a direct effect. Others have, however, failed to confirm this idea (17,28,29). Diet habits and the use of topical corticosteroids have been suggested as more plausible reasons for the reported changes in plasma phospholipid fatty acids (29).

The fatty acid composition of lesional and nonlesional skin from patients with atopic dermatitis has recently been studied (30). Arachidonic acid and n-6 fatty acids of phosphatidyl choline were decreased in lesional skin whereas free arachidonic acid was increased, suggesting an increased activity of phospholipase A_2. The long chain fatty acids ($22:0 + 24:0 + 25:0 + 26:0$) were decreased in lesions whereas the short chain fatty acids ($14:0 + 15:0 + 16:0 + 17.0 + 18:0$) were markedly increased, indicating a defective maturation of long chain fatty acids (30). Of particular interest are the fatty acids that are components of acylceramides, since these might be of great importance for the water barrier function of the epidermis.

Another interesting aspect is the finding that in human breast milk from mothers of children with atopic eczema the proportion of linoleic acid was increased and that of its metabolites such as dihomo-γ-linolenic acid was decreased (31). Breast milk from mothers without atopy would be expected to be best at preventing the manifestations of atopic dermatitis by providing sufficient metabolites, whereas mothers with affected children would be less able to exert this protective effect. Increased maternal consumption of polyunsaturated fatty acids with a reduction in saturated fats, during lactation, may influence the fatty acid composition of the milk. Since human milk contains more γ-linolenic and dihomo-γ-linolenic acid than cow's milk, prolonged breast-feeding could, despite this, still be of value. Dihomo-γ-linolenic acid serves as precursor for prostaglandin E_1, an immunomodulating and cell-differentiating role which has been suggested to play an important part in the etiology of atopy (32). Since fatty acids are necessary for fluidity of membrane lipids, defects of their incorporation into cell membranes could also be of importance.

The effect of blackcurrant seed oil rich in γ-linolenic acid was compared with grapeseed oil as placebo in 24 patients with atopic dermatitis (33). A certain improvement was seen in both groups but no effect could be attributed to γ-linolenic acid. We tried in the same way to study the effect of γ-linolenic acid in 13 patients (13–51 years of age) with atopic dermatitis. They were randomly allocated to a double blind study taking identical-looking capsules each with either 400 mg of blackcurrant oil or 400 mg of grapeseed oil (Table 1). Two hundred parts per million of d-α-tocopherol were added to both types of capsule. The study started in December–January and lasted for 3 months. Four capsules were taken twice daily with food. The total amount of γ linolenic acid intake was thus similar to the evening primrose studies. Blackcurrant oil also contains only a small proportion of α linolenic acid (the study preparation provided 0.55 g/day). The patients all had severe atopic dermatitis with over 50% of the surface involved, and markedly raised IgE levels (300–8,000 kU/l). The severity of itching, skin condition and use of corticosteroids was evaluated before and three times during the study.

Two of the seven patients taking blackcurrant oil showed some improvement and used less corticosteroids, as did one of the six patients taking grapeseed oil. The skin condition of one patient taking blackcurrant oil slowly deteriorated and the

TABLE 1. Percent fatty acids in oils from terrestrial plants

Acid	Blackcurrant	Evening primrose	Grapeseed
Palmitic 16:0	7	7.0	8
Stearic 18:0	1.5	1.0	4
Oleic 18:1 cis 9	10	0.6	16
Elaidic 18:1 trans 9	0.5	—	—
Linoleic 18:2 cis 9, 12	48	72.7	71
γ-linolenic 18:3 cis 6,9,12	17	8.7	—
α-linolenic 18:3 cis 9,12,15	13	—	<1
Stearidonic 18:4	3	—	—

treatment was interrupted after 70 days. No certain effect could be detected in the other patients. External factors such as exposure to horses and cats, infections, and stress situations caused worsening during the treatment period, making the evaluation very difficult. In many the amount and type of corticosteroid used was uncertain. Laboratory routine data, including blood cell transaminases, were not affected. Cholesterol level remained unchanged within normal levels in all, while one patient on blackcurrant oil and two patients on grapeseed oil showed an increase in their total triglycerides after 2–3 months. Since no diet regimen was included in which saturated fatty acids consumed were controlled, the results were as a whole not possible to evaluate further.

Other researchers have studied the effect of dietary supplementation with n-3 fatty acids (eicosapentenoid) for 12 weeks in atopic dermatitis (34). They gave 10 g of fish oil *versus* placebo (olive oil) in a double blind study of 31 patients. Severity score showed no significant between the active and the placebo groups before and after the trial. Patients' assessment scores with fish oil were superior to placebo with regard to itch ($p < 0.05$), scale ($p < 0.05$), and total symptoms score ($p < 0.02$). No significant difference was found between the groups with regard to topical steroid use during the trial.

CONCLUSION

A moderately beneficial effect of γ-linolenic acid and eicosapentaenoic acid in patients with atopic dermatitis has been documented in some studies, and this cannot be disregarded. That others have failed to show an effect of γ-linolenic acid can be due to the fact that eczema patients' skin is sensitive to so many other factors in our environment which could easily have obscured a slight improvement caused by the fatty acids. We do not know if there is a special subgroup of atopic dermatitis where such a treatment is of particular importance. Larger doses of purer products and control of fatty acid intake in the daily diet in very well-controlled studies with an inert placebo are needed. Interrelated effects of long chain fatty acids suggest that a "balanced" intake of the n-6 and n-3 series could be important. The effects obtained currently with long chain fatty acids seem for a clinician to be in most cases quite small when compared to the improvement seen following a 2 week hospital admission or a vacation in different surroundings.

To have any chance of inhibiting the decrease in suppressor cells and the increase in IgE in atopic children it would be necessary to treat infants before the age of 3 months when such changes are seen. This means that we should consider treating the mothers during pregnancy and/or lactation. Controlled studies have to be done in the future before any recommendations can be made.

REFERENCES

1. Endres S, Ghorbani R, Kelley VE, *et al*. The effect of dietary supplementation with n-3 polyunsaturated fatty acids on the synthesis of interleukin-1 and tumor necrosis factor by mononuclear cells. *N Engl J Med* 1989; 320: 265–71.
2. Garg ML, Thomson ABR, Clandinin MT. Interactions of saturated, n-6 and n-3 polyunsaturated fatty acids to modulate arachidonic acid metabolism. *J Lipid Res* 1990; 31: 271–7.
3. Burr GO, Burr MM. A new deficiency disease produced by rigid exclusion of fat from diet. *J Biol Chem* 1929; 82: 345–67.
4. Burr GO, Burr MM, Miller ES. On the fatty acids essential in nutrition. *J Biol Chem* 1932; 97: 1–6.
5. Hansen AE. Serum lipid changes and therapeutic effects of various oils in infantile eczema. *Proc Soc Exp Biol Med* 1933; 31: 160–1.
6. Hansen AE, Knott EM, Wiese HF, Shaperman E, McQuarrie I. Eczema and essential fatty acids. *Am J Dis Child* 1947; 73: 1–18.
7. Brown WR, Hansen AE. Arachidonic and linoleic acid of serum in normal and eczematous human subjects. *Proc Soc Exp Biol Med* 1937; 30: 113–6.
8. Cornbleet T. Use of maize oil (unsaturated fatty acids) in the treatment of eczema: preliminary report. *Arch Dermatol Syph* 1935; 31: 224–34.
9. Finnerud CW, Kester RL, Wiese HF. Ingestion of lard in the treatment of eczema and allied dermatoses. *Arch Dermatol Syph* 1941; 44: 849–53.
10. Ginsberg JE, Bernstein C. Effects of oils containing unsaturated fatty acids on patients with dermatitis. *Arch Dermatol Syph* 1937; 36: 1033–35.
11. Azerad E, Grupper C. Le traitement de l'eczéma par les acides gras non saturés. *Semin Hopital Paris* 1949; 25: 684–9.
12. Epstein NN, Glick D. Unsaturated fatty acids in eczema: observations on acne vulgaris, psoriasis and xantoma palpebrarum. *Arch Dermatol Syph* 1937; 35: 427–32.
13. Taub SJ, Zakon SJ. The use of unsaturated fatty acids in the treatment of eczema (atopic dermatitis, neurodermatitis). *JAMA* 1935; 105: 1675.
14. Petit JHS. Use of unsaturated fatty acids in the treatment of eczema of childhood. *BMJ* 1954; i: 79–81.
15. Lovell CR, Burton JL, Horrobin DF. Treatment of atopic eczema with evening primrose oil. *Lancet* 1981; i: 278.
16. Wright S, Burton JL. Oral evening-primrose-seed oil improves atopic eczema. *Lancet* 1982; ii: 1120–2.
17. Schalin-Karrila M, Mattila L, Jansen CT, Uotila P. Evening primrose oil in the treatment of atopic eczema. Effect on clinical status, plasma phospholipid fatty acids and circulating blood prostaglandins. *Br J Dermatol* 1987; 117: 11–19.
18. Bordoni A, Biagi PL, Masi M, *et al*. Evening primrose oil (Efamol) in the treatment of children with atopic eczema. *Drugs Exp Clin Res* 1987; 14: 291–7.
19. Meigel W, Dettke T, Meigel E-M, Lenze U. Additive orale Therapie der atopischen Dermatitis mit ungesättigten Fettsäuren. *Z Hautkr* 1987; 62[Suppl 1]: 100–3.
20. Bamford JTM, Gibson RW, Reiner CM. Atopic eczema unresponsive to evening primrose oil (linoleic and α-linolenic acids). *J Am Acad Dermatol* 1985; 13: 959–65.

21. Skogh M. Atopic eczema unresponsive to evening primrose oil (linoleic and γ-linolenic acids). *J Am Acad Dermatol* 1986; 15: 114–5.
22. Rasmussen J. Management of atopic dermatitis. *Allergy* 1989; 44[Suppl 9]: 108–13.
23. Morse PF, Horrobin DF, Manku MS, *et al*. Meta-analysis of placebo-controlled studies of the efficacy of Epogram in the treatment of atopic eczema. Relationship between plasma essential fatty acid changes and clinical response. *Br J Dermatol* 1989; 121: 75–90.
24. Sharpe GR, Farr PM. Evening primrose oil and eczema. *Lancet* 1990; 335: 667–8.
25. Horrobin DF, Stewart C. Evening primrose oil in atopic eczema. *Lancet* 1990; 335: 664–5.
26. Manku MS, Horrobin DF, Morse NL, Wright S, Burton JL. Essential fatty acids in the plasma phospholipids of patients with atopic eczema. *Br J Dermatol* 1984; 110: 643–8.
27. Strannegård IL, Svennerholm L, Strannegård Ö. Essential fatty acids in serum lecithin of children with atopic dermatitis and in umbilical cord serum of infants with high or low IgE levels. *Int Arch Allergy Appl Immunol* 1987; 82: 422–3.
28. Nissen HP, Wehrmann W, Kroll U, Kreyser HW. Veränderungen im Plasma-Lipid-Muster bei Patienten mit Neurodermitis-Beeinflussung durch Applikation umgesättigter Fettsäuren. *Fette Wissensch Tech* (Fat Sci Technol) 1988; 90: 268–71.
29. Schäfer L, Kragballe K, Jepsen LV, Iversen L. Reduced neutrophil LTB_4 release in atopic dermatitis patients despite normal fatty acid composition. *J Invest Dermatol* 1991; 96: 16–19.
30. Schäfer L, Kragballe K. Abnormalities in epidermal lipid metabolism in patients with atopic dermatitis. *J Invest Dermatol* 1991; 96: 10–15.
31. Wright S, Bolton C. Breast milk fatty acids in mothers of children with atopic eczema. *Br J Nutr* 1989; 62: 693–7.
32. Melnik BC, Plewig G. Is the origin of atopy linked to deficient conversion of α-6-fatty acids to prostaglandin E_1? *J Am Acad Dermatol* 1989; 21: 557–63.
33. Rilliet A, Queille C, Saurat J-H. Effects of gamma-linolenic acid in atopic dermatitis. *Dermatologica* 1988; 177: 257.
34. Bjorneboe A, Soyland E, Bjorneboe G-EA, Rajka G, Drevon CA. Effect of dietary supplementation with eicosapentaenoic acid in the treatment of atopic dermatitis. *Br J Dermatol* 1987; 117: 463–9.

DISCUSSION

Dr. Cunnane: I wonder if there is a problem of linoleic acid utilization or oxidation in atopy. Kristian Bjerve (1), who has looked at patients on long-term total parenteral nutrition in whom safflower oil was the source of essential fatty acids, has seen a dramatic improvement in the dermal lesions after giving very small amounts of α-linolenic acid. I suggest that if this is a genuine effect it may partly be due to the fact that α-linolenic acid is readily oxidized and that linoleic acid may be channeled toward an oxidation route in people with insufficient α-linoleic acid, thereby causing a deficiency systemically which can be avoided or corrected by α-linolenic acid supplements. Thus in patients who respond to evening primrose oil the effect may simply be through providing additional linoleic acid.

Dr. Koletzko: In Germany it has been proposed recently that γ-linolenic acid should be used by pregnant and lactating women to prevent atopy in their babies. This seems irresponsible to me in the present state of knowledge. I appreciate that long chain fatty acids may well have a therapeutic effect on the disease, which is obviously related to immunologic mechanisms. However, I have my doubts as to whether the basic cause of the problem is really a defect of δ-6-desaturase, as you have stated, and I should appreciate a further comment on this.

Dr. Juhlin: I understand your doubts on the existence of a deficit in the δ-desaturases in atopic dermatitis since no direct measurements of the enzyme have been made. The evidence is only indirect and is based on the finding of low arachidonic acid levels despite raised levels of linoleic acid. Another explanation for the deficiency of arachidonic acid could be that its turnover in plasma is faster than in healthy subjects.

Dr. Small: Is breast milk abnormal in women who are atopic?

Dr. Juhlin: A deficiency in milk γ-linolenic acid has been shown.

Dr. Guesry: A study published in 1986 (2) showed that milk of atopic mothers had very low levels of specific antibetalactoglobulin IgA compared with control mothers, so I don't think it is likely that such milk is protective against allergy in the baby. In another study (3) two groups of lactating mothers with atopic children were compared. In one group the mothers had a diet low in allergens, in the other group the mothers were on a normal diet. There was a striking reduction in the severity of atopic eczema in the low allergen group, showing that transmission of allergens was more important than IgA or long chain polyunsaturated fatty acids.

Dr. Galli: Is there any evidence of altered eicosanoid production in atopic eczema?

Dr. Juhlin: The arachidonic acid derived inflammatory mediators are raised in affected skin of patients with atopic dermatitis, which might also indicate increased consumption of arachidonic acid. The whole cascade of prostaglandins increases in the skin in almost any inflammatory lesion.

Dr. Merrill: Skin is rich in acylglucoceramides and acylceramides which have a highly unsaturated fatty acid composition. These fatty acids are now available as creams for cosmetic purposes. It might be worth trying these formulations as a route for administering unsaturated fatty acids, since they more closely mimic the form in which such fatty acids are found in the skin.

Dr. Juhlin: The O-acylceramides are located intercellularly in the skin surface and it would be of great interest to influence them. Studies of γ-linolenic acid-rich oils have been disappointing in atopic dermatitis, but other formulations such as you suggest might certainly be worth exploring.

REFERENCES

1. Bjerve KS, Mostad IL, Thoresen L. Alpha-linolenic acid deficiency in patients on long-term gastric-tube feeding: estimation of linolenic acid and long-chain unsaturated n-3 fatty acid requirement in man. *Am J Clin Nutr* 1987; 45: 66–77.
2. Machtinger S, Moss R. Cow's milk allergy in breast fed infants. The role of antigen and maternal secretory IgA antibody. *J Allergy Clin Immunol* 1986; 77: 341–7.
3. Chandra RK, Puri S, Surarya C, *et al*. Influence of maternal food antigen avoidance during pregnancy and lactation on prevalence of atopic eczema in infants. *Clin Allergy* 1986; 16: 565–9.

Long Chain Fatty Acids and Cholesterol Metabolism

Richard J. Deckelbaum

Division of Gastroenterology and Nutrition, Department of Pediatrics, College of Physicians and Surgeons of Columbia University, New York, New York 10032, USA

Early in the 20th century it was recognized that diet could affect atherosclerosis. Anitschkow and Chalatow reported atherosclerosis in rabbits who were fed diets rich in cholesterol (1). Since then, many studies have been carried out in both animals and humans showing marked effect of dietary intake on cholesterol metabolism, morbidity, and mortality, coronary heart disease, and atherosclerosis. More recently, it has become apparent, at least in humans and some mammals, that cholesterol intake *per se* has less of an effect on blood cholesterol levels and atherosclerosis than does the quality and quantity of the type of fatty acids ingested (2,3). Most important, it is now recognized that lowering blood cholesterol levels can lead to regression of atherosclerosis in humans and reduce morbidity and mortality from coronary artery disease.

The Seven Countries study (4) showed a clear correlation between the proportion of energy ingested as saturated fats and blood cholesterol levels in a variety of populations. More importantly, these studies demonstrated a close correlation between these blood cholesterol levels and coronary heart disease cases in the populations under study, clearly showing in multiple populations a close link between saturated fat intake and coronary heart disease. People in the four locations who consumed the highest proportion of their energy intake as saturated fat also had the highest average cholesterol levels and highest rate of coronary heart disease. Conversely, people who consumed the lowest proportion of their energy intake as saturated fat had lower cholesterol levels and lower rates of coronary heart disease (4). Studies on the Japanese showed that the total intake of fat and saturated fat increased progressively when Japanese people moved to Hawaii and to San Francisco. This was associated with an increase in blood cholesterol levels and in deaths from coronary heart disease (5).

After studies in the 1950s showed that serum cholesterol related more to the quality of fat in the diet than to dietary cholesterol itself, Keys, Hegsted, and their colleagues framed equations for predicting the effects of different fats and cholesterol in the diet on changes in total serum cholesterol as follows:

Equation of Keys et al. (6)

$$\Delta \text{Cholesterol (mg/dl)} = 2.7\Delta S - 1.35\Delta P + 1.5\sqrt{\Delta C} \text{ mg/1,000 cal-day}$$

Equation of Hegsted et al. (7)

$$\Delta \text{Cholesterol (mg/dl)} = 2.16\Delta S - 1.65\Delta P + 0.068\Delta C_{mg/day}$$

Where S = saturated fatty acids (% of total energy); P = polyunsaturated fatty acids (% of total energy); C = dietary cholesterol

Both of these equations show that major emphasis is placed upon the percent contribution of saturated fats and percent of polyunsaturated fats as part of total energy intake, with a lesser input from dietary cholesterol. This has been borne out in many subsequent studies, although in defining the response to particular fatty acids and cholesterol, variations do exist. For example, stearic acid (18:0) has been reported to behave more like a polyunsaturated than a saturated fatty acid in terms of effect on the serum cholesterol levels (8). Also, it is now recognized that in human populations there may be hypo- and hyper-responders to dietary cholesterol.

More recently, there has been high interest in the potential of fish oils to modulate serum lipid levels and the atherosclerotic process (9). While these Ω-3 polyunsaturates, with their high contents of eicosapentaenoic acid (EPA) and docosahexaenoic acid (DHA), are able to reduce triglyceride levels in both normal and hypertriglyceridemic individuals, their effects on plasma cholesterol and lipoprotein cholesterol are not as well defined. Clearly, however, a high intake of marine fatty acids in Eskimos leads to a marked diminution in the incidence of coronary heart disease, although it is likely that this is determined more by the effects of fish oil fatty acids on coagulation and thrombogenesis than on serum lipid levels. Still, major questions remain as to the potential of these Ω-3 fatty acids to modulate plasma, lipoprotein and cholesterol metabolism.

In this chapter, we shall address questions relevant to the effects of fatty acids on cholesterol metabolism:

1. Does the quantity of fat intake, as compared to the quality of fat intake, have an equal or more important effect on human cholesterol metabolism?
2. Are the effects of different dietary intakes, specifically the fatty acid intakes, related more to increased synthesis of cholesterol or to increased catabolism and removal of cholesterol from tissues and the body?
3. What regulatory mechanisms of cholesterol metabolism are potentially modified by free fatty acids?

For a comprehensive review on the effects of different fatty acids on plasma lipids, the reader is referred to recent reviews by Grundy and Denke (10) and Harris (9). I shall focus herein on potential mechanisms whereby different fatty acids may affect cholesterol metabolism and review recent work of a number of investigators, as well as work in my own laboratory.

POTENTIAL MECHANISMS FOR THE EFFECTS OF FATTY ACIDS ON CHOLESTEROL METABOLISM

In simplest terms, the potential effects of different fatty acids on cholesterol metabolism can be related to changes in cholesterol synthesis and/or changes in cholesterol catabolic routes. The net result of these two pathways will be the final effect on plasma and tissue cholesterol levels. With regard to new lipid synthesis, different fatty acids have the potential to 1) increase or decrease cellular lipid synthesis, 2) modulate synthesis and release of apoproteins and lipoproteins from cells, and 3) modulate delivery of cholesterol carried in lipoproteins into cells. Fatty acids may modulate cholesterol catabolism by changing the number and activity of lipoprotein receptors, e.g., the low density lipoproteins (LDL) receptor, which will affect the clearance of lipoprotein from plasma by receptor-mediated pathways. Fatty acids also have the potential of modulating interactions and affinity between circulating lipoproteins and cell receptors. Finally, fatty acids can modulate reverse cholesterol transport by effects on the ability to remove cholesterol from peripheral tissues and deliver it to the liver, where different dietary fatty acids may also have variable effects on the excretion of cholesterol through bile, either as cholesterol itself or as bile acids.

EFFECTS OF DIFFERENT FATTY ACIDS ON PLASMA LIPID AND LIPOPROTEIN LEVELS

Recent studies indicate that the amount of saturated fat ingested may be more important than the overall percentage of dietary energy taken as fat in determining plasma cholesterol levels. As an example, we recently reported reduction of plasma cholesterol levels in normal men receiving an American Heart Association (AHA) Step 1 diet or a Step 1 diet with added monounsaturated fat (11). In this study, the plasma lipid levels in a cohort receiving the "average American" diet (38% of total energy from fat, 18% total energy from saturated fats) were compared to those in a cohort on the AHA Step 1 diet (30% of total energy from fat, 10% total energy from saturated fats), and a Step 1 diet containing 38% of total energy from fat, again with 10% from saturated fats but with added monounsaturated fats bringing the total fat intake up to 38% of total energy. We found that there was a statistically significant reduction in plasma total cholesterol levels both in the group on the Step 1 diet and in the group with the monounsaturated fat-enriched diet. At the same time there were parallel reductions in plasma and LDL-cholesterol in these two groups with no significant changes in plasma triglyceride levels or high density lipoprotein (HDL)-cholesterol levels. These results suggested that the total fat intake could be increased, but as long as the saturated fat intake was kept low, a reduction in plasma and LDL-cholesterol could be attained. Other reports by Mattson and Grundy (12) and Mensink and Katan (13) also showed that with high fat intake (that is 40% total energy) plasma cholesterol and LDL-cholesterol reductions can be attained as long as absolute intake of saturated fatty acids is maintained at low levels.

The Keys and Hegsted equations do not account for monounsaturated fat intakes, and in fact regard them as "neutral," that is, much like carbohydrates in terms of their effects on cholesterol metabolism. Recent evidence, however, suggests that monounsaturated fats may either have independent effects or behave in a similar manner to polyunsaturated fats (10). Of interest, however, is the evidence that monounsaturated fats do not lower HDL-cholesterol levels, an effect that has been repeatedly documented with diets high in polyunsaturated fats (10,11).

There is some evidence that not all saturated fats will raise plasma cholesterol levels. For example, medium chain fatty acids (which are saturated) behave much like carbohydrates and will not increase serum cholesterol levels as compared to long chain saturated fatty acids. Clearly, palmitic acid and myristic acid, and probably lauric acid, do raise plasma cholesterol levels (10). Grundy et al. have suggested that stearic acid does not have this effect, and that it does in fact have a cholesterol lowering effect (10). Mensink and Katan have recently suggested (14) that trans fatty acids (produced after hydrogenation of polyunsaturated fats) raise total blood cholesterol and LDL-cholesterol levels in a manner similar to cholesterol-raising saturated fatty acids. Therefore the types of double bond, as well as their number and position, also determine effects on cholesterol metabolism.

In a recent pilot study, we assayed plasma cholesterol levels in children before and during ketogenic diets (J. Schroeder, R. Deckelbaum, unpublished data). These diets, which provide intakes of 80–90% of total energy as fat, are sometimes used in children with seizure disorders as an adjunct to prevent convulsions. With these very high fat intakes, we were surprised to observe that while, as expected, children who received the traditional ketogenic diet with a high intake of dairy fats (which are largely saturated) raised their plasma cholesterol levels by 30%, children who received high fat intake entirely from polyunsaturated vegetable oils, in contrast, lowered their plasma cholesterol levels by 25%. Thus, at extreme levels of fat intake, plasma cholesterol levels can fall as long as saturated fat intake or the ratio of saturated fats to other fats is low.

EFFECTS OF DIFFERENT FATTY ACIDS ON LIPID AND LIPOPROTEIN PRODUCTION

Surprisingly little evidence is available to suggest that different fatty acids have marked influence on synthetic rates of lipids in humans. With the exception of the fish oil fatty acids, which show a marked ability in both cell culture and whole body turnover studies to decrease synthetic rates of triglyceride and very low density lipoprotein (VLDL) production (9,15), few data are available to suggest similar or opposite effects for other fatty acids. In isolated cells, however, it is clear that specific fatty acids can have important effects on cellular lipid metabolism. For example, oleic acid, long known to increase cellular triglyceride synthesis, has recently been shown in a preliminary report to increase rapidly apoprotein B secretion by cultured Hep G2 cells in a novel way (16). Surprisingly, this increase was not due to an increase in synthesis of the apoprotein B molecule itself, but rather to an effect of decreasing intracellular apoprotein B degradation, leaving more apoprotein B available for secretion. Such a mechanism may exist *in vivo* as an important regulator of triglyceride-rich lipoprotein release from the liver in situations where fatty acids are rapidly released into tissue, e.g., the postprandial state.

There is some evidence in humans that dietary exchange of polyunsaturates for saturates reduces the production of LDL apoprotein B, suggesting that polyunsaturates may in fact decrease the production of LDL precursors (17,18). We have shown in tissue culture systems with different cell lines that long chain, but not medium chain, saturates increase cholesterol esterification and decrease the ratio of cholesterol ester to free cholesterol within cells. This effect is different with different fatty acids, for example palmitic acid has a much greater ability to increase cholesterol esterification and total cell cholesterol than does oleic acid in cells that are being "cholesterol loaded" in the presence of pure LDL or human serum (19). It is possible that the ability of fatty acids to change the distribution between free cholesterol and cholesteryl ester in the cell (19) may affect LDL receptor synthesis, and that this can be modulated by intake of saturated *vs.* unsaturated fatty acids.

Work with fish oil fatty acids, DHA and EPA, has shown a definite effect of these Ω-3 fatty acids in inhibiting new triglyceride synthesis and VLDL release from cultured cells (15). In these experiments, secretion of VLDL-apoprotein B was also decreased, but this was likely to have been related to a decrease in the synthesis of triglyceride-rich particles in general. It is possible that DHA and EPA are poorly incorporated into triglycerides themselves, or alternatively that they inhibit synthesis of triglyceride from other fatty acids (10,15).

EFFECTS ON LIPID AND LIPOPROTEIN CATABOLISM

Dietary fatty acids have an effect on regulating clearance of both triglyceride-rich and cholesterol-ester-rich lipoproteins from plasma. Interesting recent data have shown that normal subjects chronically ingesting a diet rich in saturated fat have a decreased ability to clear exogenous fat after an oral fat load from plasma (20). In particular, this results from decreased clearance of remnant triglyceride-rich particles, and this is independent of the type of fat consumed. Conversely, individuals chronically fed a polyunsaturate-rich diet were able to clear saturated and polyunsaturated fat loads more efficiently (20). This suggests that the chronic intake of an individual will be important in determining the ability to clear triglyceride-rich particles, and this may then result in a decrease in production of HDL.

The major effect of different fatty acids, saturated *vs.* polyunsaturated, on regulating LDL plasma levels is most likely to be related to effects on LDL receptor activity. Diets high in saturated fatty acids seemingly suppress LDL-receptor-mediated clearance of LDL. This has been shown by turnover studies in man and animals (21,22). The mechanism whereby saturated fatty acids depress LDL receptor activity (whether by number or by activity of the receptor itself) is not yet known.

Studies in our own group have shown that free fatty acids have an ability to modulate interaction of lipoproteins with their cell receptors (23,24). Because of the ability of free fatty acids to displace other molecules with heparin binding sites from endothelial walls (25), we hypothesized that free fatty acids might also displace LDL from its LDL receptor. We explored this in systems where LDL was incubated with cultured fibroblasts. We found that in physiologic concentrations, free fatty acids (FFA) were able to displace LDL already bound to the receptor and inhibit binding of LDL to the LDL receptor by about 50%. The effect of FFA was not due to toxic or irreversible effects on the cultured cells nor to detergent-like effects. Of particular interest was the finding that different fatty acids had very different abilities to displace LDL. Short chain fatty acids (8–12 carbons) had little displacement ability while longer saturated fatty acids ($\geq$14 carbons) had increasing ability to modulate LDL binding to the receptor depending on their chain length. Moreover, the type and position of double bonds also had a modulating influence. The effect of the FFA is modified by the hydrophobic properties of the fatty acid, but the inhibition is directly dependent upon the presence of negative charge on the carboxyl group (23).

We then questioned whether FFA would have similar effects on the interaction of triglyceride-rich particles with cells. To study this, we used human VLDL and triolein-phospholipid emulsions with added apoprotein E (24). Unlike effects on LDL, the presence of FFA increased binding of VLDL- and apo-E-containing emulsions by two- to sixfold. These results suggest that FFA might be important physiologically in providing a rapid switch mechanism for decreasing binding and uptake of specific lipoproteins, such as LDL, and increasing that of others, e.g., apo-E-containing triglyceride-rich particles such as VLDL and remnants, in tissues with lipase-rich microenvironments. Such mechanisms may be particularly important in the postprandial state.

Different fatty acids may also have different abilities to change fecal excretion of sterols and excretion of body cholesterol. There has been some suggestion in normal and hypertriglyceridemic subjects that substituting linoleic acid for saturated fatty acids will lead to increased mass excretion of fecal steroids, although no effects were noted in hypercholesterolemic subjects (10).

Thus the interaction of fatty acids on cholesterol metabolism may be multiple and complex with a potential to interact at a variety of metabolic sites. The balance of these effects will determine whether changes will occur rapidly, with changing plasma lipid levels, and whether over longer periods they will affect the atherosclerotic process.

DOES INFANT DIET INFLUENCE CHOLESTEROL LEVELS LATER IN LIFE?

At the present time dietary modifications, with respect to fat reduction, have not been recommended for children less than 2 years old. It is of interest to consider the potential of early diet to modify cholesterol levels and perhaps atherosclerosis in adulthood. Can high cholesterol intake in infancy (e.g., in infants receiving breast milk) or high intake of polyunsaturated fats (e.g., in children receiving certain formulas) induce mechanisms that would predispose to lower cholesterol levels at older ages? In reviewing a number of studies addressing this, it is evident that the major effects on cholesterol levels, at the time when the diets are being administered and examined, are associated with the ratio of polyunsaturated to saturated fats in the diets and not to the amount of cholesterol ingested (26). A preliminary report has suggested that dietary fatty acids, and not dietary cholesterol, determine LDL- and HDL-cholesterol in infants, and perhaps LDL receptor activity, as well (27). These studies therefore suggest the hypothesis that the type of fat ingested in infancy rather than the amount of cholesterol could be the more important determinant of the effect of early diet on cholesterol metabolism in later life (26).

CONCLUSION

In summary, it is clear that the type of fatty acid ingested can have a major role in regulating cholesterol metabolism in humans, and that the effects of fatty acids are likely to be more important than the ingestion of cholesterol itself. The potential for different fatty acids to modify atherosclerosis acts not only via cholesterol metabolism but also by their integration with other contributors to the atherosclerotic plaque, such as the coagulation and thrombosis systems, and perhaps the immune response as well.

Future research on the effects of different fatty acids on cholesterol metabolism needs to address mechanisms whereby free fatty acids modulate receptor lipoprotein interaction, cell cholesterol synthesis, esterification and deposition, and cell cholesterol elimination. Particular attention should be directed toward whether fatty acids affect receptor function and lipid metabolism by alterations in physical properties of membranes, by changes in pre- or posttranslation regulatory pathways of apoprotein synthesis and degradation, and/or by effects on enzymes involved in cellular lipid metabolism. Clinically, and of particular interest to those caring for children, do changes in cholesterol metabolism ascribed to effects of different fatty acids in adults have similar, greater, or lesser effects in infants and children? And, are these alterations important in normal growth and development?

REFERENCES

1. Anitschkow N, Chalatow S. Veber experimentelle Cholesterinseatose und ihre Bedeutung für die Entstehung einiger pathologischer Prozesse. *Zentralbl Allg Pathol Pathol Anat* 1913; 24: 1–9.
2. Mott GE, McMahan CA, Kelley JL, Farley CM, McGill HC Jr. Influence of infant and juvenile diets on serum cholesterol, lipoprotein cholesterol, and apolipoprotein concentrations in juvenile baboons (Papio sp). *Atherosclerosis* 1982; 45: 191–202.
3. Slater G, Mead J, Dhopeshwarkar G, Robinson S, Alfin-Slater R. Plasma cholesterol and triglycerides in men with added eggs in the diet. *Nutr Rep Int* 1976; 14: 249–60.
4. Keys A. Coronary heart disease in seven countries. *Circulation* 1970; 41: 11–211.

5. Conference on the Health Effects of Blood Lipids: Optimal distribution for populations. *Prev Med* 1979; 8: 612–78.
6. Keys A, Anderson JT, Grande F. Serum cholesterol response to changes in the diet. IV. Particular saturated fatty acids in the diet. *Metabolism* 1965; 14: 776–87.
7. Hegsted DM, McGandy RB, Myers ML, Stare FJ. Quantitative effects of dietary fat on serum cholesterol in man. *Am J Clin Nutr* 1965; 17: 281–95.
8. Bonanome A, Grundy SM. Effect of dietary stearic acid on plasma cholesterol and lipoprotein levels. *N Engl J Med* 1988; 318: 1244–8.
9. Harris WS. Fish oils and plasma lipid and lipoprotein metabolism in humans: a critical review. *J Lipid Res* 1989; 30: 785–807.
10. Grundy SM, Denke MA. Dietary influences on serum lipids and lipoproteins. *J Lipid Res* 1990; 31: 1149–72.
11. Ginsberg HN, Barr SL, Gilbert A, *et al*. Both an American Heart Association Step 1 Diet and a Step 1 Diet with added monounsaturates decrease plasma cholesterol levels in normal males. Results of a randomized, double-blind trial. *N Engl J Med* 1990; 322: 574–9.
12. Mattson FH, Grundy SM. Comparison of effects of dietary saturated, monounsaturated, and polyunsaturated fatty acids on plasma lipids and lipoproteins in man. *J Lipid Res* 1985; 26: 194–202.
13. Mensink RP, Katan MB. Effect of a diet enriched with monounsaturated or polyunsaturated fatty acids on levels of low-density and high-density lipoprotein cholesterol in healthy women and men. *N Engl J Med* 1989; 321: 436–41.
14. Mensink RP, Katan MB. Effect of dietary trans fatty acids on high-density and low-density lipoprotein cholesterol levels in healthy subjects. *N Engl J Med* 1990; 323: 439–45.
15. Wong S, Nestel PJ. Eicosapentaenoic acid inhibits the secretion of triacylglycerol and of apoprotein B and the binding of LDL in HepG2 cells. *Atherosclerosis* 1987; 64: 139–46.
16. Dixon JL, Furukawa S, Ginsberg HN. Oleic acid stimulates secretion of apolipoprotein B-containing lipoproteins from HepG2 cells by reducing intracellular degradation of apolipoprotein B. *Atherosclerosis* 1990; 10: 763a.
17. Grundy SM. Effects of polyunsaturated fats on lipid metabolism in patients with hypertriglyceridemia. *J Clin Invest* 1975; 55: 269–82.
18. Chair A, Onitiri A, Nicoll A, Rabaya E, Davies J, Lewis B. Reduction of serum triglyceride levels by polyunsaturated fat. Studies on the mode of action and on very low density lipoprotein composition. *Atherosclerosis* 1974; 20: 347–64.
19. Lipschitz B, McIntosh RA, Galeano NF, Gleeson AM, Carpentier YA, Deckelbaum RJ. Medium chain as compared to long chain fatty acids decrease cell cholesteryl ester accumulation from LDL or serum. *Atherosclerosis* 1990; 10: 841a.
20. Weintraub MS, Zechner R, Brown A, Eisenberg S, Breslow JL. Dietary polyunsaturated fats of the ω-6 and ω-3 series reduce postprandial lipoprotein levels. *J Clin Invest* 1988; 82: 1884–93.
21. Spady DK, Dietschy JM. Dietary saturated tricylglycerols suppress hepatic low density lipoprotein receptors in the hamster. *Proc Natl Acad Sci (USA)* 1985; 82: 4526–30.
22. Nicolosi RJ, Stucchi AF, Kowala MC, Hennessy LK, Hegsted DM, Schaefer EJ. Effect of dietary fat saturation and cholesterol on LDL composition and metabolism. *Atherosclerosis* 1990; 10: 119–28.
23. Bihain BE, Deckelbaum RJ, Yen FT, Gleeson AM, Carpentier YA, Witte LD. Unesterified fatty acids inhibit the binding of low density lipoproteins to the human fibroblast low density lipoprotein receptor. *J Biol Chem* 1989; 264: 17316–21.
24. Yen FT, Bihain BE, Gleeson AM, Vogel T, Gorecki M, Deckelbaum RJ. Free fatty acids increase the binding of apoprotein E-containing particles to the cultured human fibroblast. *Atherosclerosis* 1989; 9: 719a.
25. Peterson J, Bihain BE, Bengtsson-Olivecrona G, Deckelbaum RJ, Carpentier YA, Olivecrona T. Fatty acid control of lipoprotein lipase: a link between energy metabolism and lipid transport. *Proc Natl Acad Sci (USA)* 1990; 87: 909–13.
26. Deckelbaum RJ. Long term effects of diet in the first year of life on cholesterol metabolism and atherosclerosis. In: Heird WC, ed. *Nutritional needs of the six to twelve month old infant*. Carnation Nutrition Education Series, Vol. 2. Glendale: Carnation Co. New York: Raven Press; 1991: 297–302.
27. Uauy R, Mize C, Grundy S. Effect of early diet on plasma lipoproteins and LDL receptor activity at one year of age. *Pediatr Res* 1989; 25: 126a.

DISCUSSION

Dr. Hernell: I have a comment. It is interesting that human milk triglycerides are secreted as globules enveloped by a membrane. Pancreatic lipase, even in the presence of colipase and bile salts, will not attack that globule. The best way to overcome the inhibition is to add free fatty acids, since FFA enforce binding between the lipase and the substrate surface. The best binders are the long chain and unsaturated fatty acids such as oleic and linoleic. Medium chain fatty acids have no effect.

Dr. Spector: Does oleic acid have a direct effect on apo B degradation?

Dr. Deckelbaum: It is possible that when we increase triglyceride synthesis in the cell, apo B is more stable attached to a triglyceride globule than just sitting on a membrane. Thus putting apo B on a triglyceride droplet may make it less susceptible to degradation.

Dr. Spector: I agree with this interpretation. This is a critical point now because we are thinking about fatty acids affecting gene expression or directly affecting the turnover and degradation of an apolipoprotein. The simplest explanation is that as more triglyceride is produced the apo B is needed to secrete this triglyceride, binds to the particle, and is less available for degradation.

Dr. Heim: You mentioned several times that LDL oxidation is stimulated by many substances. For those working on intermediary metabolism, oxidation means end-oxidation to carbon dioxide and water, or during the intermediate process, oxidation of a substrate and excretion in another form. I think LDL is too complex a molecule to investigate in this respect and I wonder if you have any evidence that the protein part is oxidized to urea, or the carbon skeleton to carbon dioxide and water. What happens to the cholesterol and triglyceride fatty acids?

Dr. Deckelbaum: I think what is meant by LDL oxidation is still being defined, but it is not end-oxidation, nor is it the using up of LDL as an energy source. It is a "peroxidation" and involves oxidation changes in both lipid and protein molecules. With oxidation the LDL particle does not disappear under the microscope, nor does it change its density in the centrifuge. What it does is change the properties of these lipids and proteins. It might change surface properties in terms of binding of other apoproteins or affect the protein itself in terms of an oxidized group on the amino acid or carbohydrate groups on the protein.

Dr. Van Biervliet: In our studies on neonatal development of lipoprotein metabolism we show low LDL and relatively high HDL at birth in humans (1,2). However, at birth and before birth, a very important HDL fraction is present, rich in apolipoprotein (apo) E that we call HDL_E. This HDL_E could be one of the mechanisms by which fat and among others long chain polyenoic acids are delivered to E receptors, before birth (3). We showed furthermore that after birth the apo E is shifted from HDL to VLDL. Chylomicrons become the main fatty acid transporting mechanism, once the umbilical cord is cut. After birth LDL concentrations increase drastically with HDL increasing at a steadier rate until 30 days. Nutrition, however, rules over this phenomena (2,4). To study this phenomena we took comparative measures in four groups of neonates on different diets. The first group being the human milk group (HM), the second group receiving a standard formula supplemented with γ-linoleic acid (F+γLA), the third group supplemented with cholesterol (F+Chol) to half the values of cholesterol in human milk, and the fourth group receiving a standard formula (F). At birth total serum cholesterol is relatively low, it increases very rapidly soon after birth with differences in the four groups, the highest increase being in the human milk group (see post workshop reply). HDL levels showed also increases at four different levels; an increase of 8.3 mg/dl in the standard formula group, of 20.3 and 23.2 mg/dl in the cholesterol and the γ linoleic supplemented groups, and of 29.9 mg/dl in the HM group. The main HDL fractions separated by gradient ultracentrifugation technique were the HDL_{2b}, the most mature particles, and HDL_{2a+3a} and HDL_{3b+3c} (5). Here again we have the four levels of HDL_{2b}: it is the highest in the HM group, then comes the F + γLA, then the F + Chol supplemented group, and then the F group. The differences between the four groups were examined from birth to age 30 days. In the SF group HDL_{2b} cholesterol levels almost did not increase, but in the F + Chol group and the F + γLA group, there was an increase of HDL_{2b} apo A-I which increases the most in human milk. Both dietary cholesterol and γ linoleic acid increase HDL levels and play a role in the maturation of HDL particles as some constituents of human milk do.

Dr. Small: I think it is very interesting, there is quite a big difference between the formula and human milk. Do you know about the fatty acid composition of the cholesterol esters and phospholipids in the HDL fraction.

Dr. Van Biervliet: We have performed all these analysis and indeed found differences, but I don't have the data with me.[1]

Dr. Deckelbaum: If I recall correctly your previous work (6) comparing breast milk to formula milk did not show such big differences in the effects of cholesterol intake on HDL. Do you think that this is an effect specifically of an interaction of γ-linolenic acid with cholesterol in changing cholesterol metabolism?

Dr. Van Biervliet: I don't have the data now.

Dr. Widhalm: The data you presented support the suggestion I made yesterday that the addition of long chain fatty acids in infant nutrition should not be discussed without the addition of cholesterol because your data show clearly that cholesterol has an obviously beneficial effect on the HDL_{2b} fraction of mothers milk.

Dr. Van Biervliet: I fully agree.

Dr. Heim: I wonder how many of you read the paper of Dr. Trude Forte from Berkeley in California (7) in which she described abnormal HDL in a large number of premature infants. She could normalize the HDL_2 and HDL_3 levels by giving breast milk to these infants. But she could also normalize the HDL pattern in many of these infants by giving them an intravenous lipid infusion. Since the latter does not contain much cholesterol (70 mg/dl) but large amount of dietary essential fatty acids (58% of total fatty acids) it implies that the abnormal HDL can be normalized with dietary essential fatty acids without much cholesterol intake.

Dr. Spielman: I should like to add to your data some additional data on the use of γ-linolenic acid in adults. It has to be given without at the same time giving a lot of linolenic acid. If you manage to give concentrated amounts of γ-linolenic acid (a high γ-linolenic to linoleate ratio), as was done in three clinical trials, you can show that HDL is raised by γ-linolenic acid. There is also some kind of preferential esterification of cholesterol ester by γ-linolenic acid. We don't know what it means but each time you give γ-linolenic acid you can see a significant rise in this fatty acid in cholesterol esters.

Dr. Deckelbaum: This is a valuable point. When different fatty acids are bound to these various lipids, it is important to consider that you form a cholesterol ester with fatty acid attached to the cholesterol molecule. Thus different fatty acids are going to have the potential to modify the accumulation of cholesterol esters in the cells and in different lipoprotein

---

[1] The corresponding data were provided after the workshop and is mentioned at the end of this discussion.

particles. We have evidence that with γ-linolenic acid feeding the cholesterol ester content and the fatty acid composition of LDL is markedly changed.

Dr. Small: I should like to add one comment about HDL cholesterol. Most of the epidemiology done in adults shows that HDL levels correlate quite well with decreased risk of atherosclerosis. But the simplest way to raise HDL in animals is to give them cholesterol. When you do this, HDL continues to increase until you give massive amounts of cholesterol, at which point the animals can develop atherosclerosis because the LDL also goes up. I think that simply suggesting that increases in HDL are always good could be dangerous.

Dr. Heim: One can increase HDL cholesterol separately from LDL by supplementing the diet with moderate amounts of alcohol, both in experimental animals and in humans. So I think there is a distinct mechanism for HDL increase and perhaps for the prevention of atherosclerosis.

REFERENCES

1. Van Biervliet JP, Vercaemst R, De Keersgieter W, Vinaimont N, Rosseneu M. Evolution of lipoprotein patterns in newborns. *Acta Paediatr Scand*. 1980; 69: 593–6.
2. Van Biervliet JP, Caster H, Vinaimont N, Vercaemst R, Rosseneu M. Plasma apoprotein and lipid patterns in newborns. Influence of nutritional factors. *Acta Paediatr Scand* 1981; 70: 851–6.
3. Van Biervliet JP, Rosseneu M, Bury J, Caster H, Stul M, Lamote R. Apoprotein and lipid composition of plasma lipoproteins in neonates during the first month of life. *Pediatr Res* 1986; 20: 324–8.
4. Van Biervliet JP, Rosseneu M, Caster H. Influence of dietary factors on the plasma lipoprotein composition and contents in neonates. *Eur J Pediatr* 1985; 144: 489–3.
5. Rosseneu M, van Biervliet JP, Bury J, Vinaimont N. Isolation and characterisation of lipoprotein profiles in newborns by density gradient ultracentrifugation. *Pediatr Res* 1983; 17: 783–94.
6. Van Biervliet JP, Rosseneu M, Caster H. Influence of dietary factors on the plasma lipoprotein composition and contents in neonates. *Eur J Pediatr* 1986; 144: 489–93.
7. Forte TM, Genzel-Boroviczeny O, Austin MA, *et al*. Effect of total parenteral nutrition with intravenous fat on lipids and high density lipoprotein heterogeneity in neonates. *J Ent Parent Nutr* 1989; 13: 490–500.

Post Workshop Reply

We studied the effects of cholesterol supplementation, and also of γ-linolenic acid supplementation (1) to infant formula on the distribution of cholesteryl esters and the serum cholesterol concentration, compared to an unsupplemented formula and to human milk in 40 full-term infants during the 1st month of life. Breast feeding results in significantly higher levels of serum cholesterol, cholesteryl arachidonate oleate and palmitate (Table 1). Although all the cholesterol esters increased during the 1st month of life, the most pronounced increase of the cholesteryl linoleate concentration reflects the dietary composition. The cholesterol ester distribution was calculated as the percentage of the sum of cholesteryl arachidonate, linoleate, oleate and palmitate. At birth the cholesteryl arachidonate percentages are identical for all groups (Fig. 1) However after 30 days the percentage is significantly higher in the cholesterol-supplemented group and in the γ-linolenic acid supplemented groups than in the unsupplemented (9.1 ± 1.1 and 10.8 ± 3.7 *vs.* 7.4 ± 1.7%; $p < 0.05$). In the breast-fed babies it was significantly higher than in those fed the adapted formula (11.6 ± 1.7; $p < 0.05$).

These data suggest a positive relation between increased nutritional cholesterol intake and serum cholesteryl arachidonate levels. Moreover they suggest that the supply of exogenous cholesterol, enhancing the production of cholesteryl esters, especially those of the long-chain

TABLE 1.[a]

	F mg/dl	F + Chol mg/dl	F + γLA mg/dl	HM mg/dl
day 0				
Total Cholesterol	60.1 ± 12.7	53.1 ± 9.3*	65.4 ± 15.1	68.5 ± 11.3
CE 20:4(ω6)	10.7 ± 1.5	9.7 ± 2*	12.2 ± 3.4	12.8 ± 2.6
CE 18:2(ω6)	16.4 ± 3	14.9 ± 3.7	18.6 ± 5.1	17.6 ± 3
CE 18:1(ω9)	24.4 ± 8.2	20.7 ± 4.8	27.4 ± 7.8	28.1 ± 8.2
CE 16:0	9.9 ± 1.9	9.2 ± 2.4	11.9 ± 3.2	13.9 ± 1.9
day 7				
Total Cholesterol	109.4 ± 25.9	110.3 ± 17.3	102.2 ± 16.5*	132.5 ± 21.6
CE 20:4(ω6)	11 ± 2.4**	11.6 ± 2.4*	13.6 ± 1.9*	21.2 ± 5.4
CE 18:2(ω6)	40.7 ± 7.5	44.1 ± 8.8	40.3 ± 7.8	44.3 ± 13.3
CE 18:1(ω6)	44.4 ± 13.8	40.8 ± 8.4	40.3 ± 8.9	52.4 ± 14.5
CE 16:0	16.6 ± 3.8	16.1 ± 3.5*	14.1 ± 3.2*	21.6 ± 5.6
day 30				
Total Cholesterol	103.4 ± 16.2**	115.3 ± 18.2**	118.5 ± 21**	145.1 ± 19
CE 20:4(ω)	8.6 ± 8.6**	10.5 ± 2.1**	13.8 ± 5.6*†	18.2 ± 4.2
CE 18:2(ω6)	54.8 ± 11.9*	53.6 ± 10.6**	56.8 ± 8.2	63.2 ± 6.4
CE 18:1(ω9)	36 ± 8.1*	35.9 ± 6.9*	42.8 ± 12.2	51.7 ± 12.2
CE 16:0	14.9 ± 2.8**	15.4 ± 3.4*	15.1 ± 4.3*	23.3 ± 6.4

[a] Evolution of the concentrations of serum total cholesterol, cholesteryl arachidonate (CE20:4(ω-6), cholesteryl linoleate C18:2(ω-6), cholesteryl oleate CE18:1(ω-9), cholesteryl palmitate CE 16:0, mean ±1 SD in mg/dl in the 4 groups formula-fed (F), cholesterol supplemented (Chol), γ-linolenic acid supplemented (γLA), and human milk-fed (HM). Values at birth, 7 and 30 days.
Significance vs. HM ** $p < 0.01$
* $p < 0.05$; Significance vs. F † $p < 0.05$.

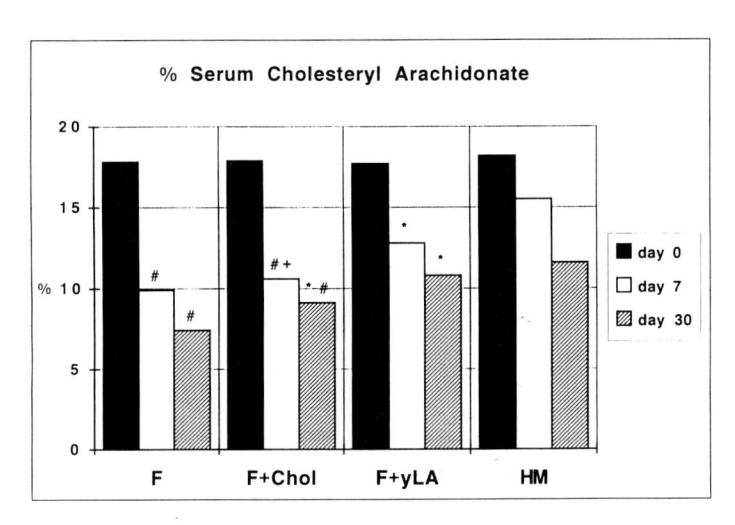

FIG. 1. Percent distribution of serum cholesteryl arachidonate at birth, day 7, and day 30 after birth in the 4 groups.
F: standard formula, containing 5 mg/dl cholesterol; F+Chol: cholesterol supplemented formula containing 10 mg/dl cholesterol; F+γLA: formula supplemented with 0.7% of the fatty acids as γ-linolenic acid; HM: human milk.
Significance vs. HM * $p < 0.05$; Significance vs. F †$p < 0.05$; Significance vs. F+γLA: + $p < 0.05$

polyenoic acids, could represent a role for the high cholesterol concentrations of human milk. An increased supply of cholesteryl arachidonate could be beneficial during the period of brain growth and myelinization (2).

Arachidonate levels increase after γ-linolenate supplementation. Apparently the desaturase-elongation steps are not efficient enough in the unsupplemented formula to provide arachidonate levels of the supplemented formula and of the human milk fed babies. By providing γ-linolenic acid we bypass the apparently difficult Δ6 desaturation step. These data could suggest that even full-term infants benefit from γ-linolenic acid supplemented formula.

REFERENCES

1. Van Biervliet JP, Vinaimont N, Vercaemst R, Rosseneu M. Serum cholesterol, cholesteryl ester, and high-density lipoprotein development in newborn infants: Response to formulas supplemented with cholesterol and γ-linolenic acid. *J Pediatr* 1992; 120: S101–8.
2. Bourré JM, Faivre A, Dumont J, *et al*. Effect of polyunsaturated fatty acids on fetal mouse brain cells in culture in a chemically defined medium. *J Neurochem* 1983; 41: 1234–42.

Subject Index

A

Abetalipoproteinemia, 118
Acatalasemia, 72
Acceptors, competition for, 37–38
Acetic acid, solubility of, 25
Acid soap, 27–28
Acylceramides, in atopic dermatitis, 214, 218
Acylcoenzyme A
  deficiency of, 70
  in fatty acid utilization, 3
Acylglucoceramides, for atopic dermatitis, 218
Adipocytes, in fatty acid utilization, 2
β-Adrenergic response, arachidonic acid and, 161
Adrenoleukodystrophy (ALD)
  neonatal, 68–69
  pseudo-neonatal, 70
  X-linked, 65, 69–70, 72, 73–75, 79
Albumin
  fatty acid bound to, 2–3
  interactions in blood with, 28–33, 34, 38–39
1-Alkyl-2-acylglycerols (EAG), in signal transduction pathways, 42
Allergic hyperreactivity, 172
American Heart Association (AHA) Step 1 diet, 118–119, 221
Animal fats, in chronic disease and cancer, 175
Anorexia nervosa, 184
Antioxidants
  for fish oils, 153–155
  PUFA and, 87–89
Apolipoprotein B, oleic acid and, 222–223, 227

Apolipoprotein E
  at birth, 227
  in DHA metabolism, 130
  and lipid uptake in retina, 133
Arachidonate
  γ-linolenate supplementation and, 231
  in liver and extrahepatic tissues, 84, 85–87, 91–92
  in long chain fatty acid metabolism, 21
  and parturition, 188
Arachidonic acid, 2
  at birth, 103, 104, 105, 109
  in breast milk vs. formula, 118, 155–156
  in cord blood and umbilical artery, 93, 99
  in cystic fibrosis, 160–162, 163
  deposition in photoreceptor cells of, 124
  eicosapentaenoic acid and, 23–24
  in endothelial cells, 11, 12
  GLA and, 158
  hydroxylated forms of, 7
  linoleic acid in maternal diet and, 145
  metabolism of, 41–42
  plasma levels of, 118
Arrhythmias, 92
Ascorbyl palmitate, 158
Atherosclerosis, HDL cholesterol and, 229
Atopic dermatitis, 211–216
Atopic diathesis, 211
Atopy, 211
Autoimmune disease, 208
Auto-immune response, in peroxisomal disorders, 79

233

B

Barter syndrome, 166
Behavior, effect of α linolenic acid on, 170–172, 177–178
Bifunctional enzyme deficiency, 70
Bile salts, in utilization of triglycerides, 58, 60
Bile salt-stimulated lipase (BSSL), 55, 56–58
Birthweight, low. *See* Low birthweight infants
Blackcurrant oil
  analysis of, 149
  for atopic dermatitis, 214–215
  chromatographic cleaning of, 153, 154
Blood, interactions of fatty acids with components of, 28–33, 34, 38–39
Blood-brain barrier, for long chain polyunsaturated fatty acids, 12
Brain
  fatty acid accretion in, 112–113
  fetal development of, 97, 112
  growth spurts in, 111
  integrity and function of, 96
  LCPUFA and, 113–116
  α linolenic acid and, 170–172, 177–178
  liver in supply of docosahexanoic acid to, 124–127
  minimum required amount of n-3 fatty acids for, 171–172
  myelination of, 111, 113
  phospholipid biosynthesis in, 18
Breast cancer, 185
Breast milk
  and atopic dermatitis, 214, 218
  and cell membrane composition, 10–11
  cholesteryl arachidonate with, 229–231
  essential fatty acids in, 53–54, 103
  fatty acid content of, 113, 117–118
  LCPUFAs in, 53–63
  LDL and HDL levels with, 227–228
  linoleic acid intake and arachidonic acid composition of, 145
  for preterm infants, 146
  triglycerides in, 53, 54–58, 227
  uptake of LCPUFA from, 138
  variability of, 11

BSSL (bile salt-stimulated lipase), 55, 56–58
Bulimia, 184
Butyric acid, solubility of, 25

C

Calcium-linked potassium channels, 92
Cancer, 174–175, 177, 185
Cardiolipin, 92
Cardiomyocytes, fatty acid biosynthesis by, 17
Catalase, in peroxisomal disorders, 66, 67–68
Catfish oil, 119
Cell function, polyunsaturated fatty acids and, 89–90
Cell membranes
  fatty acid composition of, 6, 9–11
  interactions in blood with, 29–33, 34, 38–39
Ceramides
  in signal transduction pathways, 42
  structure of, 45
Cerebral palsy, 93, 97
Cerebrosides, in brain development, 113
CF. *See* Cystic fibrosis (CF)
CFTR (cystic fibrosis transmembrane conductance regulator), 159, 162
Chain elongation
  in fatty acid biosynthesis, 15–16
  to provide 20-carbon HUFA, 169–170
Chain melting temperatures, 26–28
Chloride transport, arachidonic acid and, 161
Cholesterol
  at birth, 227–228
  in brain, 116
  breast milk vs. formula and, 227–228
  in diet vs. serum, 219–224
  fatty acids in metabolism of, 221
  fecal excretion of, 224
  in infant diet, 224–225
  γ linolenic acid and, 228–229
  and partitioning into membranes, 38
  for premature infants, 144–145
Cholesterol esters, in peroxisomal disorders, 79

Cholesteryl arachidonate, 229–231
Choline phosphoglycerides (CPG)
  at birth, 103
  fatty acid composition of, 15–16
Chronic diseases, 173, 174–175
Chylomicrons
  in fatty acid utilization, 1, 2
  phospholipids in, 63
Cisparinaric acid, 7
Clofibrate, for peroxisomal disorders, 78
Colipase-dependent lipase, 55, 56–58, 60, 63
Compartmentalization
  desaturation and, 95
  and placental delivery, 95
Competition, for acceptors, 37–38
Conception, nutrition prior to, 96–97, 98–99, 100, 110
Conservation, of fatty acid profiles, 94, 95
Cord blood, as diagnostic tool, 93, 99–102
Corn oil, for atopic dermatitis, 212
Coronary heart disease, saturated fat intake and, 219–220
CPG (choline phosphoglycerides)
  at birth, 103
  fatty acid composition of, 15–16
Crazy chick disease, 96
Cyclo-oxygenase, 13
Cyclo-oxygenase products, 41–42
Cystic fibrosis (CF), 159
  arachidonic acid release in, 160–162, 163
  essential fatty acid deficiency in, 159, 160, 162, 167
  future research on, 162–164
  hypotheses of pathophysiology in, 160–163
  lipid parenteral emulsion for, 166–167
  primary symptoms in, 160–162
  prostaglandins in, 166
  secondary symptoms in, 162, 163
  steatorrhea in, 167
  and zinc deficiency, 166
Cystic fibrosis transmembrane conductance regulator (CFTR), 159, 162

D

DAG (diacylglycerols)
  alteration of acyl moiety of, 51
  in signal transduction pathways, 42
Deacylation-reacylation cycle, 18–19
Dermal application, 145
Dermatitis, atopic, 211–216
Desaturases
  in atopic dermatitis, 213, 217
  in fatty acid biosynthesis, 14, 23
Desaturation
  and compartmentalization, 95
  competition between substrates in, 83
  in fatty acid biosynthesis, 14–15
  to provide 20-carbon HUFA, 169–170
DHA. See Docosahexaenoic acid (DHA)
Diabetes mellitus, 185, 187, 194
Diacylglycerols (DAG)
  alteration of acyl moiety of, 51
  in signal transduction pathways, 42
Diathesis, atopic, 211
Dihydroxycholestanoic acid, in peroxisomal disorders, 68
Dihydrosphingosine, 45
Docosahexaenoic acid (DHA), 2
  accumulation in photoreceptor cells of, 122–124
  availability to brain of, 6–7
  at birth, 103, 104, 109
  in breast milk vs. formula, 118
  dietary supply of, 127–130
  in ethanolamine plasmalogens, 6, 9
  interorgan metabolism of, 127–130
  liver in supply of, 85, 124–127
  in phospholipid biosynthesis, 24
  and rhodopsin, 132, 133
  role of, 6
  in testes, 132
  uptake of, 130
  vitamin E and, 132
Docosahexaenoyl-coenzyme A synthetase, 127

E

EAE (experimental allergic encephalomyelitis), 96

EAG, in signal transduction pathways, 42
Eczema, atopic, 211–216
EFA. *See* Essential fatty acid(s) (EFA)
EFAD. *See* Essential fatty acid deficiency (EFAD)
Eicosanoid(s)
  in atopic dermatitis, 218
  in cystic fibrosis, 161
  formation of, 180
  in thymus, and tolerance to self, 195–206
Eicosanoid-independent mechanisms, 13
Eicosanoid-mediated events, 13
Eicosapentaenoic acid (EPA), 2, 6
  absorption of, 150
  and arachidonic acid, 23–24
  for atopic dermatitis, 215
  in premature infants, 140
Encephalomalacia, nutritional, 96
Encephalomyelitis, 96
Endocytosis, of plasma lipoproteins, 5
Endometrial cancer, 185
Endothelial cells
  linoleic acid in, 11–12
  low density lipoproteins in, 12
EPA. *See* Eicosapentaenoic acid (EPA)
Erucic acid, for peroxisomal disorders, 74, 78–79
Essential fatty acid(s) (EFA), 53–54
  and allergic hyperreactivity, 172
  in atopic dermatitis, 212
  and cancer, 174
Essential fatty acid deficiency (EFAD)
  in cystic fibrosis, 159, 160, 162, 167
  and HUFA in liver and extrahepatic tissues, 84, 92
Esterification, and uptake in lipoproteins, 38
Estrogens
  and lipid metabolism, 181
  and prostaglandin synthesis, 182
Ethanolamine phosphoglycerides, fatty acid composition of, 15–16
Ethanolamine plasmalogens, docosahexaenoic acid in, 6, 9
Evening primrose seed oil, for atopic dermatitis, 212–213

Experimental allergic encephalomyelitis (EAE), 96

F

FABPs (fatty acid binding proteins), 3, 35
Fasting, and parturition, 187
Fat intake
  chronic, 223
  recommendations to prevent cancer and chronic diseases, 175, 178
  and serum cholesterol, 221–222, 223
Fat store, at birth, 105, 109
Fatty acid(s)
  competition for acceptors of, 37–38
  distribution within cells of, 33–36
  future research on, 7–8
  interactions with components of blood, 28–33, 34, 38–39
  oxidation by peroxisomes of, 65–66
  physical properties in water of, 25–28
  as precursors of eicosanoids, 180
  signal transduction mechanisms and membrane properties of, 182–183
  and steroid hormones, 180–181
  utilization of, 1–6
Fatty acid analogs, 7
Fatty acid binding proteins (FABPs), 3, 35
Fatty acid biosynthesis
  cellular specificities for, 17–18
  chain elongation and retroconversion in, 15–17
  desaturation in, 14–15
Fatty acid pathways, genetic variation in, 9
Fatty acyl-carnitines, 44
Fatty acyl-coenzyme A, 44
Fecal steroids, 224
Fetal development
  of brain, 97, 112
  diagnostic technique for, 99–102
  nutrition during, 97–98
FFA (free fatty acids)
  and lipoprotein catabolism, 224
  utilization of, 1, 2
Fish oils

absorption of fatty acids from, 150, 151
antioxidant systems for, 88, 153–155
and arachidonic acid metabolism, 42
and atherosclerosis, 220
chromatographic cleaning of, 153, 154
risk of bleeding with, 140, 144
to supplement formula fed premature infants, 138–140
and triglyceride synthesis, 223
Flip flop mechanism, 10
Formula
   adding LCPUFAs to, 61, 140–142, 155
   alternative methods of supplementation of, 145
   arachidonic acid in, 118, 155–156
   cholesterol as supplement to, 144–145, 229–231
   encapsulation of lipids in, 158
   fatty acid content of, 113, 118
   fish oils as supplement to, 138–140, 144
   LDL and HDL levels with, 227–228
   for preterm infants, 146, 157
   technological approach to new lipid ingredients for, 153–156
   uptake of LCPUFA from, 138
Free fatty acids (FFA)
   and lipoprotein catabolism, 224
   utilization of, 1, 2

G

Ganglioside G_{M3}, 45
Gastric lipolysis, 55
GLA, 158
Glial cells, in peroxisomal disorders, 79
Glycosphingolipids, 4
GTE-GTO diet, for peroxisomal disorders, 74
GTO diet, for peroxisomal disorders, 74
Gynecological cancers, 185

H

Head circumference, nutritional markers and, 101, 102
Heart, uptake of fatty acids by, 92
Helper T cells, 204

HETE, 7
High density lipoproteins (HDL)
   and atherosclerosis, 229
   at birth, 227–228
   fat intake and, 221–222
   fatty acid bound to, 29, 32
   fatty acid composition of, 38
   in premature infants, 228
Highly unsaturated fatty acids (HUFA)
   and fat intake, 87, 88
   formation from 18-carbon PUFA of, 81, 169–170
   in hypercholesterolemia, 87
   intake of preformed, 81–82
   in liver and extrahepatic tissues, 84–87
HODE, 7
Human milk. *See* Breast milk
Hydroxy fatty acids, 10
Hypercholesterolemia, HUFA in plasma and cell lipids in, 87
Hyperoxaluria type 1, 71–72
Hyperpipecolic acidemia, 68
Hyperreactivity, 172
Hypertension, pregnancy-induced, 185–186

I

I-FABP, 35
Impotence, 184–185
Infant(s), 18-carbon vs. long chain fatty acids in, 103. *See also* Newborns
Infertility, 183–185
Inositol-containing phosphoglycerides, 20
Inositol phosphate (IP), 89–90
Interleukin-2 (IL-2), and tolerance to self, 195, 201–203, 205–206
Interphotoreceptor retinoid-binding protein, 130
Intestinal fatty acid binding protein (I-FABP), 35
Intestinal lipolysis, 55
Intestinal lymphangiectasia, 118
Intestinal mucosa, modification of dietary fat by, 63
Intracellular distribution, of fatty acids, 33–36

Intralipid, 103
Ionized fatty acids
  distribution in plasma of, 38
  solubility of, 26
IP (inositol phosphate), 89–90

K

Kennedy pathway, 18
Ketogenic diets, cholesterol level with, 222

L

Lactosylceramide, structure of, 45
Lands pathway, 18–19, 20
LCPUFA. *See* Long chain polyunsaturated fatty acids (LCPUFA)
LDL. *See* Low density lipoprotein (LDL)
Learning ability, α linolenic acid and, 170–172, 177–178
Lecithin, 158
Leukotriene B4 (LTB4), and tolerance to self, 195–196, 201–206
L-FABP, 35
Lignoceroyl-CoA, 70
Linoleate, 20
Linoleic acid, 2
  and allergic hyperreactivity, 172
  in atopic dermatitis, 217
  in breast milk, 11, 53
  in cancer, 174, 175
  and chronic disease, 175
  conversion to 20-carbon HUFA of, 169–170
  in endothelial cells, 11–12
  as essential fatty acid, 53
  hydroxylated derivatives of, 7
  in liver and extrahepatic tissues, 85–87, 91–92
  maternal intake of, 145
  transfer to fetus of, 109
α-Linolenic acid
  and arachidonic acid metabolism, 42
  in brain and nerve functions, 170–172
  in breast milk, 53
  conversion to 20-carbon HUFA of, 169–170
  as essential fatty acid, 53
γ Linolenic acid
  and arachidonate levels, 231
  for atopic dermatitis, 214–215, 217
  in blackcurrant oil, 149
  and cholesterol level, 228–229
Lipid(s)
  catabolism of, 223–224
  plasma levels of, 221–222
  production of, 222–223
  sex hormones and metabolism of, 181
  structural function of, 93–94
Lipid second messengers, 41, 42
  long chain bases as putative, 44–47
Lipolysis
  gastric, 55
  intestinal, 55
Lipolysis products, physical-chemical behavior and absorption of, 58–60, 61
Lipoprotein(s)
  catabolism of, 223–224
  charge of, 38
  endocytosis of, 5
  interactions in blood with, 29–33, 34, 38–39
  plasma levels of, 221–222
  production of, 222–223
Lipoprotein lipase (LPL)
  estrogens and, 181
  in fatty acid utilization, 1, 2
Lipoxygenase, in thymus, 197, 204
Lipoxygenase products, long chain fatty acids and, 41–42
Liver
  in fatty acid biosynthesis, 17–18, 23
  HUFA in, 84–87
  PUFA metabolism in, 82–83
  supply of docosahexaenoic acid by, 85, 124–125
Liver fatty acid binding protein (L-FABP), 35
Long chain bases, as new class of lipid second messengers, 44–47
Long chain dicarboxylic acid urea, in peroxisomal disorders, 79

Long chain fatty acids
  biologically important, 1, 2
  and lipoxygenase/cyclo-oxygenase products, 41–42
  and other signaling pathways, 44
  and protein kinase C, 43
  structure and biological value of, 148–150, 151
Long chain polyunsaturated fatty acids (LCPUFA)
  blood-brain barrier for, 12
  and brain development, 113–116
  18-carbon vs., 94–95, 103
  as essential fatty acids, 53–54
  intrauterine supply of, 137–138
  major pathway for synthesis of, 136
  newborn absorption of, 53–63
  newborn synthesis of, 136–137, 141
  postnatal intake of, 138
  in premature infant diet, 135–142
  reactivity of, 150–153
  release from triglycerides of, 55–56
  sources of, 148, 157
  synthesis of, 54
Low birthweight infants
  arachidonic acid level in, 104, 109
  cerebral palsy in, 93, 97
  diagnostic technique for, 99–102
  maternal intake and, 98–99, 100, 109–110
  neurodevelopmental distortions in, 97, 146
  pentaene/tetraene ratio in, 101
  placental growth in, 99–102
  preconceptional nutrition and, 98–99, 100
  social class and, 98
  triene/tetraene ratio in, 100–101
Low density lipoprotein (LDL)
  at birth, 227–228
  in endothelial cells, 12
  fat intake and, 221–222, 223–224
  free fatty acids and, 224
  oxidation of, 227
LPL (lipoprotein lipase)
  estrogens and, 181
  in fatty acid utilization, 1, 2

LTB4, and tolerance to self, 195–196, 201–206
Lymphangiectasia, intestinal, 118
Lysine, loss during storage of, 151, 152
Lysophospholipids, 44

M

Macrophage, in self-tolerance, 208–209
Malonyl CoA, in chain elongation, 15
Maternal intake
  and birthweight, 97, 98–99, 100, 109–110
  of linoleic acid, 145
MaxEPA, 88
Mead acid, in umbilical arteries, 100, 101, 109
Medium chain fatty acids, 222
Methionine, loss during storage of, 151, 152
Micelles, 26
  solubilization of lipolysis products by, 58–60, 62–63
Monounsaturated fats, 222
Mucus production, arachidonic acid and, 161
Myelination, 111, 113
Myristic acid, 1, 2
  in arteriosclerosis, 10
  and cholesterol level, 222

N

Neonatal adrenoleukodystrophy, 68–69
Neonates. *See* Newborns
Nerve functions
  α linolenic acid and, 170–172
  minimum required amount of n-3 fatty acids for, 171–172
Neural damage
  in low birthweight infants, 97, 146
  in premature infant, 105–106, 146
Neuronal migration, in peroxisomal disorders, 79
Neutrophils, fatty acid biosynthesis by, 17

Newborns
  bile salts in, 58, 60
  brain development of, 112–113
  capacity for LCPUFA biosynthesis in, 136–137
  18-carbon vs. long chain fatty acids in, 103
  LDL and HDL in, 227–228
  long chain fatty acid absorption in, 53–63
  maternal transfer of LCPUFA to, 137–138
Nonsteroidal anti-inflammatory drugs (NSAID), and cancer, 185
Nose bleeds, from fish oil, 140, 144
n-6 fatty acids, 147
  in allergic hyperreactivity, 172
  in chronic disease, 173
  in formula, 147, 158
  in premature infant diet, 140–142
  sources of, 148
n-3 fatty acids, 6–7, 147
  in allergic hyperreactivity, 172
  for brain and nerve functions, 170–172
  in cancer, 174, 175
  in chronic disease, 173, 175
  and eicosanoid production, 42
  in formula, 147, 158
  in premature infant diet, 140–142
  sources of, 148
n3/n6 ratio, 172–174, 175
Nutritional encephalomalacia, 96

O

Obesity, and infertility, 184
Oleic acid, 2
  and apoprotein B, 222–223, 227
  and lipoprotein production, 222–223
  for peroxisomal disorders, 74, 78–79
Ω-6 fatty acids. *See* n-6 fatty acids
Ω-3 fatty acids. *See* n-3 fatty acids
Ovulation, 184
Oxidation
  of LCPUFA, 150–153
  of low density lipoproteins, 227

Oxidative pathways, in fatty acid utilization, 3–4, 16–17
3-Oxo-coenzyme A thiolase deficiency, 70

P

Palmitic acid, 2
  and cholesterol level, 222, 223
  solubility of, 25
Partial degradation, 14, 16–17
Parturition, 186–188
Pentaenes, synthesis in brain of, 115
Pentaene/tetraene (P/T) ratio, in umbilical artery, 93, 101, 104
Perilla oil, 170–171, 173, 177
Peroxidation, nutritional encephalomalacia and, 96
Peroxisomal disorders
  biochemical consequences of, 67–68
  biogenesis defects in, 67
  cholesterol esters in, 79
  classification of, 66
  diagnosis of, 72, 73
  of fatty acid oxidation, 70–71
  future research on, 75
  glial cells in, 79
  immunologic dysfunction in, 79
  involving single enzyme, 69–70
  long chain dicarboxylic acid urea in, 79
  neuronal migration in, 79
  other, 71–72
  phenotype-genotype correlations in, 68–69
  structural organelle defect in, 66–67
  treatment of, 72–75, 78–79
  very long chain fatty acids in, 68
Peroxisomes, 66
  oxidation of fatty acids by, 4, 65–66
  and very long chain fatty acids, 65–66
PGE_2 (prostaglandin E_2)
  in cancer, 174
  in endothelial cells, 11–12
pH, and partitioning in blood, 29, 38–39
Phosphatidic acid
  in phospholipid biosynthesis, 18
  in signal transduction pathways, 42

Phosphatidylcholine
  in brain, 116
  and rhodopsin, 132–133
Phosphatidylcholinetransferase, in brain, 116
Phosphatidylethanolamine, uptake of, 92
Phosphatidylethanolamine methyltransferase, in brain, 116
Phosphatidylinositol, 20
Phosphoglycerides
  ethanolamine, 15–16
  inositol-containing, 20
  transfer to fetus of, 109
Phospholipase A_2 (PLA_2), in signal transduction pathway, 42
Phospholipase C (PLC), in signal transduction pathway, 42, 182
Phospholipase D (PLD), in signal transduction pathway, 42
Phosphilipid(s)
  in brain development, 113
  in chylomicrons, 63
  fatty acid turnover in, 5–6
  molecular species of, 4–5
Phospholipid biosynthesis
  in brain and retina, 18
  specificities in, 18–20
Photoreceptor cells
  accumulation of docosahexaenoic acid in, 122–124
  deposition of arachidonic acid in, 124
  postnatal development of, 121, 122
  vitamin E and, 132
Physical properties, of fatty acids in water, 25–28
Phytanic acid, 7
  in peroxisomal disorders, 68
Phytosphingosine, 45
PIH (pregnancy-induced hypertension), 185–186
"Ping-pong" mechanism, in phospholipid biosynthesis, 19
PIP (porcine intestinal peptide), 35
Pipecolic acid, in peroxisomal disorders, 68
pKa, and partitioning in blood, 29, 38–39
PKC. See Protein kinase C (PKC)

PLA_2 (phospholipase A_2), in signal transduction pathway, 42
Placenta
  prostaglandin synthesis by, 188, 194
  thrombosis of, 194
Placental delivery, compartmentalization and, 95
Placental growth, diagnostic technique for, 99–102
Plasma, interactions with components of, 28–33, 34, 38
Plasmalogens
  ethanolamine, 6, 9
  in peroxisomal disorders, 68, 72
Platelet(s), fatty acid biosynthesis by, 17
Platelet activating factor (PAF)
  in allergic hyperreactivity, 172
  in signal transduction pathways, 42, 44
  and tolerance to self, 208
PLC (phospholipase C), in signal transduction pathway, 42, 182
PLD (phospholipase D), in signal transduction pathway, 42
PMS (premenstrual syndrome), 186
Polyunsaturated fatty acids (PUFA)
  and antioxidants, 87–89
  and cell function, 89–90
  long chain. See Long chain polyunsaturated fatty acids (LCPUFA)
  metabolism in liver of, 82–83
  sources of, 148, 157
Porcine intestinal peptide (PIP), 35
Pre-eclampsia, 185–186
Pregnancy, nutrition during, 97, 98–99, 100, 109–110
Pregnancy-induced hypertension (PIH), 185–186
Premature infants
  breast milk vs. formula for, 146, 157
  cerebral palsy in, 93
  cholesterol supplements for, 144–145
  docosahexaenoic acid and, 104, 109
  essential fatty acids for, 53, 54, 103–105
  fat store in, 105
  fish oil supplements for, 138–140, 144

Premature infants (*contd.*)
    HDL in, 228
    inability to synthesize LCPUFA by, 145
    LCPUFA in diet of, 135–142
    linoleic acid in, 11
    neural damage in, 105–106, 146
Premenstrual syndrome (PMS), 186
Preterm infants. *See* Premature infants
Progestogens
    and lipid metabolism, 181
    and prostaglandin synthesis, 182
Propionic acid, solubility of, 25
Prostacyclin, in umbilical arteries, 101
Prostaglandin(s)
    in breast cancer, 185
    in cystic fibrosis, 166
    formation of, 180
    hormonal control of, 181–182
    in parturition, 186–188
    in pregnancy-induced hypertension, 186
    in sperm function, 184–185
    synthesis by placenta of, 188, 194
Prostaglandin E_2 (PGE$_2$)
    in cancer, 174
    in endothelial cells, 11–12
Prostanoids, in cystic fibrosis, 161
Protein kinase C (PKC)
    dietary fat and, 51
    long chain fatty acids and, 43
    in signal transduction, 182–185
    sphingosine and, 45–46
Protonated fatty acids
    distribution in plasma of, 38
    solubility of, 25
Pseudo-neonatal adrenoleukodystrophy, 70
Pseudo-Zellweger syndrome, 70
P/T ratio, in umbilical artery, 93, 101, 104
PUFA. *See* Polyunsaturated fatty acids (PUFA)

R

Refsum disease, infantile, 68–69
Reproductive processes
    future research in, 188–189
    gynecological cancers, 185
    infertility, 183–185
    parturition, 186–188
    pregnancy-induced hypertension, 185–186
    premenstrual syndrome, 186
    prostaglandin synthesis in, 181–182
    signal transduction mechanisms in, 182–183
    steroid hormone-fatty acid interactions in, 180–181
Retina
    liver in supply of docosahexaenoic acid to, 124–127
    nutrition and development of, 116
    phospholipid biosynthesis in, 18
Retroconversion, 14, 16–17
Rhizomelic chondrodysplasia punctata, 72
Rhodopsin, 132, 133
Rinoleic acid, 10

S

Safflower oil, 170–171, 173
Saturated fat intake
    and coronary heart disease, 219–220
    and lipoprotein catabolism, 223–224
    and lipoprotein levels, 221–222
Self-tolerance, 195–206
Seminal fluid, 184–185
Sex hormones, and lipid metabolism, 181
Signal transduction genes, 146
Signal transduction mechanisms, 182–183
Signal transduction pathways, 42
Social class, and low birthweight, 98
Solubility, 25–28
Sperm function, 184–185
Sphinganine, 45
Sphingomyelin, 45
Sphingosine
    agonists for, 51
    formation of free, 46–47, 51
    growth-inhibitory vs. growth-stimulatory effect of, 51–52
    for psoriasis, 51
    as second messenger, 42, 44–47
    structure of, 45

Starvation, 184, 187
Stearic acid, 2
  and cholesterol level, 220, 222
Steroid hormones, interaction with fatty acids, 180–181
Suppressor T cells, 204, 205
Supraenoic molecular species, 122

T

T cells, 195, 204, 205
Testes, docosahexaenoic acid and, 132
Tetraenes, synthesis in brain of, 115
Thromboxanes, formation of, 180
Thymocytes, and tolerance to self, 195–206
Thymus eicosanoids, and tolerance to self, 195–206
Tocopherols, 88
Tolerance to self, 195–206
Trans fatty acids, 222
Triene/tetraene (T/T) ratio, in umbilical artery, 93, 101, 104, 109
Triglycerides
  absorption of, 150
  in breast milk, 53, 54–58, 227
  digestion of, 54–58
  release of LCPUFA from, 55–56
  splitting of fatty acids from, 149–150
  utilization of, 1, 2
Trihydroxycholestanoic acid, in peroxisomal disorders, 68
T/T ratio, in umbilical artery, 93, 101, 104, 109

U

Umbilical artery, as diagnostic tool, 93, 99–102
Usher syndrome, 132

V

Very long chain fatty acids (VLCFA)
  in peroxisomal disorders, 68, 69–75, 78–79
  peroxisomes and, 65–66
Very low density lipoproteins (VLDL), in fatty acid utilization, 1, 2
Visual acuity, 116, 127
Vitamin C, 153–155, 158
Vitamin E, 88, 132, 153–155, 158

W

Water, physical properties of fatty acids in, 25–28

X

X-linked adrenoleukodystrophy, 65, 69–70, 72, 73–75, 79

Z

Zellweger syndrome, 66
  biochemical consequences of, 68
  biogenesis defect in, 67
  phenotype-genotype correlations in, 68, 69
  pseudo-, 70
  structural organelle defect in, 66–67
  very long chain fatty acids in, 65
Zinc deficiency, 166